The
Medicine Show

The
Medicine Show

Patients, Physicians and the Perplexities
of the Health Revolution
in Modern Society

Patricia Branca
EDITOR

Science History Publications/USA
New York   1977

Science History Publications/USA
a division of
Neale Watson Academic Publications, Inc.
156 Fifth Avenue, New York, New York 10010

Library of Congress Cataloging in Publication Data

Main entry under title:

The Medicine show.

    Includes bibliographies.
    1. Medicine--History. 2. Medicine--United States--
History. 3. Social medicine--United States--History.
4. Medicine--France--History. 5. Social medicine--
France--History. I. Branca, Patricia.
R149.M37   362.1'09   77-17146
ISBN 0-88202-179-6

Designed and manufactured in the U.S.A.

Contents

PREFACE

The story of how we came to be what we are today in terms of how we look, how we feel, how we care for our bodies is a history that is both personal and universal. We all know and boast with pride that we are healthier than our ancestors. The continuing increase in life expectancy is hailed as a key to our "good" living. However, there has yet to be written a history of the cosmic nature of the health revolution which dramatically altered the shape of Europe and America starting in the eighteenth century. The absence of an in depth study of the workings of the health revolution is certainly not due to a lack of interest. The multitude of medical histories written attest to the constant effort to understand the process by which men and women struggled against awesome fate to gain control over their personal destiny. The reason lies more with the enormous difficulty of the task. To capture in one piece the multi-dimensional phenomenon of the health revolution is extremely complex. Where does one start?

For too long the history of medicine has focused on the great discoveries and individuals (the stories of mold and Pasteurs). The purpose of this book was to show that medical history is much more. Taken as a whole the essays here illustrate well the multi-faceted phenomenon – the health revolution. Each essay in itself attests to the new sophistication of medical history through the use of a variety of novel sources, the application of social scientific techniques, particularly the use of quantitative analysis, plus the integration of disciplines. New questions are being pursued.

The essays in Part I introduce the reader to the new methodologies and themes being pursued in the history of medicine. Gerald Grob's overview of the state of medical history hits upon the important problems that face the interested scholar. He believes that to date American scholarship in the field has been too provincial and applauds the French for their innovative methodologies. While one must admit that he is correct largely in this assessment it is important to note that the work of the Kiples, Starr, Morantz and Tylor is breaking new grounds. The French scholars continue to pursue the very narrow as seen in the work of Lemay, Faure and Goubert. The general usefulness of these findings they themselves question. Grob's call for an integration of social and medical history in pursuing historical epidemiology is a most vital challenge. The contribution made by Kenneth F. Kiple and Virginia H. Kiple is unique in that it applies present day knowledge of nutrition and related disease problems to an historical context thereby enlightening us to the condition of life in the past. Paul Starr also relies heavily upon the benefits of an interdisciplinary approach in his work. His intorduction of economic theory into the history of medicine sheds new light on the history of doctors and their evolution in modern America. Edward Shorter's essay delves into the internal dynamics of the workings of the body and the mind. Shorter's suggestion that there is much to be learned about the human condition through employing psychological as well as physiological measures in studying trauma is most promising.

Parts II and III of the collection deal with the agents of change in the health revolution. Part II tries to relate the experiences of the patient in history. There can be no social history of medicine without coming to terms with the patient. My essay is an attempt to present a conceptual framework that would focus upon the patient as a primary actor in promoting and maintaining the health revolution. The essay explains in more detail the multi-dimensional levels of the health revolution. Regina Morantz's essay illustrates the importance of lay health reformers, particularly women, in stimulating the process of the health revolution in nineteenth century America. The three essays on patients in institutions by Arthur Imhof, Charles Rosenberg and Peter Tylor demonstrate that changing expectations determined who would go to the hospital. Imhof and Rosenberg, particularly, show that the hospital changed from a place for the indigent and needy to a place where one went to get better. The use of quantitative techniques by Imhof and Tylor presents a very detailed picture of the patient population.

The last sections deals with the question of doctors as agents of change and their professionalization. As the essays show there was no one method of professionalization, a variety of internal and external factors dictated a multitude of patterns as shown by Olivier Faure and Nancy Frieden. Edna Lemay and Pierre Goubert and Mattew Ramsey's works show that the experience of the doctor cannot be generalized – it was greatly dependent upon location and class.

*While the collection gives us a wealth of new information, it at the same time raises a host of questions. Much work remains to be done as most of the authors note. This collection is designed to make medical history intelligible and fun to the nonspecialist. It was exciting to put together. For this I wish to express my sincerest appreciation to all the authors whose cooperation was grand and whose fine works will speak for themselves. My thanks also to the **Journal of Social History** for permission to reprint the articles which appeared in Vol. 10 #4 Summer 1977 under my editorship (This includes Grob, Starr, Goubert, Morantz, Rosenberg, Imhof, Tyor, Ramsey, Lemay, Faure, Frieden); and the Kiple and Kiple article which appeared in Vol. 10 #3 Spring 1977.*

A personal note of thanks to C.H. and J.K. for taking care of things so that I could do my own thing.

Patricia Branca
Pittsburgh, Pa.
July 1977

Gerald N. Grob

THE SOCIAL HISTORY OF MEDICINE
AND DISEASE IN AMERICA:
PROBLEMS AND POSSIBILITIES

I

In the past ten or fifteen years, American historians have become increasingly fascinated with social history. Although defined in various ways, the so-called "new social history" is distinguished by its concern with describing the precise nature of social structures and the changes they undergo over long periods of time.[1] Methodologically, contemporary social historians employ quantitative techniques in the hope of avoiding generalizations that rest on impressionistic and idiosyncratic evidence, and are receptive — at least in theory — to the systematic testing of broad conceptual hypotheses developed in the social and behavioral sciences. Their hope is to illuminate the history of an entire society, including its social, political, and economic structures. Indeed, some of the most imaginative and significant work in American history during the recent past has been done by younger scholars familiar with the characteristic methodology of the social and behavioral sciences.

Despite the quality of recent work in social history, its scope has remained somewhat narrow and circumscribed. The most significant studies have focused on individual communities, demographic changes, social structure and mobility, and the social bases of politics.[2] Equally important, however, are the topics that have been ignored or neglected. There are as yet no systematic studies of morbidity and mortality patterns and their influence. The size and structure of a population, after all, are determined by forces other than just rates of mobility or the distribution of wealth.

When placed within an international context, the contributions of these American social historians shrink in their impressiveness. European, and especially French, scholars are more than a generation ahead of their American counterparts in raising new questions and employing novel methodologies in this field. The most significant outlet for the work of European scholars has been the *Annales,* a French journal which commenced .publication in 1929. The goal of this distinguished journal was both extraordinarily simple and complex: to break down traditional disciplinary distinctions and to create a new and unified way of understanding the totality of human activity within a given society or geographical region. Under the editorship of Lucien Febvre and Marc Bloch, the *Annales* become the acknowledged leader in creating the new field of social history or historical sociology. Continuing its innovative beginnings after the Second World War, the *Annales* increasingly served scholars employing quantitative and demographic techniques and resorting to multidisciplinary approaches.

Contemporary American social historians, for the most part, have largely ignored the examples set by European scholarship. It may be that the inevitable parochialism of a nationalistic approach inhibited cross-fertilization; perhaps the linguistic shortcomings of American historians caused many to overlook the *Annales*. Moreover, American scholarship — partly because of its scale, diversity, and organizational structure — has not been especially receptive to cross-fertilization between disciplines. Hence relatively few historians have defined their special fields in ways that facilitated the blurring of disciplinary distinctions (the same generalization holds true for the social and behavioral sciences as well). Most scholars pay homage to multidisciplinary studies; few practice what they preach. No recent social historians in the United States, for example, have undertaken detailed studies of population changes from the seventeenth to the twentieth centuries comparable to those of Thomas McKeown of the University of Birmingham in England and his colleagues. Whether or not one accepts McKeown's conclusions is beside the point; what is impressive are the ways in which he attempts to relate morbidity and mortality patterns to environmental, nutritional, economic, technological, and medical factors.[3]

Whatever the reasons, there can be no doubt that American social history has remained confined within narrow boundaries. In the United States the history of medicine and disease has drawn relatively little attention among social historians, whose names rarely or never appear in the table of contents of publications such as the *Bulletin of the History of Medicine* or the *Journal of the History of Medicine and Allied Sciences*. Much of the significant work has come from members of departments of the history of medicine, which are usually housed in medical schools rather than colleges or liberal arts faculties. The field, moreover, has been traditionally limited to studies which generally emphasize the internal development of medicine; the changing patterns of diseases, their impact upon society, and the ways in which people respond to health-related problems have been neglected despite clear evidence that medical practice until very recently had little influence over morbidity and mortality.

The failure of recent social historians to deal with disease is understandable. Few of them have mastered the minimum technical knowledge which is an indispensable prerequisite for research. Still fewer are acquainted with the source materials that have survived or understood fully the possibilities and limitations of research in the field. Moreover, an excessive preoccupation with socioeconomic determinants has served to blunt any comparable concern with the complex relationships between disease patterns, social structure, and environmental conditions. It is all too common for most historians to infer that disease is simply a function of class. Too often the history of medicine and disease has been neglected or subordinated to other admittedly legitimate problems, as indicated by the recent publication of studies dealing with sex-related biases within the medical profession.[4] Finally, the absence of epidemics that were capable of decimating the nation's population and lasting for decades seemed to make disease less pressing a topic as compared with the experiences of fourteenth-century Europe. Although epidemics of smallpox, yellow fever, and cholera appeared sporadically in the United States between the seventeenth and nineteenth centuries, their effects on the size of the population were not so devastating as to make them seem historically significant.

This is not to imply in any way that the history of medicine and disease is a barren field of specialization. Such is assuredly not the case, as an even cursory examination of the historical literature would immediately demonstrate. It is only to say that few social historians have attempted to integrate an older, and, in many ways, a distinguished body of material into their own work. Consequently, medical and social history (with some significant exceptions) remains isolated from each other. The few historians who managed to combine the two approaches were exceptions to the rule. Their contributions remained marginal, however, when compared with the growing number of quantitative studies concerned with communities which emphasized social structure, mobility patterns, distribution of wealth, and similar problems. One has only to look at recent works by Philip D. Curtin and Peter H. Wood to recognize the uniqueness of their studies of morbidity and mortality patterns among populations in the Caribbean and on the American mainland.[5]

II

In recent years, interest in health-related problems has intensified. One reason for this new-found concern is the changing age structure of the American population, which has created considerable interest in the social and medical problems associated with aging. In 1900 only four % of the population was sixty-five years of age or older; by 1970 this proportion had risen to ten %. As the number of older persons continues to increase both relatively and absolutely, the United States (like most industrial societies) will confront a series of relatively novel problems. To what degree, for example, can a society afford to allocate its resources to a group whose economic productivity is rapidly shrinking? There is little doubt that the monetary costs of social security and medical care will continue to escalate. Moreover, the care of the aged will undoubtedly become an increasingly politicized issue. In the future greater expenditures for dependent older persons must be drawn from a limited number of policy alternatives, including income-transfer programs, reallocations of current priorities, and the surplus generated by an ever-expanding economy. The first and second alternatives are bound to intensify political conflict, given the magnitude of the problem and the rising costs of medical care; the last exacerbates certain kinds of environmental problems resulting from industrial growth.[6]

Another source of concern about health-related problems are fears of adverse consequences that often seem to follow economic and technological development. To a considerable extent the debates over nuclear energy and other novel technologies are dominated more and more by a preoccupation with their relative dangers to the public health. And the existence of glaring differential morbidity and mortality patterns among various socioeconomic, ethnic, racial, and occupational groups adds another element of controversy to American politics.

If past precedent holds true, a heightened concern over a contemporary problem will sooner or later stimulate historical endeavors. The twentieth-century preoccupation with social and economic "realities" helped to shift the focus of historians' interests in very different directions as compared with their nineteenth-century predecessors.[7] There is every reason to believe, therefore, that social historians will increasingly turn their attention to health-related problems in much the same way they began to examine the relationships between ideology and social structure, childhood experiences, family history, and mobility patterns. Indeed, what is surprising is that so few American social historians have shown any interest at all in morbidity patterns and what they might reveal about the quality and length of life in different periods.

III

If the social history of medicine and disease in America as a specific field of specialization is destined to grow, it is clear that its practitioners cannot ignore an extensive and important body of literature written during the last fifty years or so. Granted that this literature may have, at least from the viewpoint of the newer social history, certain drawbacks. It also, however, possesses certain strengths, an understanding of which is indispensable for further work.

The most important characteristic of the traditional literature of the history of medicine and diseases, perhaps, was the emphasis placed on the internal logic and theory of medicine. This approach stressed the assumptions and objectives of physicians, their approaches to disease, their methodology, and the progressive development of particular patterns of thought in the treatment of disease. To a considerable degree, the internal history of medicine lead to an emphasis on the role of key individuals, or the evolution of beliefs and ideas regarding given diseases entities. Defined in this way, the history of medicine was closely related to intellectual history and the history of science; the goal was to explain how certain concepts and ideas developed and how they changed over time.

The traditional emphasis on the internal development of medicine, however, did not necessarily imply an unwillingness to deal with the relationships between medicine and society, or the social and demographic consequences of disease. Even a quick perusal of the existing literature demonstrates that medical historiography never fit a narrow mold. There are a number of specialized monographs that analyze both the patterns and social perceptions of disease. Other studies deal with the evolution of medicine as a profession, the development of medical education, and the rise of medical sectarianism. Nor have political dimensions been ignored, particularly in regard to the financing and organization of health care services, and the subsequent emergence of government as a major source of funding for medical and scientific research.[8] Indeed, Richard H. Shryock, the distinguished historian of medicine, insisted repeatedly that scholars had an obligation to study the interplay between external and internal factors in writing about the history of medicine.[9]

Well before Americans became preoccupied with the role of environmental factors in the etiology of disease, medical historians had already developed a sophisticated understanding of some of the underlying issues. In an often neglected but important study of malaria in the Upper Mississippi Valley in the nineteenth century, Erwin H. Ackerknecht traced the subtle relationship between population migration movements, land use patterns, and the appearance and eventual decline of a disease the etiology of which became known at a later date and at a time when specific antimalarial measures were unknown. Malaria, he pointed out, did not make its appearance in the Upper Mississippi Valley until after 1800. It then reached a high endemic-epidemic level in the half century following 1820, declined after 1870, and all but disappeared shortly after the turn of the twentieth century. The initial appearance of the disease in this region was instigated by the movement of people up the Mississippi River, which brought both the anopheles mosquito and a sizeable number of persons already infected with the malaria plasmodia. Settlement along rivers, combined with land clearing practices, created conditions conducive to the mosquito's breeding habits. The construction of crude dwellings without adequate ventilation or lighting during the initial stages of settlement provided still another habitat for the mosquito. The result was a rapid increase in the incidence of malaria.

But, as Ackerknecht also demonstrated, environmental changes likewise created conditions that hastened the disappearance of malaria. Railroads shifted the pattern of settlement away from waterways; intensive cultivation brought drainage problems under control; the growth of urban areas helped to eliminate ponds of stagnant water because of the paving of streets; better ventilated homes with larger windows became more common in older communities; screening for purposes of comfort came into general use; the introduction of cattle raising produced a counterattraction because many insects prefer animals to human beings; and a rising standard of living probably increased resistance to diseases like malaria. All of these factors combined to eradicate a disease that as late as 1945 affected from one-third to one-sixth of the world's population.[10]

Nor was Ackerknecht alone in stressing the mutual interdependence of disease patterns, environmental changes, and social structure. In *The Cholera Years,* Charles E. Rosenberg analyzed the relationship between social and religious values on the one hand and attitudes toward disease on the other. Taking the cholera epidemics of 1832, 1849, and 1866, he sought to relate community reaction to ideology and social structure. Similarly, Elizabeth W. Etheridge showed how a specific disease — pellagra — grew out of environmental and living patterns in the early twentieth-century South. She, too, demonstrated how the responses of a particular region to a disease were conditioned by its culture and social structure.[11] Other scholars attempted to show how developments within particular medical specialties were related to broader social forces.[12]

The traditional approach to disease and medicine admittedly contained shortcomings. Too many studies were limited either by chronology or the narrowness of the topic. Nor was there any serious attempt to synthesize the monographic literature and to develop broad conceptual frameworks that might shed light on the social history of a disease and the human responses to it.[13] The literature dealing with the seventeenth and eighteenth centuries tends to focus on specific colonies, specific diseases, individual physicians, isolated health-related crises, or the origins of public health. In dealing with the nineteenth and twentieth centuries, historians emphasized the struggle between orthodoxy and sectarianism, medical education, professionalization, and the supposed triumph of "scientific medicine." Although all of these subjects are important, their focus is necessarily restricted by the preoccupation with the evolution of medical thought and practice.

IV

Clearly, there are compelling reasons why social historians, building upon the work of earlier scholars, should turn their attention to the history of disease and medicine in America. Disease, however defined, is one of the most fundamental factors in human affairs. It affects not only the size and structure of a population, but influences and reflects a society's social structure, technology, and living and cultural patterns. Indeed, a knowledge of disease patterns can shed much light on the nature of a given society, if only because of the obvious relationship between environment and health. Moreover, the manner in which people respond to disease can illuminate the underlying values that hold a society together and give it a sense of coherence.

If the social history of medicine and disease as a specific field of specialization is destined to grow, what direction should it take? Which problems require intensive study? What conceptual frameworks and methodologies are most appropriate? Any answers to these questions can only be tentative; scholarly research into the sources invariably dictates the direction, framework, and questions in any newly developing field. Nevertheless, certain lines of inquiry are clearly worth pursuing, if only because they have been somewhat neglected in the past.

Although scholars have long been aware of the importance of disease in human history, they have yet to study in a *systematic* way the changing pattern of disease over time and the reasons for such changes. Epidemiologists have long been concerned with this subject, but they have rarely undertaken detailed retrospective studies. Their unfamiliarity with historical techniques and primary sources inhibited the development of what might well be referred to as historical epidemiology.

The literature dealing with morbidity and mortality in seventeenth and eighteenth century America illustrates both the strengths and weaknesses of traditional medical historiography. A good deal is known about the general pattern of diseases in the various colonies and the periodic epidemics that affected their people. Yet relatively little is known about the actual demographic impact of disease. Mortality rates obviously tended to be spectacular during the early years of settlement because of exposure to the elements, malnutrition, and the problem of adapting to a new physical environment. One half of those who came to Plymouth perished during the first year. Nearly two-thirds of those who migrated to Virginia between 1606 and 1618 perished either during the voyage to the New World, or upon their arrival in the colony.[14] But what happened to mortality rates after the initial stages of settlement had passed? In what ways did disease influence the size and structure of the population? How did the American experience with disease compare with that of England and Western Europe during the same period? What was the relationship between disease patterns and the nature of the colonial environment? How did social attitudes toward life and death, family relationships, and children change as the pattern of disease changed? What were the economic costs of disease, and in what ways did morbidity and mortality patterns influence economic and social development? The answers to these and to similar questions can help us to understand better the nature of colonial society.[15]

In spite of the fact that data regarding disease patterns are more readily available for the nineteenth and twentieth centuries, our knowledge regarding such patterns remains sketchy. In general terms, it is clear that infectious diseases began to decline in importance. The data from Massachusetts — which kept more systematic records than most other states — is particularly revealing in this respect. Between 1860 and 1956 mortality from diptheria fell from 89.2 to 0.1 per 100,000 of population, measles from 16.9 to virtually zero, and typhoid and paratyphoid fever from 79.9 to 0. Undoubtedly the decline in mortality from infectious diseases — especially those that had their greatest incidence among children — contributed to the general increase of life expectancy at birth. But the decline in importance of infectious diseases as a major factor in mortality did not result in a decrease in disease per se; it simply indicated a shift among diseases. By the twentieth century, for example, the incidence of other than strictly infectious diseases had grown dramatically. Whereas tuberculosis, syphilis, typhoid and paratyphoid fever, diptheria, whooping cough, and measles were significant factors in pre-1900 mortality patterns, other diseases — many of which were related to the changing age structure of the population and novel environmental factors — increasingly assumed their place. In 1900 the death rate from malignant neoplasms was 64 per 100,000; by 1969 it had risen to 160. During this same period mortality from diabetes mellitus rose from 11 to 19.1 and from the major cardiovascular-renal diseases from 345.2 to 501.7. Deaths from cirrhosis of the liver, bronchitis, emphysema, and asthma also began to rise, the last three, for example, going from 5 in 1950 to 15.4 in 1969. Moreover, some entirely new causes of death entered the picture. In 1900 there were virtually no fatalities from automobile accidents; in 1969 the death rate from this cause alone reached 27.6 per 100,000.[16]

Such data, however, conceal far more than they reveal. They tell us little about the complex relationships between disease patterns, on the one hand, and socioeconomic, educational, cultural, geographical, demographic, and occupational variables on the other hand. Nor can we safely infer from aggregated data definitive explanations about the decline of specific diseases. In the cases of cholera and typhoid fever there was undoubtedly a causal link between the incidence of the disease and changes in water supplies and sanitation facilities, particularly in the larger urban areas. Similarly, the decline in smallpox may have been due, at least in part, to the widespread use of vaccination. Tuberculosis, on the other hand, presented an entirely different problem. During the first half of the nineteenth century this disease was known as the "Great White Plague;" it has been estimated that nearly half of the population of England had the disease. In the United States scattered data indicates that tuberculosis was the single most important cause of death before 1900. Some evidence suggests that the mortality rate from tuberculosis in Boston, New York, and Philadelphia was about 400 per 100,000 of population in 1830. By 1900, when more reliable figures became available, the rate for the United States as a whole had fallen to 194.4; twenty-five years later the comparable figure was 84.8.[17]

Yet surprisingly little is known about tuberculosis, a disease whose importance may well have rivalled the plague of earlier centuries. What groups and geographical regions were most susceptible? What was the economic and social impact of tuberculosis? An even more intriguing question is: how can the decline of the disease be accounted for? Curiously enough, the decline in mortality from tuberculosis commenced long before any specific interventionist measures were made available. The tubercule bacillus was not isolated until 1882; the confinement of patients in sanitoriums – the effectiveness of which is questionable – did not commence until after 1900; and drugs and surgery were not introduced until long after the disease lost the paramount position it once occupied. It may very well be the case that the decline of this disease was related to the rise in the general standard of living and to changes in housing and occupational patterns rather than to interventionist measures. Mortality from tuberculosis among New York City Jews living in the older and more congested Gouverneur District in the 1920's was 83 per 100,000; in the newer and more open Bronx-Tremont District the comparable figure among Jews was only 52.[18] Similarly, there is some evidence that susceptibility increased dramatically when people altered their way of life; the incidence of tuberculosis increased sharply during periods of extended war. Whatever the case, historians have yet to study diseases like tuberculosis in order to illuminate in concrete terms the relationship between environment/social structure, and morbidity/mortality patterns.[19]

In studying the evolution of disease processes, social historians – by virtue of their holistic approach – have much to contribute. Indeed, what is astonishing is the absence of systematic inquiries into health-related problems. A whole host of significant problems come quickly to mind. How did disease patterns vary by class, race, sex, or ethnicity? What was the role of urbanization in altering disease processes? How did technology and new occupational structures transform disease patterns, to say nothing about changes in diet and housing? Is there evidence that changes in morbidity may have occurred because of changes in bacterial organisms and viruses rather than in human susceptibility? To what degree have disease patterns been altered by the changing age distribution of the population? Have interventionist policies minimized or maximized pathological processes?

Nor are novel methodological approaches required to answer such questions. Social historians already employ a variety of qualitative and quantitative techniques; there is no reason why these same techniques could not be applied to the study of disease. With some ingenuity, for example, it might be possible to study disease patterns by matching manuscript census schedules with death certificates, registration reports, and other sources that provide detailed information about age, sex, race, occupation, ethnicity, education, and religion. Hospital records, which in many cases preserve relatively complete pictures of patient populations, still await systematic use. It is true that surviving sources present formidable problems, particularly in terms of the identification of diseases, but this generalization applies to all historical inquiry.

V

The systematic study of disease, however significant, should not be permitted to obscure another important problem, namely, the social response to disease. How did the social and political response to disease change over time? In what way was the reaction to disease a function of group and community values rather than prevailing medical and scientific knowledge? Why were communities more fearful of certain kinds of diseases and less fearful of others which often had a far greater impact upon their people? In dealing with such issues historians could profitably compare community reaction to disease with comparable reactions to crises engendered by natural or human forces (e.g., flood, earthquake, fire, war).

Although historians have studied community reaction to epidemics,[20] they have not yet systematically analyzed the sources and nature of group perceptions of disease. The recent upsurge in interest in attitudes toward aging and death has not yet been matched by similar concern with the changing perceptions toward disease. Yet there are compelling reasons why more should be known about social perceptions, if only because of their presumed relationship to public and private policy. What is especially interesting is the manner in which large segments of the population can elevate relatively unimportant diseases into major health issues. During the 1930's and 1940's, for example, poliomyelitis became one of the more feared diseases in the United States despite its relative statistical insignificance. The result was a national crusade to eliminate a disease of only limited importance.[21] In this respect we also need to know more about the role of private organizations created to deal with specific diseases. Given their public, political, and financial importance, a good case can be made for studying their activities in detail. We need to know more about their sources of support, the reasons for their popularity, and the ways in which they influence or reflect public policy and attitudes.

No comprehensive social history of medicine and disease can avoid dealing with the development of medicine as a profession. Indeed, historians as well as scholars in the social and behavioral sciences have long been aware of the crucial role of professionalization of modern industrial societies. In his penetrating study of the late nineteenth and early twentieth centuries Robert Wiebe

made professionalization one of his central themes. He argued that the professions served as a source of stability at a time when new forces were destroying
older structures and behavioral patterns. Similarly, business and economic
historians have made organizational change central to their interpretation of
the past century.[22]

Despite widespread agreement on the central role of the professions in
contemporary society, surprisingly little has been done in the way of historical
analysis. The extensive body of literature on professionalization in the social
and behavioral sciences is extraordinarily present minded; very little of it
incorporates historical data based upon extensive research in primary sources.
Moreover, too many scholars treat professionalization in deterministic terms;
that is, they assume a straight line of development from the early nineteenth
century to the present. A recent sociological study of nineteenth-century
American physicians, for example, attributed the changes that took place in
medicine to the triumph of "science," which created objective standards and
definitions and thus undermined sectarian and unorthodox (or "empirical")
practitioners.[23]

In point of fact, however, the development of professionalization was
neither as clearcut nor simple as much of the literature suggests. Indeed, the
very meaning of the term underwent some basic changes. At the present time
the term profession implies certain specific attributes: the existence of a
systematic body of special knowledge; authority derived from the possession
of specialized knowledge not understood by laypeople; community sanction,
often in the form of a legal grant of powers and privileges; a definable
clientele; an implicit or explicit code of ethics; and a sense of unity and
corporateness in the membership.[24] It is true that many regular physicians in
the early nineteenth century sought the enactment of licensing laws, thus
making it appear that they were intent upon creating a profession in the
modern sense of the word. But those states that enacted such laws often did
not intend to prohibit the practice of medicine by unlicensed physicians; a
license was regarded simply as a badge of honor or commendation given to
certain individuals in recognition of their contributions. Although supporters
of licensing hoped that the public would drive out irregular physicians by
withholding patronage, they did not seek to establish a legal monopoly
through the enactment of exclusionary laws. Moreover, nineteenth-century
debates among physicians offered convincing evidence that the concept of a
profession differed in fundamental respects from the contemporary meaning
of the term; it is instructive to note that professionalization is a modern word
with but little relevance to earlier periods. When nineteenth-century physicians
debated the qualities desirable for medical practice, they emphasized the
importance of "character" rather than the mastery of a formal body of
knowledge. They insisted that the legitimacy of medicine as a profession was
derived from its intimate relationship with philanthropy and religion.

After 1880, of course, the meaning of the terms "profession" and "professionalization" underwent some marked changes. The changing structure of
medicine itself undoubtedly was related to a variety of determinants, including
new theories of disease, a technology that altered traditional medical practice,

changing social perceptions of the role of physicians, new avenues of recruitment, and the creation of a novel system of medical education. But we need to know much more clearly what these changes were and how they came about. Comparative studies of the process of professionalization might also be useful in illuminating not only the development of medicine as a profession, but also how a society reacts as it enters a bureaucratic and organizational phase. Nor should professionalization be studied in a social or political vacuum; it is important to understand the relationship between the professionalizing process and the role of women and blacks. Internally, professionalization was accompanied by the rapid proliferation of medical subspecialties that ultimately made the structure of health care services in the United States quite different from those of England and other Western European nations. Historians have yet to account for some of these profound structural differences.

Finally, social historians would do well to turn their attention to an analysis of health care institutions. There are innumerable histories of hospitals and similar organizations that offered a variety of services. Most of these studies, however, focused on the institution and its staff, the changing practice of medicine, structural differentiation, and modes of support. Such concerns are by no means unimportant, but they do neglect a crucial element, namely, the clientele. Clearly, there is much to be learned by studying *patients* as well as physicians. Using patient records, historians might then be in a position to ask important questions about the ways in which groups perceived physicians and hospitals, the changing incidence of disease, differential care and treatment, and the ways in which users (as compared with suppliers) influenced the shape and configuration of health care services. Moreover, patient records can be profitably used by scholars interested in the experiences of a variety of groups irrespective of whether these groups are defined by age, sex, race, ethnicity, class, or occupation.[25]

Systematic exploration of patient populations would also help us understand much more clearly the actual role of various kinds of institutions. Some of my own preliminary investigations into the history of mental hospitals in the United States from 1875 to 1940, for example, reveal an increasing percentage of admissions of older groups. In 1912 13.3% of all first admissions to mental hospitals in New York State were diagnosed as psychotic either because of senility or cerebral arteriosclerosis; by 1940 this figure had risen to 30.8%. The experiences of other states were by no means dissimilar. Why were aged persons committed to state mental hospitals? There is no evidence that communities perceived of them as threats to their security. Nor can it be argued that the function of institutionalization was to alter the behavior of such persons or to provide restorative therapy. In point of fact, the mental hospital assumed responsibility of caring for older people because of the absence of other alternatives. For all of the nineteenth and much of the twentieth century, American society was unable to resolve the problems associated with taking care of the aged. The decline in mortality rates among younger groups also led to a relative and absolute increase in the size of older

groups, thereby exacerbating the social problems arising from an aged population. Older persons ended up in mental hospitals for a variety of reasons.
Some had no family to provide basic care; others were institutionalized
because of the inability or unwillingness of relatives to assume responsibility.
Although psychiatrists and public officials were aware of this practice, they
could offer no easy alternative. One hospital superintendent defined the issue
in simple but moving terms:

> We are receiving every year a large number of old people, some of them very old,
> who are simply suffering from the mental decay incident to extreme old age. A
> little mental confusion, forgetfulness and garrulity are sometimes the only
> symptoms exhibited, but the patient is duly certified to us as insane and has no
> one at home capable or possessed of means to care for him. We are unable to
> refuse these patients without creating ill-feeling in the community where they
> reside, nor are we able to assert that they are not insane within the meaning of the
> statute, for many of them, judged by the ordinary standards of sanity, cannot be
> regarded as entirely sane.[26]

If the mental hospital was serving in part as a home for the aged, what
functions were other medical institutions actually performing? Which groups
were more (or less) likely to avail themselves of different institutional roles?
And how did institutions take on functions that were largely nonmedical in
character?

VI

If social historians are faced with opportunities in studying disease and
medicine, so too are they confronted with certain dangers. To begin with, the
training of most social historians takes place within history departments rather
than schools of medicine. Since few historians are familiar with medical
theory and practice, there is a danger that their students will be inadequately
trained in the "internal" history of medicine (as distinguished from the
"external" factors that influenced the medical profession). Such a situation is
fraught with danger, particularly if primary sources are misused because of
ignorance. Any serious work on the social dimensions of medicine and disease,
therefore, must begin with a firm understanding of the evolution of medical
theory, if only because primary sources reflect a particular generation's understanding of pathological processes.

Since social historians will presumably use medical sources, it is indispensable that they understand its language and rationale. Otherwise they will
either misuse or ignore data because of their conviction that the literature of
"prescientific" medicine is flawed by superstition and ignorance. The latter
view rests upon a simplistic understanding of modern medicine, which itself
has by no means resolved basic scientific and philosophical problems concerning the nature of disease.[27] Even in the case of the infectious diseases
where the most significant therapeutic advances have occurred, it cannot be
argued that the presence of a particular organism "explains" or "causes" the
disease. It is by no means uncommon, for example, for an individual carrying
the tubercule bacillin to develop the characteristic symptoms of tuberculosis

while another individual harboring the very same organism remains free from disease. Nor is it at all clear whether disease, abstractly defined, is a specific entity or an outward constellation of various symptoms of as yet poorly understood processes. And although contemporary medicine refers to both genetic and environmental factors in etiology, the fact of the matter is that little is known about each, to say nothing about the ways in which they presumably interact. Moreover, diseases are by no means constant. Changes in the immunities of host populations may very well lead to changes in viruses and bacteria. Given a constantly shifting equilibrium between human susceptibility and invading organisms, it is dangerous to assume that disease patterns are fixed. An understanding of the development of medical thought and theories of disease, in other words, can help social historians to avoid the use of inappropriate methodologies or to reach conclusions by a flawed process of reasoning.

Nowhere are the pitfalls that arise out of inadequate knowledge of the history of medicine better illustrated than in works dealing with the history of psychiatry and mental hospitals. Recent critics of psychiatry — including some historians — have pointed to the absence of an empirically validated relationship between physiological processes and behavior as "proving" that persons designated as insane were in fact being punished for their violation of conventional social norms. It then follows that mental hospitals performed a penal function in isolating deviants from the rest of society.[28] Neither the premise nor the conclusion, however, is necessarily valid. The fact of the matter is that the way in which psychiatry historically defined mental illness was not fundamentally different from the way in which medicine defined disease. Viewed in this light, there may be fewer differences between the definitions of somatic and mental diseases than is commonly assumed.

A brief discussion of the history of medical thought may help to clarify the problem. By the late eighteenth century medicine was influenced by the prevailing receptivity toward taxonomy, which in turn reflected the Baconian conviction that general laws could be derived from the collection and analysis of particular facts. The underlying assumption of taxonomical science was that genera and species had a natural and independent existence apart from the subjective perceptions of the human observer. Just as plants and minerals could be classified, so too could diseases. The goal of nosological medicine, therefore, was twofold: first, to give clear and precise definitions of diseases; and secondly, to exhibit the relationships and inner nature of disease states by grouping together states with similar characteristics.[29] Once this process was accomplished, it might then become possible to identify the conditions that determined health and disease, and then to alter them. Unable to establish the etiology of disease, physicians developed a nosology based on external symptoms in the belief that they would be able to infer causation, usually by employing a statistical methodology.

Thus prior to the specific germ theory of disease, all physicians — psychiatrists and generalists — defined pathological states by describing them in terms of external and visible symptoms. This process was inevitable, if only because neither the prevailing technology nor theory could establish a relationship between biological mechanisms and external symptoms. To be sure, a classification system based on external symptoms created serious intellectual and scientific problems. Was fever, for example, one disease state or many? While often disagreeing on specifics, few physicians questioned the practice of defining disease by observing symptoms; no other alternative was available. Nor was there any tendency to argue that individuals with a high fever were social deviants because their immediate condition (mental as well as physical) differed significantly from the population at large. Indeed, there are numerous examples in medicine where physicians identify pathological states even when patients appear to be in perfect health. The classic illustration, of course, is hypertension; an individual with high blood pressure may be designated as being sick even in the absence of any other conscious symptoms.

To argue that the difference between psychiatric and more general medical definitions of disease are not fundamentally dissimilar is not in any way to reject the view that the concept of disease is dependent partly on a series of nonscientific or external variables. With the possible exception of a number of infectious diseases, most pathological states are still described in terms of symptoms rather than etiology. Admittedly, psychiatry faces perhaps more difficult and complex problems than most medical specialties. Although there are large areas of agreement in general medicine on certain diagnostic categories — virtually no one, for example, would deny the reality of diabetes or smallpox or pneumonia — such agreement is generally lacking in psychiatry. If physiological processes are responsible for psychiatric diseases, we cannot identify them. Nor is it possible at present to specify the role played by either genetic or environmental factors in producing what is designated as mental disease.[30] Although these generalizations can be applied in some degree to all branches of medicine, past and present, they are particularly applicable to psychiatry. Only a lack of comprehension of medical theory, therefore, could lead to a denial of the reality of mental illness and an insistence that psychiatry was fundamentally different from other branches of medicine.[31]

Social historians interested in the history of medicine and disease also run the risk of imposing personal beliefs upon data, thereby giving rise to questionable conclusions. In general, social history — especially as it is now written — tends to emphasize the primacy of socioeconomic determinants. An affinity for quantitative procedures merely reinforces this tendency. But it must be remembered that categories are not given; they are selected either because the data is readily available or the individual is already convinced of its relevancy to a particular problem. Few historians are aware of the philosophical difficulties of developing a taxonomy based on the subjective perceptions of the observer; many also tend to identify correlation with causality (disclaimers to the contrary). Nor is there any awareness that the classification of a fact is not the same as knowing the fact in a scientific sense. The unsophisticated application of methodologies characteristic of social history, therefore, can lead to erroneous or uninformed conclusions. A recent study that matched death certificates with population schedules for 1960, for example, concluded that the most effective way of decreasing urban death rates was to reduce differentials in socioeconomic status.[32] Yet this very same study made no mention whatsoever of the possibility that genetic or other now unknown variables might also play a role in influencing mortality rates. Indeed, if socio-economic factors are the crucial variables, it might be possible – to use a patently absurd illustration – to eliminate Tay-Sachs disease (an inherited disease found among children of Jewish parents of East European origin) by converting all Jews to Christianity, since the disease is unknown among the latter! Given our tenuous knowledge of most disease processes, social historians must avoid the dangers of beginning their work with certain assumptions, and then interpreting their data as though these assumptions were a mirror of reality.

Finally, it is imperative that historians working with primary data become aware of its strengths *and* deficiencies. This is especially true of census materials, and manuscript schedules in particular. While a detailed analysis of the census is impossible within the confines of a brief article, suffice it to say that the statistics collected were often imprecise, inaccurate, and incomplete. To use this body of data without building in reliability checks or making provision for error, causes, from the very beginning, a flawed analysis. Yet too many social historians have employed data without a critical examination of its reliability; to do the same with source materials bearing upon morbidity and mortality would be nothing short of an unmitigated disaster.[33]

If the problem of writing the social history of medicine and disease are great, so too are the opportunities. But these opportunities can be realized only if scholars first master the "internal" history of medicine and evince a willingness to avoid the temptation to impose their own beliefs upon their data. They must also become far more familiar with related work in other disciplines that are also concerned with health-related issues. If these conditions are met, the result would be a valuable and exciting addition to our knowledge of the role of disease in human history as well as the development of a more sophisticated conceptual framework to deal with the evolution of society.

Rutgers University   Gerald N. Grob

FOOTNOTES

The author wishes to acknowledge that the research for this paper was supported by a grant from the Public Health Service (HEW), National Library of Medicine, No. 2306.

1. See Samuel P. Hays, "A Systematic Social History," *American History: Retrospect and Prospect,* ed. by George A. Billias and Gerald N. Grob (New York, 1971), 315-66.

2. For typical examples see Stephan Thernstrom, *The Other Bostonians: Poverty and Progress in the American Metropolis, 1880-1970* (Cambridge, 1973); Philip J. Greven, *Four Generations: Population, Land, and Family in Colonial Andover, Massachusetts* (Ithaca, 1970); Eric H. Monkkonen, *The Dangerous Classes: Crime and Poverty in Columbus, Ohio, 1860-1885* (Cambridge, 1975); Paul Kleppner, *The Cross of Culture: A Social Analysis of Midwestern Politics, 1850-1890* (New York, 1970). For a general analysis of the literature dealing with the social bases of American politics see Richard L. Mc-Cormick, "Ethno-Cultural Interpretations of Nineteenth-Century Voting Behavior," *Political Science Quarterly,* 89 (June, 1974), 351-77.

3. See Thomas McKeown, R.G. Brown, and R.G. Record, "An Interpretation of the Modern Rise of Population in Europe," *Population Studies,* 26 (November, 1972), 345-82; McKeown, "Medical Issues in Historical Demography," in *Modern Methods in the History of Medicine,* ed. by Edwin Clarke (London, 1971), 57-74; McKeown and Brown, "Medical Evidence Related to English Population Changes in the Eighteenth Century," *Population Studies,* 9 (November, 1955), 119-41; McKeown and Record, "Reasons for the Decline of Mortality in England and Wales During the Nineteenth Century," *Population Studies,* 16 (November, 1962), 94-122.

4. See Carroll Smith-Rosenberg and Charles Rosenberg, "The Female Animal: Medical and Biological Views of Woman and Her Role in Nineteenth-Century America," *Journal of American History,* 60 (September, 1973), 332-56; John S. and Robin M. Haller, *The Physician and Sexuality in Victorian America* (Urbania, Il., 1974); Ann Douglas Wood, "'The Fashionable Diseases': Women's Complaints and Their Treatment in Nineteenth-Century America," *Journal of Interdisciplinary History,* 4 (Summer, 1973), 25-52; Regina M. Morantz, "The Perils of Feminist History," *Journal of Interdisciplinary History,* 4 (Spring, 1974), 649-60; Martha H. Verbrugge, "Women and Medicine in Nineteenth-Century America," *Signs: Journal of Women in Culture and Society,* 1 (Summer, 1976), 959-72.

5. Philip D. Curtin, "Epidemiology and the Slave Trade," *Political Science Quarterly,* 83 (June, 1968), 190-216; Peter H. Wood, *Black Majority: Negroes in Colonial South Carolina from 1670 Through the Stono Rebellion* (New York, 1974), 63-91. See also Alfred W. Crosby, *The Columbian Exchange: Biological and Cultural Consequences of 1492* (Westport, Ct., 1974).

6. U.S. Bureau of the Census, *Historical Statistics of the United States: Colonial Times to 1970,* 2 vols. (Washington, D.C., 1975), Pt. I, 15. For a general discussion of the problems of an aged population see Kingsley Davis, "Population and Welfare in Industrial Societies," *Population Review,* 6 (January, 1962), 17-29.

7. See John Higham, *History* (Englewood Cliffs, 1965), and Morton White, *Social Thought in America: The Revolt Against Formalism* (New York, 1949).

8. For example see Joseph F. Kett, *The Formation of the American Medical Profession: The Role of Institutions, 1780-1860* (New Haven, 1968); William F. Norwood, *Medical Education in the United States before the Civil War* (Philadelphia, 1944); Martin Kaufman, *Homeopathy in America: The Rise and Fall of a Medical Heresy* (Baltimore, 1971); William G. Rothstein, *American Physicians in the Nineteenth Century: From Sects to Science* (Baltimore, 1972); James H. Young, *The Toadstool Millionaires: A Social History of Patent Medicines in America before Federal Regulation* (Princeton, 1961), and *The Medical Messiahs: A Social History of Health Quackery in Twentieth-Century America* (Princeton, 1967); Richard H. Shryock, *Medical Licensing in America, 1650-1965* (Baltimore, 1967), and *American Medical Research, Past and Present* (New York, 1947); George Rosen, *Preventive Medicine in the United States 1900-1975: Trends and Interpretations* (New York, 1975); Oscar E. Anderson, Jr., *The Health of a Nation: Harvey W. Wiley and the Fight for Pure Food* (Chicago, 1958); James H. Cassedy, *Charles V. Chapin and the Public Health Movement* (Cambridge, 1962); Rosemary Stevens, *American Medicine and the Public Interest* (New Haven, 1971); Stephen P. Strickland, *Politics, Science, and Dread Disease: A Short History of United States Medical Research Policy* (Cambridge, 1972); Daniel S. Hirschfield, *The Lost Reform: The Campaign for Compulsory Health Insurance in the United States from 1932 to 1943* (Cambridge, 1970).

These examples, of course, are only selective. For additional listings see Gerald N. Grob, compiler, *American Social History before 1860* (New York, 1970), 88-96, and Robert H. Bremner, compiler, *American Social History Since 1860* (New York, 1971), 98-101. For recent literature the most useful guide is the volumes published by the National Library of Medicine entitled *Bibliography of the History of Medicine* (1964-   ).

Every five years the Library publishes a cumulative volume; the first in this series covers 1964-1969; the second, 1970-1974.

9. Richard H. Shryock, *Medicine in America: Historical Essays* (Baltimore, 1966), 307-32.

10. Erwin H. Ackerknecht, *Malaria in the Upper Mississippi Valley 1760-1900* (Baltimore, 1945).

11. Charles E. Rosenberg, *The Cholera Years: The United States in 1832, 1849, and 1866* (Chicago, 1962); Elizabeth W. Etheridge, *The Butterfly Caste: A Social History of Pellagra in the South* (Westport, Ct., 1972).

12. Barbara G. Rosenkrantz, *Public Health and the State: Changing Views in Massachusetts, 1842-1936* (Cambridge, 1972), and "Cart Before Horse: Theory, Practice and Professional Image in American Public Health, 1870-1920," *Journal of the History of Medicine and Allied Sciences,* 29 (January, 1974), 55-73; Gerald N. Grob, *Mental Institutions in America: Social Policy to 1875* (New York, 1973), and *The State and the Mentally Ill: A History of Worcester State Hospital in Massachusetts, 1830-1920* (Chapel Hill, 1966).

13. Richard H. Shryock's *Medicine and Society in America, 1660-1860* (New York, 1960) is one of the few works that attempts a synthesis of the monographic material. While useful, Shryock's work is indicative of what remains to be accomplished.

14. John Duffy, *Epidemics in Colonial America* (Baton Rouge, 1953), 13.

15. For a discussion of the impact of mortality in colonial Virginia see Edmund S. Morgan, *American Slavery, American Freedom: The Ordeal of Colonial Virginia* (New York, 1975), 158-79. One of the neglected classics of colonial historical epidemiology is Ernest Caulfield's *A True History of the Terrible Epidemic Vulgarly Called the Throat Distemper, Which Occurred in His Majesty's New England Colonies Between the Years 1735 and 1740* (New Haven, 1939).

16. Data on disease taken from U.S. Bureau of the Census, *Historical Statistics of the United States,* Pt. I, 58-59, 63, and U.S. Department of Health, Education, and Welfare (Health Resources Administration), *Mortality Trends for Leading Causes of Death: United States – 1950-69* (Washington, D.C., 1974), 59-63.

17. U.S. Bureau of the Census, *Historical Statistics of the United States,* Pt. I, 58; Rene and Jean Dubos, *The White Plague: Tuberculosis, Man, and Society* (Boston, 1952), 185, 231.

18. Dubos, *White Plague,* 94-110, 131-81, 193.

19. *Ibid.,* 194-95, 234-35. Richard H. Shryock's *National Tuberculosis Association, 1904-1954: A Study of the Voluntary Health Movement in the United States* (New York, 1957), while a useful study of one of America's national health organizations, does not deal with the history of the disease.

20. John H. Powell, *Bring Out Your Dead: The Great Plague of Yellow Fever in Philadelphia in 1793* (Philadelphia, 1949); John Duffy, *Sword of Pestilence: The New Orleans Yellow Fever Epidemic of 1853* (Baton Rouge, 1966), and *Epidemics in Colonial America;* John B. Blake, *Public Health in the Town of Boston, 1630-1822* (Cambridge, 1959); Rosenberg, *Cholera Years;* Alfred W. Crosby, *Epidemic and Peace, 1918* (Westport, 1976).

21. See Aaron E. Klein, *Trial by Fury: The Polio Vaccine Controversy* (New York, 1972), 3-23, and Thomas M. Rivers, *Tom Rivers: Reflections on a Life in Medicine and*

Science (an oral history memoir prepared by Saul Benison) (Cambridge, 1967).

22. Robert H. Wiebe, *The Search for Order, 1877-1920* (New York, 1967): Alfred D. Chandler, Jr., *Strategy and Structure: Chapters in the History of the Industrial Enterprise* (Cambridge, 1962); Louis Galambos, *The Public Image of Big Business in America, 1880-1940: A Quantitative Study in Social Change* (Baltimore, 1975).

23. Rothstein, *American Physicians in the Nineteenth Century*, 298-326.

24. Ernest Greenwood, "Attributes of a Profession," *Social Work*, 2 (July, 1957), 45-55. A convenient sampling of the social science literature dealing with professionalization can be found in Howard M. Vollmer and Donald L. Mills, eds., *Professionalization* (Englewood Cliffs, 1966). For some examples of the historical treatment of professionalization see Daniel H. Calhoun, *Professional Lives in America: Structure and Aspiration, 1750-1850* (Cambridge, 1965); Paul H. Mattingly, *The Classless Profession: American Schoolmen in the Nineteenth Century* (New York, 1975); and Roy Lubove, *The Professional Altruist: The Emergence of Social Work as a Career, 1880-1930* (Cambridge, 1965).

25. For an example of the use of aggregated data on admissions to mental hospitals over a century see M. Harvey Brenner, *Mental Illness and the Economy* (Cambridge, 1973).

26. New York State Commission in Lunacy, *Annual Report*, 12 (1900), 29-30. Data and practices regarding the confinement of aged groups in mental hospitals was taken from the following sources: New York State Department of Mental Hygiene, *Annual Report*, 52 (1939-1940), 174-75; Ohio Department of Public Welfare, *Annual Report*, 15 (1936), 303-304; Massachusetts State Board of Insanity, *Annual Report*, 2 (1900), 32; Michigan State Board of Corrections and Charities, *Biennial Report*, 15 (1898-1900), 210; New York State Commission in Lunacy, *Annual Report*, 19 (1907), 161-68; Oklahoma Commissioner of Charities and Corrections, *Biennial Report*, 6 (1917-1918), 41; Colorado State Board of Charities and Corrections, *Biennial Report*, 11 (1911-1912), 29-30; Maryland Board of Welfare, *4* (1926), *62-63;* Kentucky Department of Public Welfare, *Biennial Report*, 1931-1933, 36, 70; Pennsylvania Committee on Lunacy, *Annual Report*, 22 (1904), 8-9, in Pennsylvania Board of Commissioners of Public Charities, *Annual Report*, 35 (1904).

27. See the series of articles on "Concepts of Health and Disease," edited by F.C. Redlich, in the *Journal of Medicine and Philosophy*, 1 (September, 1976), and Rene Dubos, *Mirage of Health: Utopias, Progress, and Biological Change* (New York, 1959), and *Man Adapting* (New Haven, 1965).

28. The most mature statements of this position are included in the following: Michel Foucalt, *Madness and Civilization: A History of Insanity in the Age of Reason* (New York, 1965); Thomas S. Szasz, *The Myth of Mental Illness: Foundations of a Theory of Personal Conduct* (New York, 1961), and *The Manufacture of Madness: A Comparative Study of the Inquisition and the Mental Health Movement* (New York, 1970); David J. Rothman, *The Discovery of the Asylum: Social Order and Disorder in the New Republic* (Boston, 1971).

29. Lester F. King, *The Medical World of the Eighteenth Century* (Chicago, 1958), Chap. VII.

30. For a perceptive analysis of psychiatry see Charles E. Rosenberg, "The Crisis in Psychiatric Legitimacy: Reflections on Psychiatry, Medicine, and Public Policy," *American Psychiatry: Past, Present, and Future*, ed. by George Kriegman, Robert D. Gardner, and D. Wilfred Abse (Charlottesville, Va., 1975), 135-48.

31. In point of fact we know relatively little about what is designated as mental illness, making it difficult to prove or to disprove its existence. The assertion that there is no such entity as mental illness represents as much an act of faith as its opposite, and those who accept either viewpoint often do so because of their own commitment to particular interpretations. Historians who begin with an acceptance of either proposition are developing interpretations which are at best a form of social criticism.

32. Evelyn M. Kitagawa and Philip M. Hauser, *Differential Mortality in the United States: A Study in Socioeconomic Epidemiology* (Cambridge, 1973), 180 *et passim.*

33. For a discussion of the origins of the modern census and some of its defects see Gerald N. Grob, "Edward Jarvis and the Federal Census: A Chapter in the History of Nineteenth-Century American Medicine," *Bulletin of the History of Medicine,* 50 (Spring, 1976), 4-27.

Kenneth F. Kiple and Virginia H. Kiple

SLAVE CHILD MORTALITY:
SOME NUTRITIONAL ANSWERS TO A PERENNIAL PUZZLE

One of the many controversies spawned by Robert Fogel and Stanley Engerman's upstream plunge against the current of slavery's traditional historiography concerns slave nutrition.[1] The cliometricians portrayed the slave diet as not only substantial calorically, but as actually exceeding "modern (1964) recommended daily levels of the chief nutrients."[2] This portrayal stands in sharp contrast to a more accepted view that had the slave diet "of sufficient bulk but improper balance,"[3] a view which has also found cliometric support. Richard Sutch, after reworking the Fogel and Engerman calculations, concluded that *Time on the Cross* claimed too much, that the caloric intake of slaves was "neither excessive nor generous," and the diet, far from being balanced, was dangerously deficient in many of the chief nutrients.[4]

This clash of cliometricians over nutrients and nutriments has had the heuristic effect of introducing students of the South to such novel preoccupations as livestock slaughter rates and conversion ratios, the kinds of sweet potatoes consumed, and the proper way to cook cowpeas (with Sutch supplying his own recipe). Unquestionably cliometric calorie counting has elevated an old argument to a higher level of sophistication. But as far as the nutritional adequacy of the slave diet is concerned, the debate has generated more methodological heat than qualitative light.

Bio-history may help to shed that light. The major reason diet is important is because it speaks to the larger question of slave health. Conversely slave health speaks to matters of nutritional adequacy, which suggests the fallacy of considering either in isolation. Examined in tandem, the one should always act as a check on the other. If blacks were well-nourished, then diseases with a nutritional etiology should be conspicuously absent in the slave quarters. If, on the other hand, specific nutrients seem lacking in the slave diet, then diseases whose etiologies include these dietary lacunae should be in evidence and a "match" of deficiencies and diseases achieved.

This study is a search for such matches in the diet and diseases of slave children — children whose physical well-being should be indicative not only of the level of health and nutrition of their own generation, but reflective of their parents' generation as well. The attempts to couple nutritional deficiency and disease however do not rely on serendipity. Rather differing biological heritages which dictate differing nutritional requirements and disease susceptibilities are employed to point the way.

I

The contestants in the nutritional debate have become so enmeshed in questions of methodological purity that they have forgotten the ultimate subject of the debate – the Negro and more specifically his nutritional needs, different in many respects from those of whites because of a difference in geographic and environmental background.

In the case of the Negro adaptation to the unique disease, climatic, and ecological circumstances of West Africa has resulted in an array of special biological equipment which insured survival there.[5] Yet much of this equipment becomes a distinct liability once its possessor is removed from that environment. Undoubtedly the best known example is the sickling trait, a balanced polymorphism that protects against the deadly falciparum malaria hyperendemic in the region.[6] Heterozygous individuals (those who inherit the trait from one parent only) develop sickle-shaped blood cells which discourage proliferation of the falciparum parasite.

There is a price for this protection however which is paid by the homozygous individual (inherits the trait from both parents) who develops sickle cell anemia. Today one individual in roughly 500 Negro births has his lifetime shortened some two-thirds by sickle cell anemia.[7] Yesterday on the plantation (because the trait is slowly dying in the United States) the incidence of sickle cell anemia, as well as the sickling trait, must have been higher.[8] Obviously then some morbidity and mortality among slave youngsters was a consequence of homozygous inheritance of the trait, but even more important from a nutritional standpoint heterozygous possession of the trait produces a mild anemia which in turn heightens the blacks' requirement (as opposed to the whites) for iron and folic acid.[9] Other less lethal hemoglobin abnormalities which appear in the black with unusual frequency include more blood disorders – hemoglobin C and β-thalassemia for example, along with enzyme deficiencies such as glucose-6-phosphate dehydrogenase.[10] These too can create anemia and therefore imply increased dietary requirements of the nutrients just noted.

A second nutritional liability for U.S. blacks stemming from their West African origin has to do with their high frequency of lactose intolerance. Lactose intolerance is occasioned by the absence of the lactase enzyme (an autosomal recessive trait) which metabolizes milk sugars into absorbable monosaccharides. In the United States today some 70 to 77 % of the black population manifest symptoms of lactose intolerance, as opposed to 5 to 19 % of the whites.[11] It seems probable that the development of the lactase enzyme among early residents of northern Europe was genetically encouraged by the prevalence of late rickets and osteomalacia, due to a lack of sunshine.[12] In West Africa, by contrast, there was no lack of sunshine; moreover, the tsetse fly made the raising of cattle virtually impossible. These twin factors then created a historical situation of low milk consumption, and no need for developing a lactase enzyme.[13]

The result is that in the United States (whose climate more closely approximates northern Europe than West Africa) most blacks discover sometime after infancy (all infants are lactose tolerant obviously, else none would live) that if they drink milk they can expect gastrointestinal complaints within thirty to ninety minutes; continued use brings on severe abdominal cramps, bloating and diarrhea. A natural response then is to eliminate milk from the diet.[14]

A final (for our purposes) characteristic of West Africans with nutritional significance concerns the skin. The darker pigmentation of the Negro helped to keep his body cool in Africa and protected against sun damage.[15] But pigment also reduces the synthesis of vitamin D by the skin.[16] Ultraviolet light from a fairly intense sun activates bodily mechanisms to produce cholecalciferol (D3), which means a dietary source of the vitamin is not requisite. Thus the black transplanted to more northerly latitudes found himself deficient in vitamin D, especially during the winter and spring months of pale sunlight and overcast skies. Whites, in other words, because of a lack of pigment, have access to sufficient vitamin D in North America; but blacks frequently do not.

To summarize then, West Africa endowed her sons with marvelous mechanisms of protection for survival in that region. However these same mechanisms contained the potential for provoking severe nutritional difficulties once their possessor was removed from West Africa's specialized environment – a potential which must have been realized after the blacks' forced migration to the United States. Therefore the important question concerning slave nutrition which should have been asked in not whether the slave diet was adequate, but rather – was it adequate for persons of West African descent?

II

Understandably, given the propensity for quantification among the participants, the debate over slave nutrition has for the most part centered on quantities of foods available to slaves. But it is not enough to simply calculate the potential yield of vitamins and minerals that nutriments contain, multiply this by the quantity supposedly consumed, and pronounce a diet satisfactory or unsatisfactory. The chemical relationships between nutrients is vital to good nutrition, and in the case of the slave diet some of the unfortunate relationships which occurred render questions of quantity irrelevant.

For example, both sides agree that the core of the slave diet was composed of fat pork and cornmeal. The yield of phosphorus from this core (the higher the quantity, the higher the yield) while not extraordinarily high by itself is overwhelmingly high in relation to the low calcium offering of the diet. Lactose intolerant slaves would have derived little calcium from milk, while the greens, sweet potatoes, etc., which supplemented the core, although a source of some calcium, could not have yielded enough to overcome a year-round imbalance because of their seasonal appearance on tables. This excessive amount of phosphorus in relation to calcium in turn would have hindered the absorption of the little calcium and magnesium the slaves did receive, and therefore increased their requirements for both minerals. Similarly, the fatty acids flowing from fat pork also interfere with the bodily absorption of calcium and magnesium, as do the oxalic acids contained in greens which form insoluable salts to impair absorption of the pair of minerals in question.[17]

If calcium and magnesium did not already have a difficult time playing a proper nutritional role in the slave regimen, they were further frustrated by the peculiar nature of the proteins inherent in that regimen. High quality protein promotes efficient absorption of these minerals (high quality defined as a protein containing all eight essential amino acids in sufficient amounts to support and maintain life). Yet the slave diet was dismally lacking in this kind of protein. Cornmeal, the chief source of protein for the slaves, is extremely low in three amino acids (tryptophan, lysine, and methionine) meaning it is of very poor quality, while pork is likewise low in these same amino acids.[18]

Clearly then the slave diet was hostile to a full nutritional participation of calcium and magnesium, yet even at this point that hostility might have been blunted had it not been for two more factors which irreparably "stacked" the slave diet against its consumers. An adequate source of vitamin C would have increased the absorption of what calcium was available; but ascorbic acid cannot be stored by the body, and no one seriously argues that slaves received a year-round supply of this vitamin. Finally, the one remaining factor which could have enhanced the absorption of calcium is vitamin D (the reason milk is fortified with this vitamin today), but as already noted pigment which was kindly to blacks in their West African homeland militated against an adequate year-round supply of this vitamin in temperate North America.

Iron presents very much the same case. Although the Fogel and Engerman diet apparently provides slaves with a sufficient supply of iron,[19] there are four reasons for believing that the supply was far from adequate. First, the iron requirements employed as a standard were those for a population whose composition is overwhelmingly white. Yet as we have pointed out, hemoglobin abnormalities mean that blacks are prone to anemia and therefore need more iron than whites.[20] Second, the cliometricians calculated a diet for *male* slaves aged 18-35 whose requirements are relatively low for the mineral in comparison with children and women, especially when the latter are pregnant or lactating.[21] Third, as in the case of calcium, the absorption of iron is retarded by phosphorus and enhanced by lactose, vitamin C and meat protein — none of which abounded in slave victuals.[22] Finally, the assumption has been that most iron in the slave diet derived from cornmeal, which would appear to have a rich yield of iron. Yet this is deceptive for iron is poorly absorbed from cereal grains.[23] In fact, research has revealed that only 5% of the iron in maize is absorbed.[24]

A similar chemical case can be constructed against the slave intake and utilization of vitamins in the B complex, but that is beyond the scope of this study.[25] For our purposes, particularly since the major concern is with the health of children, it is enough to know that a significant portion of the slave population appears to have been seriously deprived of calcium, magnesium, and iron which, if true, means that many slave children were in serious nutritional difficulty — in some cases even before birth.

III

During the prenatal period, the fetus will do its best to satisfy its own needs for minerals, even if the mother is deficient, by drawing on her skeletal stores. However, assuming a deficiency to begin with, the high fertility of the slave mother would have meant something akin to bankruptcy of those stores long before she produced her last child, unless she received a special diet to replace depleted mineral supplies – an unlikely event on the plantation.[26] If, on the other hand, multiparous mothers tried to "eat for two" while pregnant, the result would have been an even higher intake of carbohydrates and fats which would have further increased bodily needs for vitamins and minerals already in dangerously short supply. Some slave babies then must have entered the world with serious mineral deficiencies.[27]

The baby began his dietary routine normally enough at his mother's breast, but the same factors which created mineral deficiencies – especially calcium and magnesium – for the fetus implies that in some cases the infant's sole source of nourishment, his mother's milk, would perpetuate these deficiencies. Thus the first opportunity to correct them would come with weaning.

However, for many weaning (regardless of the quality of the mother's milk) would have been a giant nutritional step backwards since the custom was to wean slave children to a diet even higher in carbohydrates and lower in proteins than that of their parents. Planters were agreed that the proper diet for children should consist mostly of cornbread, hominy and fat.[28] They believed that "clear" meat (as opposed to fat) would "debilitate" children and "until puberty meats should not enter too much into the diet."[29] Many also thought vegetables to be "not proper for them."[30]

Slave children who were the victims of this sort of nutritional theorizing therefore would have continued to be seriously deficient in iron, with bovine milk their only important source of calcium and magnesium. Fortunately because the level of lactose intolerance among blacks increases with age, proportionately more slave children than adults would have been able to use milk.[31] Unfortunately many did not enjoy the opportunity. Some authorities have insisted that what milk was produced on plantations was destined mostly for white tables,[32] while others have conceded milk to slave children during the spring and summer months only, when it was most plentiful.[33] The impression which one is left with is that some slave children enjoyed milk during some of the year, but even for them milk was merely a seasonal dietary item.[34]

Yet, assuming that a child did receive substantial quantities of bovine milk, his mineral deficiencies may still not have been "cured" because first, a child must consume three times more cow's milk than human milk to absorb the same amount of calcium;[35] second, the high phosphorus content of whole cow's milk (five times more than in human milk) lowers the serum calcium and magnesium levels of babies, while the high phosphate and fat content of the slave child's diet would have further impaired the utilization of these minerals;[36] and third, those Children who were beginning to lose the lactase enzyme could not have properly metabolized the milk sugars, which means that continued consumption would have hindered the absorption of other nutrients, including calcium.[37]

There seems little question then that those slave children who became calcium, magnesium and/or iron deficient early in life could expect little from the diet they were weaned to, which was better calculated to occasion these deficiencies than to cure them. In fact, because the slave diet was more nutritionally disastrous for children than it was for adults, one is tempted to castigate southern planters for meanness – particularly since the child's diet appears suspiciously inexpensive. Yet most masters seem to have been quite solicitous of the health of their burgeoning assets, and ironically the victuals served to them were believed to be the healthiest possible. Planters were convinced "that negroes and white people are very different in their habits and constitutions, and that while fat meat is the life of the negro it is a prolific source of disease and death among the whites."[38] For slave children fat and corn were "perculiarly appropriate"[39] and "negroes who are freely supplied with them grow plump, sleek and shiny."[40] Masters on the whole took much pride in the "plump, sleek and shiny" pickaninnies.

However, as will be seen later, they were often deceived by this "plumpness" which can be as symptomatic of bad nutrition as it can good nutrition. Indeed a regimen high in carbohydrates and low in proteins will produce precisely this kind of physical appearance, which to the twentieth century medical eye spells protein-calorie malnutrition.

IV

If slave children were severely deficient in calcium, magnesium and iron, then evidence of this should be contained in antebellum records. To be more specific, black children should reveal a much higher incidence of morbidity and mortality than whites from diseases with an etiology which includes these nutritional deficiencies. This does not mean that all white children enjoyed a diet substantially different from and superior to that of blacks, although many undoubtedly did because the circumstances of slavery were more likely to dictate a circumscribed regimen. But our basic contention is that, even if white children were fed the same diet as slave children, the latter would have evidenced symptoms of malnourishment to a greater degree for the biological reasons already discussed.

Our evidence from antebellum sources is both statistical and impressionistic. Most of the impressionistic evidence comes from the pens of southern physicians who, as a group, entertained the belief that a "package" of largely "Negro diseases" existed — diseases blacks were far more likely to contract and die from than whites. Much of this "package" is composed of children's diseases, and the clinical descriptions of these ailments become extremely valuable when trying to match deficiency with disease. For the moment, however, the entire contents of the package are germane as they speak to the question of the nutritional heritage of black children, and we find it highly significant that physicians found blacks unusually susceptible to infectious diseases, to an appallingly high level of infant mortality, and to an unusually high frequency of dental caries and bone and skin complaints. In an age of more advanced medical knowledge, these symptoms describe a people suffering serious nutritional deficiencies.

Backing up these physicians' opinions and observations regarding black disease susceptibilities is a sample of runaway slave descriptions which are replete with references to crooked or bandy legs, knocked-knees, stooped shoulders, jaundiced complexions, splotchy skin, inflamed and watery eyes, partial blindness, and rotten, missing, or buck teeth.[41] Moreover, the records of over one hundred estates ranging from Louisiana to South Carolina, and from Florida to Arkansas suggest that these afflictions of the runaways were hardly atypical by revealing data which also point to a high incidence of blindness, lameness, deformed bones, skin lesions, and dental problems.[42]

Mortality data which narrows the focus to children's diseases has been drawn from various state manuscript census schedules of mortality for the year 1849-50[43] and from DeBow's *Compendium* of the 1850 mortality figures done in 1855.[44] Unfortunately the practice of compiling extensive mortality statistics in 1850 was not followed during the next decennial census, and those data which are available for the year 1860 are of little worth for our purposes.[45] Nor are the 1850 data as complete as one might wish,[46] and despite their invaluable nature as one of the few available comprehensive sources on the causes of slave deaths, any rates derived from them are invariably going to be low.[47] In fact, as one will quickly note from Table 1, most authorities would probably at least double the infant mortality rate of both white and black.[48] However, we have chosen to let the data "speak for themselves" because we regard the black/white differentials as more significant than the actual rates.

The census of 1850 revealed a black population in the United States of 3,638,808 individuals. Of these 2,539,617 or slightly over 75% resided in the seven states of Virginia, North Carolina, South Carolina, Mississippi, Georgia, Alabama, and Louisiana — the states from which mortality data has been drawn for this study. About 31% (786,404) of that population was aged "9-and-under." The whites residing in these states by contrast numbered 3,221,686 with 33.6% of their population (1,084,486) falling into the "9-and-under" category.

A "9-and-under" age grouping is of course an actuarially perilous category. Yet it was far more hazardous for black children than for white. Black children in this cohort accounted for fully 51% of all Negro deaths, while white children contributed only 38% of the white deaths during the twelve months spanning the years 1849-50. Table 1 presents the age specific death rates for our seven state sample.

Table 1. Race and Age Specific Death Rates Per 1,000

Age	0-1	1-4	5-9	0-9
White	61.4	11.8	5.0	12.9
Black	137.2	27.7	6.8	26.3

Clearly the disproportionate number of deaths of black children in the 0-4 age group accounts for much of the black/white differential. Black youngsters in this cohort died at a rate (44 per thousand) more than double that of their white counterparts (19 per thousand).

A glance at the diseases which caused these deaths is most revealing. From a possible 120 or so lethal afflictions contained in the census there were six maladies to which slave youngsters proved fearfully susceptible. Indeed "convulsions,"[49] "teething," "tetanus," "lockjaw," "suffocation," and "worms" were listed as the cause of almost a quarter (23%) of the black deaths for which a cause was given in the 0-9 age group, yet they accounted for only 11.7% of the white deaths exclusive of "unknown" causes in the same age cohort.[50] By total population the differential is even more impressive. Fully 45 out of every 10,000 black children in the 9-and-under age group could expect to die from one of these six diseases, while only 11 white youngsters per 10,000 faced the same prospect. Hence black children's risk of dying from one of these six diseases was more than four times that of their white counterparts, which calls for a close examination of each of the fatal maladies to discover the reasons behind this deadly color preference.

Convulsions, Teething, and Tetanus

Medical science in this century has become increasingly aware that calcium, magnesium, and vitamin D deficiencies, singularly or in combination, play an important part in the etiology of the long misunderstood children's disease called tetany — an affliction characterized by hyperirritability of the neuromuscular system, whose symptoms include convulsions and spasms of the voluntary muscles.[51] Calcium is essential to the proper contraction of these muscles, magnesium is important to their relaxation, and vitamin D is essential to calcium's absorption; thus a severe deficiency of any one may produce those tetanic symptoms, including convulsions, which can lead to death.

A vicious cycle of calcium-magnesium deficiency seems to have been inevitable for many slave families. It began with a deficient mother undergoing multiple pregnancies and her maternal calcium serum falling with each succeeding pregnancy until she herself became a candidate for maternal tetany, while simultaneously each fetus whose own bone development is dependent on its mother's mineral supply became progressively more deprived. Today this vicious cycle is known to account for the positive correlation between frequent pregnancies and hypocalcemic or hypomagnesic convulsions in infants.[52]

A shortage of vitamin D could only have compounded the problem for the fetus of a slave mother — a shortage occasioned not only by his mother's pigmentation, but also by the practice of "lying in" with her receiving little exposure to the sun during the last weeks of pregnancy.[53] Consequently the unborn child may easily have become vitamin D deficient and unable to utilize minerals he did draw from his mother's skeletal structure. Some slave babies therefore must have developed tetany while still in the womb.[54]

After birth, the infant's magnesium-calcium supply was still dependent on the extent of his mother's stores, while weaning to a high carbohydrate-low protein diet would have perpetuated the problem for the reasons already stressed. Finally even those slave infants given a plentiful supply of bovine milk could not be considered safe from tetany, for the high phosphorus content of undiluted bovine milk has lately been indicted as an important factor in the disease.[55]

In short, reason for suspecting tetany among the slaves abounds, but because it was not recognized as a disease during antebellum days, all children's ailments characterized by its symptoms demand scrutiny. Three likely possibilities become "convulsions," "teething," and "tetanus," all of which antebellum physicians believed were largely responsible for a substantially higher incidence of black as opposed to white infant mortality.[56] This collective opinion is buttressed by mortality statistics generated by the seventh census, which indicate that indeed black children were the chief victims of the diseases in question.

The lethal trio killed 2419 individuals in the seven largest slaveholding states, with blacks constituting 66.5% of the victims. Fully 204 Negroes per 100,000 live population aged nine-and-under could expect to die from one of the three, as opposed to only 74 per 100,000 white youngsters. Supporting data confirming the discriminatory nature of these diseases come from the city of Charleston, where during the years 1822-48 they killed 1738 individuals. Fully 72.4% of that total were blacks, although the white population exceeded the black throughout that period.[57]

"Convulsions" of course describe precisely those symptoms of nutritional tetany we are looking for and consequently require little explanation. Teething is suspect because nineteenth century physicians observed that the convulsions which ravaged babies often occurred during the teething process and concluded that the sprouting of teeth was somehow responsible — hence "teething" as a cause of death.[58] However, infants did not die simply because their teeth decided to make an appearance.

Rather it is at this point that some mothers, who had not yet weaned their babies, decided (often hastily) to do so, and in the process quite possibly deprived the child of his sole source of calcium. Similarly, research has revealed disturbances in calcium and phosphorus metabolism during dentition.[59] Finally, the high phosphorus content of bovine milk abruptly introduced is known to trigger convulsions.[60] Confirmation that "teething" deaths frequently represented tetany cases may be found in nineteenth century clinical descriptions of the problem. The symptoms — hurried "crouplike" breathing, crowing cough, convulsive movements of the body, constant frowning ("carp mouth"), wrist and ankle joints drawn inward and head drawn back — read like a depiction of tetany in its classic form.[61]

Tetanus presents a somewhat different problem of linkage with tetany. Convulsions and teething were not diseases by themselves but rather (we have argued) frequently symptoms of a disease whose nutritional origins only became widely known in this century. Tetanus, on the other hand, was understood to be a disease during antebellum days, was associated (albeit imperfectly) with wounds, and appears as a cause of death in the mortality schedules of the census of 1850. However, "lockjaw" also appears as a cause of death which suggests (as do the categories of "convulsions" and "teething") both a fondness of medical men for symptomatic appellations and a reluctance, despite the urgings of specialists, to regard lower jaw rigidity of the muscle and tetanus (without trismus) as selfsame.

The distinction made (although erroneous) is useful. For the symptoms of tetany and tetanus are identical, and as the former was for all practical purposes unknown during the nineteenth century, it would invariably have been diagnosed as the latter. Had patients uniformly displayed a history of wounds, one could be reasonably certain the statistics were speaking of tetanus, not tetany, yet physicians often pondered the mystery of tetanus without wounds.[62] Moreover, it was noted that tetanus "epidemics" occurred among southern blacks during the late winter months — months when milk and sunshine were in short supply.[63] Today, too, tetany deaths peak during the same months,[64] all of which suggests strongly that tetany may often have been diagnosed as tetanus, thus explaining our lumping of tetanus deaths with convulsions and teething for purposes of analysis.

That we also included "lockjaw" by subsuming it under tetanus requires even more explanation, for in this case at least one might surmise that he is confronting *bona fide* cases of tetanus. Yet it is an uneasy confrontation, again because of the uncanny awareness of color and youth that "lockjaw" revealed. Of the 398 reported victims of fatal "lockjaw" within our seven state sample, 264 or 66% were blacks, while 308 of the victims or 77.3% were under the age of five.

Common symptoms of tetany are severe and prolonged spasms of the larynx (often to the point of suffocation) and a rigid face characterized by "carp mouth" in which the corners of the mouth are turned down, causing difficulties' in speech or swallowing. Either of these symptoms may have been confused with lower jaw rigidity (particularly in the case of infants) by almost all laymen and more than a few antebellum physicians.

On the other hand, a high incidence of tetanus among southern infants would scarcely be surprising, and we are certainly not arguing that all "lockjaw" deaths were tetany. Tetanus thrives best in agrarian areas where sterile medical procedures are absent, and reveals a special affinity for infants whose umbilicus proves particularly liable to infection. Indeed, a few physicians thought umbilicus infection the chief factor in what they termed *trismus nascentium* and what midwives called the "nine day fits." The problem remains, however, of why "lockjaw" sought out black babies — the same problem which baffled one experimentally inclined doctor who used both rusty and clean scissors on the umbilical cords of black and white alike, yet saw only blacks contract "lockjaw."[65]

Rickets

Rickets, a usually non-lethal childhood disease, would not normally be included in any discussion of child mortality. However, rickets and tetany have similar etiologies, and a high incidence of one among a population is usually *prima facie* evidence of the presence of the other.[66] Thus if a high frequency of rickets can be discerned during the slave days, the case for nutritional tetany as an important killer of slave youngsters will be immeasurably strengthened. The problem is that, although rickets was known as a disease in antebellum times, its seldom fatal nature facilitated its escaping both statistical and medical attention.[67] A case for its frequency among slaves therefore must be largely inferential.

The "hardest" data comes from the seventh census which reveals 25 deaths from rickets during the year 1849-50. Of the victims 84% (21) were black children. Numerically the number of deaths seems insignificant, but because rickets is rarely fatal, 25 deaths does suggest a fairly high incidence of the disease. Certainly its attraction to blacks is obvious.

A high frequency of childhood rickets is also indicated by runaway slave advertisements in newspapers ranging geographically from New Orleans to Charleston to Memphis which frequently mention deformed bones.[68] Such descriptions identifying a runaway as "bowlegged and lame," "slightly bandy-legged," "very knock-kneed," "slightly knock-kneed" and "much knock-kneed" appeared so often in antebellum newspapers that they could not have been very useful as a distinguishing characteristic. Bowlegs and knock-knees of course are the most obvious adult signs of a bout with childhood rickets.

Finally, at the turn of this century as the medical profession became far more concerned about the problem of rickets, they "discovered" such a high frequency of the disease among blacks that many physicians became convinced that *all* black children in the cities of Washington and New York suffered from the disease, while as late as the 1920's, 87.6% of Negro children in Memphis were rachitic. It seems of some importance that these physicians who "discovered" this heavy incidence of rickets in black children concluded that it must have been widespread on the plantations as well.[69]

Smothering

The link between calcium, magnesium, and vitamin D deficiences, on the one hand, and nutritional tetany among slave children, on the other, represents the beginning of a chain to which other nutritional diseases may be joined, among them that mysterious killer of slave children — smothering. Anyone familiar with the subject of American Negro slavery has encountered and perhaps puzzled over the appalling number of instances of parents having supposedly "overlain" their child while sleeping, and the concomitant planter disgust at the carelessness of slave parents.[70]

Superficially it would seem that planters most certainly did have reason for disgust. Of the 723 deaths from suffocation recorded during the year 1849-50 in the seven largest slaveholding states, 666 or fully 92% of the victims were black. In terms of the live population under one year of age, the differential is even more staggering. For every 10,000 blacks in this age cohort, 108 succumbed to "suffocation," while less than 1 white child per 10,000 perished from the same cause.

Yet the phenomenon of infants suddenly dying during the night of no apparent cause has occurred throughout history, and is still occurring at a rate which makes these deaths collectively one of the major killers of babies during their first year of life.[71] In the past, when youngsters frequently slept with parents, it is understandable that the latter often believed they had accidentally "overlain" a child found dead in the morning. Yet experiments have demonstrated the near impossibility of an infant smothering so long as any circulating air at all reaches him,[72] and of course today, although babies rarely sleep with parents, the mysterious deaths continue.

Contemporary appellations for the disease (or diseases) in question are crib or cot deaths and, more scientifically, the Sudden Infant Death Syndrome (SIDS). There seems little doubt that most of the "smothering" deaths of the nineteenth century and the crib deaths of the present are one in the same. After studying the problem for Virginia, Professor Todd Savitt has reported that there exists not only a compelling descriptive similarity between the "smothering" deaths of slave infants and modern day crib deaths, but that there is also "a remarkable epidemiological correspondence, both in age and seasonal variation between the two."[73]

More than half of crib deaths occur during the coldest months of the year, with the majority of the victims aged between two and eight months.[74] Mortality figures from our seven states coincide with these findings by revealing that some 57% of the smothering deaths occurred during the South's chilliest months, while fully 82% of the smothering victims were less than one year of age.

Hypotheses to account for SIDS have ranged from the implication of foreign proteins in bovine milk[75] to spinal injuries,[76] airway obstruction,[77] immature neural systems,[78] and congenital anomalies of the parathyroids[79] to anaphylaxis by the house dust mite.[80] Yet none individually have proven sufficiently inclusive to account for all of the factors in the syndrome, while many are so contradictory as to constitute mutually exclusive explanatory efforts. Indeed, data generated by small experiments and questionable samples have generated findings which vary so wildly it is surprising that even the following broad generalizations regarding the "syndrome" have been agreed upon:[81] (1) the aforementioned age and seasonal factors (2) the disease kills at least twice as many blacks as whites in proportion to their respective populations (3) a breastfed baby is much less likely to become an SIDS statistic than one fed with a formula (4) a significant percentage of the victims are born prematurely or weigh under five-and-a-half pounds at birth (5) although most SIDS victims die suddenly from no apparent cause, a common thread of respiratory infections and convulsions seems to link those who manifested some premonitory signs prior to death, while (6) autopsies performed on SIDS youngsters have revealed signs of respiratory distress and circulatory collapse before death.

We would point out (at the risk of seeming presumptuous) that most medical researchers do not look for nutritional etiologies, yet these factors do fit together rather nicely if a nutritional etiology — specifically calcium and/or magnesium deficiency is assumed. The convulsions and respiratory difficulties resemble, at least to the layman, nutritional tetany — and we are impressed that the tatany syndrome reveals factors identical to those of SIDS.[82] The frequency of prematurity and low birth weights among the victims suggests that the faster than normal growth rate of premature infants[83] meant a lack of both time and opportunity for building proper mineral stores — a problem which cow's milk (breast-fed babies being far less susceptible to both SIDS and tetany) high in phosphorus cannot compensate for. Moreover most deaths occur during those coldest months when fresh vegetables containing calcium and magnesium are in shortest supply. Finally, most victims are blacks who are far more likely to be mineral deficient.

Nonetheless, almost no nutritional explanations of SIDS have been forthcoming, and nine implicate mineral deficiencies, save an ingenuous hypothesis which does account for each of the above syndrome factors. Dr. J.L. Caddell has pointed out that the magnesium deprivation growth syndrome which has occupied her attention for many years closely approximates SIDS.[84] Children on a diet poor in magnesium relative to calcium, phosphorus and protein, or relying on milk from a multiparous mother whose magnesium stores have been depleted are the most vulnerable. The deficiency in turn brings on the liberation of histamine (particularly in the early hours when the child has been asleep for some time) which in turn initiates an autonomic reflex action, putting the body in histamine shock. The latter is characterized by bronchospasm, apnea, pulmonary edema and heart hemorrhage which lead to circulatory collapse.

The similarities between nutritional tetany, the magnesium deprivation growth syndrome and SIDS do strongly indicate a nutritional etiology for the latter. Moreover, yesterday in the slave quarters black children who were magnesium and calcium deficient also exhibited a high rate of what we now know were crib deaths. We have long felt that medical researchers could make better use of historical materials, and in the case of SIDS the circumstances of slave nutrition and slave infant mortality would seem to present them with an important epidemiological laboratory.

Protein-Calorie Malnutrition

The practice of weaning plantation infants to a diet high in carbohydrates and low in proteins should have resulted in a fairly high incidence of protein-calorie malnutrition. Moreover, this problem may well have been exacerbated considerably by lactose intolerance, which some black children develop during the first year of life,[85] because the lactase enzyme is important not only for the metabolism of lactose, but indirectly for all carbohydrates. Its absence therefore means that a diet high in carbohydrates can only be partially utilized by the body, presenting the paradox of a person very nearly starving on an apparently abundant diet. Studies of African populations for example have revealed a high correlation between infant malnutrition and tribes characterized by low lactose levels. In fact, it has been hypothesized that lactose intolerance is a predisposing factor to kwashiorkor. [86]

One of the most prevalent types of protein-calorie malnutrition is kwashiorkor, whose sufferers are normally children in the five-and-under age group and whose symptoms in extreme form include those distended bellies with which the entire world has become heartbreakingly familiar since World War II. However, it was not until 1956, when enough information had accumulated on its etiology, that a protein-deficient diet could be established as the culprit. The disease was first observed clinically on the Gold Coast (now Ghana), hence the Ga word which means "the sickness of the deprived child." [87]

In this sense of the word, antebellum plantations must have abounded with somewhat deprived children who exhibited mild cases of kwashiorkor.[88] Their diet was not completely devoid of protein (which produces extreme edema) but was seriously deficient because it (1) centered around corn, a low quality protein, and (2) contained too little protein in proportion to total caloric intake. Either or both of these conditions can be responsible for kwashiorkor.[89] Edema is a result of a low intake of tryptophan or methionine (the slave diet, particularly the children's, was deficient in both) essential amino acids which among other things stimulate the production of the blood protein albumin. When this process is retarded a reduction in serum albumin and hence water retention (edema) occurs.

Some evidence of widespread kwashiorkor ironically enough comes from the records of self-satisfied masters who took pride in the sleek plump pickaninnies of their plantations and from the pens of travelers who accepted the little pot-bellies as evidence of planter largess.[90] Physicians, however, were not fooled by this appearance of health and pondered at some length the distention of slave children's stomachs.[91]

Another form of protein-calorie malnutrition, symptomatically on the opposite pole from kwashiorkor, is marasmus, which is quite simply starvation. It is caused by an inadequate intake of calories, with a resulting general emaciation and growth retardation. Infants who have been weaned to a nutritionally inadequate diet are among its chief victims.[92]

A Mississippi doctor writing on "The Negro and His Diseases" described the disease vividly in 1853 as one "to which Negro children are liable between the second and the fifth year. ... It is literally a 'wasting away' – a tabes ... styled provincially [as] 'the drooping disease of negro children.'" It begins with "languor, fretfulness and loss of strength. The child gradually becomes emaciated ... diarrhea supervenes ... [soon] fever complicates the case" and perhaps "convulsions."[93]

Both kwashiorkor and marasmus puzzled physicians, who blamed it alternately on prolonged lactation and premature weaning (both in many cases were probably correct assessments), on unsanitary conditions, diet, worms, and dirt-eating.[94] Yet this shotgun approach pathologically may have scored important hits, for a diet which produces kwashiorkor or marasmus in children will also create problems with worms, and very possibly a craving for pica. Moreover, the symptoms of all can be remarkably similar which suggests an examination of the remaining two disorders.

Pica

Cachexia africana and dirt-eating were two of the most common antebellum sobriquets for pica, an exotic disease which fascinated physicians and terrified planters because it seemed to appear almost solely among Negroes.[95] Certainly our seven state sampling of mortality statistics from the 1850 census tends to confirm the predilection of Africans for geophagy, while at the same time suggesting the normally non-lethal nature of the malady. For despite the fearsome reputation of dirt-eating only 86 deaths were attributed to it. Almost all (83) of the victims however were blacks.

Symptoms of adult "dirt-eating" first manifested themselves in dyspepsia, then in acute diarrhea, heart palpitations and a jaundiced or ash-colored skin. Advanced cases became emaciated and anemic, developing swellings and "dropsical effusions." Children, on the other hand, often developed only edema, exactly as in the case of kwashiorkor. Antebellum authorities disagreed wildly over the reasons for pica usage, but they did agree that although geophagy seemed to be practiced by all age and sex groups, those most susceptible were children and pregnant and lactating women.[96]

If southern physicians were baffled by the origin of pica, they were no less perceptive than modern authorities who have grouped themselves into three identifiable schools of thought. The oldest would have pica a response to hook-worm infection;[97] a second insists that clay-eating was essentially a cultural trait or habit passed along from generation to generation;[98] while a third has concentrated on a nutritional explanation.[99] The schools are not however mutually exclusive and all concede that nutritional deficiencies play at least some part in the etiology of pica.

Indeed there exists an impressive number of both statistical and clinical studies which testify t o a connection between pica and nutrition. Their major conclusions may be categorized and summarized as follows: 1) geophagy is practiced, with few exceptions, by the malnourished who have a high incidence of physical ailments;[100] 2) among the most serious deficiencies in the diet of these people are the minerals calcium, magnesium, potassium, and iron;[101] 3) the soils consumed by pica users have been analyzed and found to contain high concentrations of these minerals;[102] 4) pica users who have been treated clinically with the minerals in question have lost interest in "substitute" or non-foods, while others who were given placebos instead of the actual mineral supplements did not abandon "non-foods."[103]

Thus it seems likely that dirt-eating among slaves was in many cases symptomatic of severe mineral deficiencies, particularly in light of the evidence which indicates a dietary lack of iron, calcium, and magnesium — the minerals most often associated with the practice. Interestingly such a possibility did not escape antebellum medical authorities, some of whom observed that better and more varied slave diets constituted the best insurance planters could have against pica outbreaks on their plantations.[104] Significant also is their collective warning that youngsters and pregnant and lactating women were most liable to acquire the pica habit — precisely those groups whose requirements for iron, calcium and magnesium are the highest.

Worms

Worms proved extraordinarily deadly to the under-ten age group of the slaves. Of 1708 deaths due to worms recorded during the year 1849-50 in our seven state sample, 77% of the victims were listed as black, while 96% of the total were aged 9-and-under. In terms of live population, 16 out of every 10,000 black youngsters under ten years of age could expect to die of worms as opposed to only 3 out of every 10,000 white children. Small wonder that antebellum authorities viewed worms as one of the most terrible maladies to affect the slave population.[105]

What they could not know is that the high incidence of worm mortality among slave children is by itself potent evidence of serious malnutrition. Worms are color blind and find their way into black and white bodies with equal facility. For the reasonably well-nourished person, they present no problems. Yet they obviously gave slave youngsters problems of a very serious and frequently fatal nature. As Professor Josué Castro put it, with perhaps more poetry than worms deserve:[106]

> There can no longer by any doubt that, with good nutrition . . . worms become quite inoffensive, sharing the regime of abundance like peaceful fellow boarders. They become quiet domestic animals, like any other. . . . All that is necessary is to furnish enough food for both man and worm.

That food should include particularly substantial doses of proteins, iron, and vitamins A, B-12, and C. Only when enough food containing these nutrients is not forthcoming, do worms begin to abuse their host by interfering with the digestion and absorption of those nutrients they do encounter.[107]

Protein-Calorie Malnutrition — Pica — Worms and their Interrelationships

Protein-calorie malnutrition, pica, and worm ravages are so interrelated as to constitute a syndrome of their own.[108] The poor quality diet which begets kwashiorkor or marasmus can also produce a general hunger (as carbohydrates are metabolized faster than proteins) and, especially in the young, the impulse to fill the stomach with non-foods or pica. It can also breed specific hungers. For example, if a diet is low in protein, it is very difficult for the body to satisfy its iron requirements. Hence again the pica impulse is noted, although this time for specific materials containing iron or calcium or magnesium, etc.

Pica, on the other hand, while normally the result of mineral deficiencies, is also capable of generating these deficiencies, both by decreasing the practitioner's interest in real foods and, it has been theorized, by actually binding up minerals inside the body, thus making them unusable.[109] Finally, of course, pica usage frequently adds worms to the body. Worms in turn become harmful to their hosts when they are forced to share a diet sufficiently low in quality to produce protein-calorie malnutrition. And their abuse very often results in anemia, including iron-deficiency anemia which heightens the craving for pica.[110]

Because of this interaction between the diseases, it seems reasonable to hypothesize that slave children were not infrequently victims of all three. The net effect of this was not only to increase considerably their chances of dying from any one of them, but also to leave their bodies depleted and to raise their susceptibility to infectious disease.

Conclusion

A high incidence of slave child, and particularly slave infant, mortality relative to their white antebellum counterparts has proved to be a continuing source of frustration for students of the peculiar institution. Those who depicted slavery as paternalistic, along with those who viewed it as capitalistic, have both been confounded with infuriating impartiality by the phenomenon of planters who seemed to tolerate a situation where as many as three infants out of every ten died before reaching their first birthday, and close to half perished before age ten.[111]

This study however suggests that slave child mortality was largely beyond the control of paternalist and capitalist alike. Black children were victims of a conspiracy of nutrition, African environmental heritage, and North American climatic circumstances rather than planter mistreatment.

Bowling Green State Univ.

Kenneth F. Kiple
Virginia H. Kiple

The authors wish to thank the Bowling Green Faculty Research Committee for their generous support and the Interlibrary Loan Services of the BGSV Library for locating many rare volumes which we could not.

FOOTNOTES

1. Robert W. Fogel and Stanley L. Engerman, Vol. 1: *Time on the Cross; The Economics of American Negro Slavery* and Vol. 2: *Time on the Cross; Evidence and Methods – A Supplement* (Boston, 1974), 1:109-15, 2:90-99.

2. *Ibid.,* 1:115.

3. Kenneth M. Stampp, *The Peculiar Institution: Slavery in the Ante-Bellum South* (New York, 1956), 282.

4. Richard Sutch, "The Treatment Received by American Slaves: A Critical Review of the Evidence Presented in *Time on the Cross,*" *Explorations in Economic History,* 12 (1975), 386.

5. Excellent studies which point up the importance of this survival equipment by juxtaposing the disease experience of blacks and whites in West Africa are Michael Gelfand, "Rivers of Death in Africa," *Central African Journal,* Supplement, 11 (1965), 1-46; Philip D. Curtin, "Epidemiology and the Slave Trade," *Political Science Quarterly,* 83 (1968), 190-216, and K.G. Davies. "The Living and the Dead: White Mortality in West Africa, 1684-1732," in Stanley L. Engerman and Eugene D. Genovese, eds., *Race and Slavery in the Western Hemisphere: Quantitative Studies* (Princeton, 1975), 83-98.

6. It is the sickling trait, of course, which made instant malariologists out of geneticists and has focused so much attention on the African disease environment. A good recent summary of *The Clinical Features of Sickle Cell Disease* is by Graham R. Serjeant (New York, 1974).

7. Robert B. Scott, "Health Care Priority and Sickle Cell Anemia," American Medical Association, *Journal,* 214 (1970), 731-34; Arno G. Motulsky, "Frequency of Sickling Disorders in U.S. Blacks," *New England Journal of Medicine,* 288 (1973), 31-33.

8. P.L. Workman, B.S. Blumberg and A.J. Cooper, "Selection, Gene Migration and Polymorphic Stability in a U.S. White and Negro Population," *American Journal of Human Genetics,* 15 (1963), 429-37.

9. Roger A. Lewis, *Sickle States: Clinical Features in West Africans* (Accra, Ghana, 1970), 62.

10. For a full discussion of *Genetic Polymorphisms and Diseases in Man,* see Bracha Ramot, *et. al.,* eds. (New York, 1974).

11. John M. Hunter, "Geography, Genetics, and Culture History: The Case of Lactose Intolerance," *Geographical Review,* 61 (1971), 606, whose figures may be on the conservative side. David M. Paige, Theodore M. Bayless, and George G. Graham, "Milk Programs: Helpful or Harmful to Negro Children?" *American Journal of Public Health,* 62 (1972), 1487, found that 60-85% of the black *children* they studied in Baltimore manifested symptoms of lactose intolerance. Theodore M. Bayless and Norton S. Rosenzweig discovered from their look at "A Racial Difference in Incidence of Lactase Deficiency" (American Medical Association, *Journal,* 197, 1966, 139), that 19 out of 20 Negro males were lactase deficient, while only 1 in 20 white males had this condition.

12. It has been hypothesized that vitamin D was undersupplied both dietarily and by the low ultraviolet irradiation in northern Europe, thus rickets and its adult counterpart, osteomalacia, were very prevalent. The result was a reduction in reproductivity of females suffering pelvic deformation. The lactose tolerant trait was therefore encouraged because milk provided its consumer with both a rickets preventative (calcium) and a substitute for vitamin D (lactose), which facilitates the absorption of calcium. Gebhard Flatz and Hans W. Rotthauwe, "Lactose Nutrition and Natural Selection," *Lancet,* 2 (1973), 76-77.

13. Robert D. McCracken, "Lactase Deficiency: An Example of Dietary Evolution," *Current Anthropology,* 12 (1971), 484.

14. J. Kocián, I. Skála, and K. Bakos, "Calcium Absorption from Milk and Lactose-Free Milk in Healthy Subjects and Patients with Lactose Intolerance," *Digestion,* 9 (1973), 322; Theodore M. Bayless, *et. al.,* "Lactose and Milk Intolerance: Clinical Implications," *New England Medical Journal,* 292 (1975), 1158.

15. Winthrop D. Jordan, *White over Black: American Attitudes Toward the Negro, 1550-1812* (Chapel Hill, 1968), 583-85, is technically correct when he points out in his excellent "Note on the Concept of Race," 585, that the "precise adaptive value of the Negro's skin is not as yet known." However, see C.D. Darlington, *The Evolution of Man and Society* London, 1969, 43-44) for a concise summary of the question.

16. W.F. Loomis, "Skin-Pigment Regulation of Vitamin D Biosynthesis in Man," *Science,* 157 (1967), 505.

17. The following sources have been employed for the ensuing discussion of calcium and magnesium absorption. D.M. Hegsted, "Calcium, Phosphorus and Magnesium," in Michael G. Wohl and Robert S. Goodhart, eds., *Modern Nutrition in Health and Disease* (4th ed.; Philadelphia, 1971), 325-26; R.J.C. Stewart, "Bone Pathology in Experimental Malnutrition," *World Review of Nutrition and Dietetics,* 5 (1965), 293-298; Abraham Cantarow, "Mineral Metabolism," in Duncan G. Garfield, ed., *Diseases of Metabolism* (3rd ed., Philadelphia, 1952), 240-42, 285; Margaret S. Chaney and Margaret L. Ross, *Nutrition* (8th ed.; Boston, 1971), 125-28, 132.

18. Martha L. Orr and Bernice K. Watt, *Amino Acid Content of Foods,* Home Economics Research Report No. 4 (Washington, 1957), 50,56; R.C. Miller, L.W. Aurand, and W.R. Flach, "Amino Acids in High and Low Protein Corn," *Science,* 112 (1950), 57.

19. See Figure 34, Fogel and Engerman, *Time on the Cross,* 1:114.

20. It is in large part for this reason that iron deficiency anemia is "nearly universal" in much of Africa today. Virgil F. Fairbanks, John L. Fahey and Ernest Beutler, *Clinical Disorders of Iron Metabolism* (2nd ed.; New York, 1971), 238.

21. While the 1964 Recommended Dietary Allowances employed by Fogel and Engerman suggest 15 mg. of iron for women and children (as opposed to 10 for men), the 1973 revised figures have increased that allowance for women to 18 mg. daily. Helen S. Mitchell, "Recommended Dietary Allowances up to Date," American Dietetic Association, *Journal,* 64 (1974), 149.

22. Fairbanks, Fahey, and Beutler, *Clinical Disorders of Iron Metabolism,* 84, 88, 161; Chaney and Ross, *Nutrition,* 146-47.

23. Sheila T. Callender, "Fortification of Food with Iron – is it Necessary or Effective?" in Dorothy Hollingsworth and Margaret Russell, eds., *Nutritional Problems in A Changing World* (New York, 1973), 207.

24. Ann Ashworth, P.F. Milner, and J.C. Waterlow, "Absorption of Iron from Maize and Soya Beans in Jamaican Infants," *British Journal of Nutrition,* 29 (1973), 269,272.

25. See Kenneth F. Kiple and Virginia H. Kiple, "Black Tongue and Black Men: Pellagra in the Antebellum South," forthcoming in the *Journal of Southern History.*

26. There is general agreement among demographers that black fertility was substantially higher than white during the late antebellum period, with most putting the black fertility

rate at about 250, and endowing slave mothers with an average of at least seven children. Reynolds Farley, "The Demographic Rates and Social Institutions of the Nineteenth-Century Negro Population: A Stable Population Analysis," *Demography,* 2 (1965), 388, 395. Moreover, for the argument that black fertility was even higher during the early decades of the century see Melvin Zelnick, "Fertility of the American Negro in 1830 and 1850," *Population Studies,* 20 (1966), 77-83.

27. Derrick B. Jelliffe, *Infant Nutrition in the Subtropics and Tropics* (2nd ed.; Geneva, 1968), 113; B.S. Platt and R.J.C. Stewart, "Reversible and Irreversible Effects of Protein-Calorie Deficiency on the Central Nervous System of Animals and Man," *World Review of Nutrition and Dietetics,* 13 (1971), 68-70.

28. See for example the J.H. Hammond Plantation Manual (South Carolina Library, University of South Carolina); Solon Robinson, "Negro Slavery at the South," *DeBow's Review,* 7 (1849), 380-82; John B. Cade, "Out of the Mouths of Ex-Slaves," *Journal of Negro History,* 20 (1935), 300; and William D. Postell, *The Health of Slaves on Southern Plantations* (Gloucester, 1970), 123.

29. Jules Cartier, "Observations on First Dentition, and the Attentions which Children Require," *New Orleans Medical News and Hospital Gazette,* 1 (1854), 296.

30. Andrew Flinn, "Instructions to the Overseer" (Andrew Flinn Plantation Diary, Southern Historical Collection, University of North Carolina).

31. Lactase levels in most Africans begin to fall between the third and fourth year, yet some infants manifest low levels during the first six months of life. G.C. Cook, "Lactase Activity in Newborn and Infant Baganda," *British Medical Journal,* 1 (1967), 529. In the United States, 40% of black school children (and 60% of black teenagers) have been pronounced lactose intolerant. Theodore M. Bayless, "Milk Intolerance: Clinical, Developmental and Epidemiological Aspects," in Irving I. Gottesman and Leonard L. Heston, eds., *Summary of the Conference on Lactose and Milk Intolerance* (Washington, 1972), 14.
   Interestingly, many of the planters who do discuss serving milk to slave children caution that the milk be buttermilk or in soured form. Since the lactose intolerant have less difficulty with soured milk or buttermilk (in both cases some of the milk sugars have been removed) one wonders if these southern planters did not pioneer in recognizing and treating the problem in blacks. See Thomas Affleck, "On the Hygiene of Cotton Plantations and the Management of Negro Slaves," *Southern Medical Reports,* 2 (1850), 435; Alabama Planter, "Management of Slaves," *DeBow's Review,* 13 (1852), 193; and St. George Cocke, "Management of Negroes," *DeBow's Review,* 14 (1853), 177. Consult also Eugene D. Genovese, *Roll, Jordan, Roll: The World the Slaves Made* (New York, 1974), 508, who states that the milk children received was "usually in soured form," and Baird U. Brooks, "A Study of Infant Mortality in the Southern States," *Southern Medical Journal,* 23 (1930), 869, who believes buttermilk feedings "drastically reduced the death rate of colored infants" in the South.

32. Consult for example Postell, *Health of Slaves,* 35; Vernie A. Moody, "Slavery on Louisiana Sugar Plantations," *Louisiana Historical Quarterly,* 7 (1924), 264; and Lewis C. Gray, *History of Agriculture in the Southern United States to 1860* (2 vols.; 2nd ed.; New York, 1941), 2:838.

33. Gray, *ibid.;* Harry Toulmin, "A Sketch of the District of Mobile," *American Register,* 6 (1810), 338; Ebenezer Starnes, *The Slave-holder Abroad* (Philadelphia, 1860), 503; Richard O. Cummings, *The American and his Food: A History of Food Habits in the United States* (Chicago, 1940), 20.

34. This is a factor overlooked by Fogel and Engerman *(Time on the Cross,* 1: 113) who have slaves enjoying about 8 ounces of milk daily. Even with this amount of milk available which Sutch ("The Treatment Received by American Slaves" 372) makes clear is very

doubtful it would not have been available on a year-round basis, but rather for a few months only.

35. A nursing infant requires 45 mg. of calcium per kg. daily of which 50-70% will be absorbed, while the artificially fed infant needs about 150 mg. per kg., for he absorbs only 30-35% of the calcium in bovine milk. Cantarow, "Mineral Metabolism," 239.

36. Samuel J. Foman, *Infant Nutrition* (2nd ed.; Philadelphia, 1974), 284.

37. David M. Paige, "Milk Intolerance: Field Studies and Practical Considerations," in Gottesman and Heston, eds., *Summary of the Conference on Lactose and Milk Intolerance,* 35; A. Stewart Truswell, "Carbohydrate and Lipid Metabolism in Protein-Calorie Malnutrition," in Robert E. Olsen, ed., *Protein-Calorie Malnutrition* (New York, 1975), 120.

38. John S. Wilson, "The Negro – His Diet, Clothing, etc.," *American Cotton Planter and Soil of the South,* 3 (1859), 197.

3 0
39. Wilson, *ibid.* See also 'Tattler,' "Mangagement of Negroes," *Southern Cultivator,* 8 (1850), 162; Agricola, "On the Management of Negroes," *ibid.,* 13 (1855); J. Hume Simons, *The Planter's Guide and Family Book of Medicine* (Charleston, 1848), 209; Samuel A. Cartwright, "Philosophy of the Negro Constitution," *New Orleans Medical and Surgical Journal* (hereinafter cited as NOMSJ), 9 (1852), 197; and M.W. Philips, "More Meat," *American Cotton Planter and Soil of the South,* 2 (1858), 96-97.

40. Wilson, "The Negro," 197.

41. Advertisements in our files have come from the following antebellum newspapers: *Washington Republic, Alexandria Advertiser, American Beacon, Virginia Gazette, Carolina Centinel, Tennessee Gazette, Raleigh Register, Norfolk Gazette and Public Ledger, Mississippi Republican, The Mississippian, Arkansas State Gazette and Democrat, The Supporter and Scioto Gazette, The Daily Journal, The Memphis Daily Appeal, The Telegraphical Texas Register, The Daily Picayune, The Charleston Courier, Georgia Journal and Messenger, Arkansas State Democrat,* and *Gazette and Democrat.*

42. Plantation records have been examined in the following archives, libraries, and historical societies: South Caroliniana Library, University of South Carolina; Georgia Historical Society; Florida State University Library; William R. Perkins Library, Duke University; Southern Historical Collection, University of North Carolina; South Carolina Historical Society; South Carolina Department of Archives and History, Columbia, South Carolina; Department of Archives and History, Raleigh, North Carolina; Virginia Historical Society; Virginia State Library, Richmond, Virginia; Alderman Library, University of Virginia; Department of Archives, Louisiana State University; Department of Archives and History, Jackson, Mississippi; Texas State Library and Archives, Austin, Texas; Fondren Library, Rice University; Alabama State Archives, Montgomery, Alabama.

43. "Seventh Census of the United States. Original Returns of the Assistant Marshalls. Third Series, persons who died during the year ending June 30, 1850" for the states of Mississippi (Dept. of Archives and History, Jackson), South Carolina (Dept. of Archives and History, Columbia, North Carolina (Dept. of Archives and History, Raleigh) and Virginia (Virginia State Library, Richmond).

44. J.D.B. DeBow, *Mortality Statistics, the Seventh Census,* H.R. Ex. Doc. No. 98, 33rd Congress, 2nd Sess. (Washington, 1855). Unless otherwise specified mortality statistics presented were recorded during the year 1849-50 and are for the seven states of Alabama, Georgia, Louisiana, Mississippi, North and South Carolina, and Virginia.

45. The little useful material which does exist was published separately as *Statistics of the United States including Mortality, Property, etc. in 1860 . . .* (Washington, 1866).

46. DeBow, *Mortality Statistics,* 8, comments that "at least one-fourth of the whole number of deaths have not been reported at all." For a study of "J.D.B. DeBow and the Seventh Census," see that by Ottis C. Skipper, *Louisiana Historical Quarterly,* 22 (1939), 479-91.

47. And some will be somewhat misleading because of the method employed to present the mortality data. Deaths in the census were listed by race and by age/sex categories, but unfortunately the two are not combined. Thus to employ a hypothetical example, one could know that 100 individuals died of "croup" in Alabama of which 80 victims were black and 70 victims were aged 5 and under. He does not however, know how many of the 80 black victims were aged 5 and under. The reader is therefore cautioned that the rates this study gives in terms of live population for an age cohort are approximations only.

48. Farley ("The Demographic Rates and Social Institutions of the Nineteenth Century Negro Population" 398) for example finds it "likely" that 30% of the slave infants born did not survive their first year of life, while Paul H. Jacobson ("An Estimate of the Expectation of Life in the United States in 1850," *Milbank Memorial Fund Quarterly,* 35, 1957, 198) has placed the white infant rate for males at 160.6 and females at 130.8 per thousand.

49. "Fits" and "seizures" appear as causes of death in the manuscript mortality schedules but presumably were lumped together as "convulsions" in DeBow's 1855 compilation of the mortality data.

50. In the seven states under consideration, there were 14,139 unknown deaths of which blacks accounted for roughly 60%. Assuming from this that 60% of the 8273 unknown deaths for those aged 9-and-under were black, blacks in this age cohort experienced 15,748 "known" deaths and 4964 "unknown" deaths, while the whites suffered 10,686 deaths with a given cause and another 3309 for which no cause was given.

51. We do not wish to leave the impression that tetany was unknown during the nineteenth century. Rather John Clarke, *Commentaries on Some of the Most Important Diseases of Children* (London, 1815) contains a chapter "On a Peculiar Species of Convulsion in Infant Children" (chaper IV) which describes the disease, although the author had no idea of its cause. In 1855 the French clinician Trousseau distinguished tetany from tetanus. However, for the painfully slow discovery of the etiology of the disease, see Arthur L. Bloomfield, "A Bibliography of Internal Medicine: Tetany," *Stanford Medical Bulletin,* 17 (1959), 1-12.

52. Cantarow, "Mineral Metabolism," 274; Jelliffe, *Infant Nutrition,* 113; Stephen A. Roberts, Mervyn D. Cohen and John O. Forfar, "Antenatal Factors Associated with Neonatal Hypocalcaemic Convulsions," *Lancet,* 2 (1973), 811.

53. Plowden Charles Jennett Weston, "Rules to be Observed by the Overseer" (Charleston, n.d.), 9-10; Wendell H. Stephenson, "A Quarter-Century of a Mississippi Plantation: Eli J. Capell of 'Pleasant Hill,'" *Mississippi Valley Historical Review,* 23 (1936), 371; William D. Postell, "Birth and Mortality Rates Among Slave Infants on Southern Plantations," *Pediatrics,* 10 (1952), 538. Genovese, *Roll, Jordan, Roll,* 497, points out however that the "ideal" of a month's confinement (or at least release from field work) prior to giving birth, and another month after, was not always realized.

54. R.J. Purvis, *et. al.,* "Enamel Hypoplasia of the Teeth Associated with Neonatal Tetany: A Manifestation of Maternal Vitamin D Deficiency," *Lancet,* 2 (1973), 811.

55. Hess, *Rickets including Osteomalacia and Tetany* (Philadelphia, 1929), 368-69; Roberts, Cohen, and Forfar, "Antenatal Factors Associated with Neonatal Hypocalcaemic Convul-

sions," 809; Max Friedman, Geoffrey Hatcher, and Lyal Watson, "Primary Hypomagnesaemia with Secondary Hypocalcaemia in an Infant," *Lancet*, 1 (1967), 704.

56. J. Cam. Massie, *A Treatise on the Eclectic Southern Practice of Medicine* (Philadelphia, 1854), 455; Samuel A. Cartwright, "Report on the Diseases and Physical Peculiarities of the Negro Race," *NOMSJ*, 7 (1851), 696; Dr. 'J,' "On Tetanus," *Medical News and Hospital Gazette*, 7 (1860-61), 526-29; S.L. Grier, "The Negro and his Diseases," *NOMSJ*, 9 (1853), 752-54; W.G. Ramsay, "The Physiological Differences between the European (or White Man) and the Negro," *Southern Agriculturist*, 12 (1839), 412; Daniel Drake, "Diseases of the Negro Population," *NOMSJ*, 1 (1845), 584; H. Perry Pope, "A Dissertation on the Professional Management of Negro Slaves" (Masters thesis, Medical College of South Carolina, 1837), 15.

57. Computed from the appropriate pages in J.L. Dawson and H.W. DeSaussure, *Census of the City of Charleston, South Carolina, for the Year 1848* (Charleston, 1849).

58. Cartier, "Observations on First Dentition," 268; Michael Underwood, *A Treatise on the Diseases of Children* (Philadelphia, 1818), 190; Massie, *A Treatise on the Southern Eclectic Practice of Medicine*, 442; Charles S. Tripler, "On the Use of Mustard in the Convulsions of Children," *NOMSJ*, 1 (1845), 75; W.H. Coffin, *The Art of Medicine Simplified* (Wellsburgh, Va., 1853), 39: Clarke, *Important Diseases of Children*, 141.

59. Cantarow, "Mineral Metabolism," 269.

60. See n. 55.

61. Clarke, *Important Diseases of Children*, 87-88; Underwood, *A Treatise on the Diseases of Children*, 78, 81, 109; Simons, *Planter's Guide and Family Book of Medicine*, 142-43; Samuel K. Jennings, *A Compendium of Medical Science* (Tuskaloosa, Ala., 1847), 576.

62. See for example W.M. Boling, "Remarks on Remittant Fever Complicated with Symptoms of Tetanus," *NOMSJ*, 3 (1847), 737; John Erichsen, "Clinical Lecture on Tetanus," *New Orleans Medical News and Hospital Gazette*, 6 (1859), 614; and L.A. Dugas, "A Lecture Upon Tetanus," *Southern Medical and Surgical Journal*, n.s., 17 (1861), 433,444.

63. 'J,' "On Tetanus," 526, 529. That one doctor stumbled onto a "cure" for tetanus by dosing patients with milk punch suggests emphatically that these victims suffered from tetany, rather than tetanus. R.H. Goldsmith, "Tetanus – Epidemic or Constitutional Among Negroes," *Practitioner*, 1 (1880), 23.

64. Roberts, Cohen and Forfar, "Antenatal Factors Associated with Neonatal Hypocal-Caemic Convulsions,"810; Hess, *Rickets, Osteomalacia and Tetany*, 367; Paul D. Saville and Norman Kretchmer, "Neonatal Tetany: A Report of 125 Cases and Review of the Literature," *Biology of the Neonate*, 2 (1960), 6-8.

65. E. Hughes, "On Trismus Nascentium," *NOMSJ*, 3 (1846), 293. See also Dugas, "A Lecture Upon Tetanus," 434, 443-44; Ramsay, "The Physiological Differences between the European and the Negro," 412; Grier, "The Negro and his Diseases," 758; 'J,' "On Tetanus," *passim;* and Drake, "Diseases of the Negro Population," 342, all of whom believed lockjaw, too, was a "Negro disease."

66. Hess, *Rickets, Osteomalacia and Tetany*, 369; Cantarow, "Mineral Metabolism," 269, 273-75.

67. Even in this century when the disease was found to be widespread and regularly diagnosed, mortality from rickets averaged only 280 deaths per year for a half century

beginning in the year 1910. Mary T. Weick, "A History of Rickets in the Unites States," *American Journal of Clinical Nutrition,* 20 (1967), 1234.

68. See n. 41.

69. Hess, *Rickets, Osteomalacia and Tetany,* 41-42; G.N. Acker, "Rickets in Negroes," *Archives of Pediatrics* 11 (1894), 894; Weick, "A History of Rickets in the United States," 1238.

70. See for example the remarks of Fogel and Engerman, *Time on the Cross,* 1:124-26.

71. In the United States today, SIDS occurs in one out of every 350 births, and is the biggest killer of infants during the first year of life. Abraham B. Bergman, "Sudden Infant Death Syndrome," *American Family Physician,* 8 (1973), 96. For statistics outside the United States, consult Abraham B. Bergman, J. Bruce Beckwith, and C. George Ray, eds., *Sudden Infant Death Syndrom: Proceedings of the Second International Conference on Causes of Sudden Death in Infants* (Seattle, 1970) and Marie A. Valdes-Dapena, "Sudden and Unexpected Death in Infancy: A Review of the World Literature, 1954-1966," *Pediatrics,* 39 (1967), 123-38.

72. Paul V. Woolley, "Mechanical Suffocation During Infancy," *Journal of Pediatrics,* 26 (1945), 572-75.

73. Todd L. Savitt, "Smothering and Overlaying of Virginia Slave Children: A Suggested Explanation," *Bulletin of History of Medicine,* 49 (1975), 402.

74. Bergman, "Sudden Infant Death Syndrome," 96.

75. W.E. Parish, *et. al.,* "Hypersensitivity to Milk and Sudden Death in Infancy," *Lancet,* 2 (1960), 1106-1110.

76. A. Towbin, "Sudden Infant Death (Cot Death) Related to Spinal Injury," *Lancet,* 2 (1967), 940.

77. K.W. Cross and Sheila R. Lewis, "Upper Respiratory Obstruction and Cot Death," *Archives of Diseases of Childhood,* 46 (1971), 211-13.

78. Richard L. Naeye, "Hypoxemia and the Sudden Infant Death Syndrome," *Science,* 186 (1974), 837-38.

79. Preben Geertinger, "Sudden, Unexpected Death in Infancy with Special Reference to the Parathyroids," *Pediatrics,* 39 (1967), 43-48.

80. P.M. Mulvey, "Cot Death Survey: Anaphylaxis and the House Dust Mite." *Medical Journal of Australia,* 2 (1972), 1240-44.

81. Since the recognition of the Sudden Infant Death Syndrome in the early 1960's, a myriad of articles has appeared on its epidemiology. For the accumulation of knowledge on the syndrome, consult Ralph J. Wedgwood and Earl P. Benditt, eds., *Proceedings of the Conference on Causes of Sudden Death in Infants* (Seattle, 1963); Valdes-Dapena, "Sudden and Unexpected Death in Infancy," and Bergman, Beckwith and Ray, eds., *Proceedings of the Second International Conference on Causes of Sudden Death in Infants.*

82. Tetany too presents a "syndrome" which is most prevalent among those aged 2 to 8 months, and reveals a much higher incidence among those born prematurely or with a low birth weight. It strikes much more often at blacks, prefers formula-fed to breast-fed, seems to be related to respiratory distress and has a definite peak season in the late winter months. .

Hess, *Rickets, Osteomalacia and Tetany,* 356, 366-68; Thomas E. Oppe' and David Redstone, "Calcium and Phosphorus Levels in Healthy Newborn Infants Given Different Various Types of Milk," *Lancet,* 1 (1968), 1045-48; Reginald C. Tsang and William Oh, "Neonatal Hypocalcemia in Low Birth Weight Infants," *Pediatrics,* 45 (1970), 773; Derek J. Pearce, "Hypocalcaemia and Breast-feeding," *British Medical Journal,* 1 (1970), 563.

83. Blacks weigh on the average at least 50g. less than whites at birth. For a study of "The Relation of Ethnic and Selected Socio-economic Factors to Human Birth-Weight" see Alfred F. Naylor and Ntinos C. Myrianthopoulos, *(Annals of Human Genetics,* 1967, 71-83).

84. Joan L. Caddell, "Magnesium Deprivation in Sudden Unexpected Infant Death," *Lancet,* 2 (1975), 258-62.

85. Cook, "Lactase Activity in Newborn and Infant Baganda," 529.

86. G.C. Cook and F.D. Lee, "The Jejunum after Kwashiorkor," *Lancet,* 2 (1966), 1263; Truswell, "Carbohydrate and Lipid Metabolism in Protein-Calorie Malnutrition," 120.

87. Cicely D. Williams, "Nutritional Disease of Childhood Associated with Maize Diets," *Archives of Disease in Childhood,* 8 (1933), 423.

88. Kwashiorkor is caused by a diet adequate calorically, but whose protein content is either insufficient or of poor quality. Symptoms of the disease include skin lesions, anemia, muscular atrophy, diarrhea, "moon face," and a fatty liver as well as edema. Consult A. von Muralt, ed., *Protein-Calorie Malnutrition* (Heidelberg, 1969).

89. Williams, "Nutritional Disease of Childhood Associated with Maize Diets," *passim.*

90. See for example William H. Russell, *My Diary North and South,* ed. by Fletcher Pratt (New York, 1954), 149, who commented on pickaninnies in Louisiana with their "glistening fat ribs and corpulent paunches." Fredrika Bremer, *Homes of the New World* (2 vols.; New York, 1853), 294, on the other hand, encountered more serious cases of edema such as the "young lad very much swollen as if with dropsy." Consult also Eugene D. Genovese, *The Political Economy of Slavery* (New York, 1965), 45, who seems to allude to this phenomenon with his remark to the effect that the slave diet was one which guaranteed "the appearance of good health."

91. James Maxwell, "Pathological Inquiry into the Nature of Cachexia Africana," *Jamaica Physical Journal,* 2 (1835), 413, says that edema was "normal" in slave children. See also Grier, "The Negro and his Diseases," 755; F.W. Craigin, "Observations on Cachexia Africana or Dirt-Eating," *American Journal of Medical Sciences,* 17 (1836), 356-57; and John Le Conte, "Observations on Geophagy," *Southern Medical and Surgical Journal,* n.s.1 (1845), 430.

92. Jelliffe, *Infant Nutrition,* 135.

93. Grier, "The Negro and his Diseases," 754-55. See also Minnie C. Boyd, *Alabama in the Fifties* (New York, 1931), 190, who discusses marasmus in slave infants, and Simons, *Planter's Guide and Family Book of Medicine,* 208, who called it "starvation."

94. Maxwell, "Pathological Inquiry into the Nature of Cachexia Africana," 413; *Southern Medical Reports,* 1 (1849), 194; Le Conte, "Observations on Geophagy," 430, 443.

95. See Cartwright, "Report on the Diseases and Physical Peculiarities of the Negro Race," 704-707, John R. Hicks, "African Consumption," *Stethoscope,* 4 (1854), 625-29, Grier, "The Negro and his Diseases," 757-63, and Drake, "Diseases of the Negro Population," 341. Craigen, "Observations on Cachexia Africana or Dirt-Eating," William Telford, "On the Mal

d'Estomac," *London Medical and Physical Journal,* 47 (1822), J. Hancock, "Remarks on the common Cachexia, or Leucophlegmasia, called Mal d'Estomac in the colonies," *Edinburgh Medical and Surgical Journal,* 25 (1831), Maxwell, "Pathological Inquiry into the Nature of Cachexia Africana," and Le Conte, "Observations on Geophagy." Dirt-eating was also called "Negro consumption" which led to a bit of semantical confusion among antebellum physicians. See Cartwright, "Philosophy of the Negro Constitution," 697, and Lunsford P. Yandell, "Remarks on Struma Africana, or the Disease Usually Called Negro Poison, or Negro Consumption," *Transylvania Journal of Medicine,* 4 (1831).

96. William Carpenter, "Observations on the Cachexia Africana, or the Habit and Effects of Dirt-Eating in the Negro Race," *NOMSJ,* 1 (1844), 148, 150-52, 166; Cartwright, "Report on the Diseases and Physical Peculiarities of the Negro Race," 704-706; Maxwell, "Pathological Inquiry into the Nature of Cachexia Africana," 413, 417; Craigen, "Observations on Cachexia Africana or Dirt-Eating," 358; Affleck, "On the Hygiene of Cotton Plantations and the Management of Negro Slaves," 435.

97. See for example Charles W. Stiles, "Soil Pollution as Cause of Ground Itch, Hookworm Disease (Ground-Itch Anemia), and Dirt-Eating" (Washington, 1910), 22, and Paul H. Buck, "The Poor Whites of the Ante-Bellum South," *American Historical Review,* 21 (1925), 45.

98. Harry A. Rosell, "Association of Laundry Starch and Clay Ingestion with Anemia in New York City," *Archives of Internal Medicine,* 125 (1970), 57-61; Robert W. Twyman, "The Clay Eater: A New Look at an Old Southern Enigma," *Journal of Southern History,* 37 (1971), 439-48.

99. Philip Lanzkowsky, "Investigation into the Etiology and Treatment of Pica," *Archives of Disease in Childhood,* 34 (1959), 140-78; Pincus Catzel, "Pica and Milk Intake," *Petiatrics,* 31 (1963), 1056; C.A. Coltman, "Papophagia and Iron Lack," American Medical *tion, Journal,* 207 (1969), 513-16.

100. Margaret F. Gutelius, *et. al.,* "Nutritional Studies of Children with Pica," *Pediatrics,* 19 (1962), 1012-23; Marcia Cooper *Pica* (Springfield, Ill., 1957), 76-77; Sydney Jacobs, ed., "The Starch Eater," Louisana State Medical Society, *Journal,* 124 (1972), 79-83.

101. O. Carlander, Aetiology of Pica," *Lancet,* 277 (1959), 569; H.L. Jolly, "Advances in Pediatrics," *Practitioner,* 191 (1963), 417; R. Ber and Valero, "Pica and Hypochromic Anemia," *Harefugh,* 61 (1961), 35.

102. John M. Hunter, "Geophagy in Africa and in the United States: A Culture-Nutrition Hypothesis," *Geographical Review,* 63 (1973), 182; Cecile H. Edwards, *et. al.,* "Effect of Clay and Cornstarch Intake on Women and Their Infants," American Dietetic Association, *Journal* 64 (1964) 111; Berthold Laufer, "Geophagy," Field Museum of Natural History Publication No. 280, *Anthropology Series,* 18 (1930), 177.

103. Man Mohan, K.N. Agarwal, I. Bhutt, and P.C. Khanduja, "Iron Therapy in Pica," Indian Medical Association, *Journal,* 51 (1968), 16-18; Coltman, "Papophagia and Iron Lack," 516; Lanzkowsky, "Investigation into the Etiology and Treatment of Pica," 148; Robert McDonald and Sheila R. Marshall, "The Value of Iron Therapy in Pica," *Pediatrics,* 34 (1964), 558-62.

104. Joseph Pitt, "Observations on the Country and Diseases near Roanoke River, in the State of North Carolina," *New York Medical Reports* (2nd Hexade, 1808), 340; James B. Duncan, "Report on the Topography, Climate and Diseases of the Parish of St. Mary, La.," *Southern Medical Reports,* 1 (1849), 195; Carpenter, "Observations on the Cachexia Africana," 158, 166-67; Le Conte, "Observations on Geophagy," 441-44; Craigin, "Observations on Cachexia Africana or Dirt-Eating," 361-62; Telford, "On the Mal D'Estomac," 450, 458; Hancock, "Remarks on the Common Cachexia," 71. Interestingly more than one physician recommended iron treatment for the affliction and claimed cures. See H.V.

Wooten, "On the . . . Diseases of Luwndesboro . . . *Southern Medical Reports,* 2 (1850), 333; Maxwell, "Pathological Inquiry into the Nature of Cachexia Africana," 435; Grier, "The Negro and his Diseases," 758; while McGown, *(A Practical Treatise on the Most Important Diseases of the South,* Philadelphia, 1849, 89-90, 93)believed that calcium-deficient soils in Georgia, Mississippi and Florida, where corn was the principal "bread-stuff," meant that children and pregnant women were "urged by nature to supply the deficiency" by dirt-eating.

105. Tidyman, "A Sketch of the most Remarkable Diseases of the Negroes of the Southern States," *Philadelphia Journal of the Medical and Physical Sciences,* 12 (1826), 332; Affleck, "On the Hygiene of Cotton Plantations and the Management of Negro Slaves," 435-36; Grier, "The Negro and his Diseases," 756-57; Cartwright, "Report on the Diseases and Physical Peculiarities of the Negro Race," 702; Drake, "Diseases of the Negro Population," 341.

106. Jasue Castro, *The Geography of Hungery* (Boston, 1952) 46.

107. *Ibid.;* Williams "Varieties of Unbalanced Diet and their Effect on Nutrition," 94.

108. Certainly jaundice, edema, anemia, diarrhea and apathy are symptoms of all three afflictions.

109. V. Minnich, *et. al.,* "Effect of Clay upon Iron Absorption," *American Journal of Clinical Nutrition,* 21 (1968), 78-86.

110. Castro *The Geography of Hunger,* 86, 135; Aaron E.J. Masawe, Josephina M. Muindi and Godfrey B.R. Swai, "Infections in Iron Deficiency and Other Types of Anaemia in the Tropics," *Lancet,* 2 (1974), 316.

111. Demographers have disagreed rather wildly about the death rates of slave children largely because of the antebellum mortality data which is available is unquestionably biased on the low side (see for example Table I), and consequently estimates must supplement the data. In the case of infant mortality, Farley ("The Demographic Rates and Social Institutions of the Nineteenth Century Negro Population," 398) has stated that "It is likely that three out of every ten [slave] babies died before age 1." Jack Eblen ("New Estimates of the Vital Rates of the United States Black Population During the Nineteenth Century," *Demography,* 2, 1974, 306) has estimated a slave infant mortality rate ranging between 222 and 237 per thousand for females and 261 to 278 per thousand for males.
    Plantation records tend to confirm these higher estimates. On one of Alexandre de Clouet's plantations in St. Martin parish, for example, infants died at the rate of 194 per thousand (Alexandre Etienne De Clouet Paters, L.S.U.) while J.H. Hammond's slave infant on Silver Bluff plantation in South Carolina perished at an incredible 338 per thousand during their first year (Hammond Papers). Franklin L. Riley, ed., "Diary of a Mississippi Planter, January 1, 1840 to April, 1863," *Publications of the Mississippi Historical Society,* 10 (1909), 462 and *passim,* James H. Easterby, ed., *The South Carolina Rice Plantation as Revealed in the Papers of Robert F.W. Allston* (Chicago, 1945), 101, 113, 145, 269, 271, Guion G. Johnson, *A Social History of the Sea Islands* (Chapel Hill, 1930), 98, all present evidence of high infant mortality rates on the plantations they examined; while Affleck ("On the Hygiene of Cotton Plantations and the Management of Negro Slaves," 435) suggested that in Mississippi as many as half the slave infants perished during their first year, and the survivors continued to die at rapid rates until the age of five or six. High rates of infant mortality are also discussed by such southern physicians as Grier, "The Negro and his Diseases," 753-55, and William L. McCaa, "Observations on the Manner of Living and Diseases of the Slaves on the Wateree River" (Master Thesis, University of Pennsylvania, 1823), 4.

Paul Starr

MEDICINE, ECONOMY AND SOCIETY
IN NINETEENTH-CENTURY AMERICA

The economic history of medicine, especially before the 20th century, remains almost entirely to be written. Curiously, this is not for neglect of either the history or the economics of medical care, which separately have received abundant attention, but because those who have cultivated one subject have rarely thought about the other. Medical historians have had little taste for economics, and medical economists have had less for history. The character of contemporary economic thought, as few economists would deny, is vigorously ahistorical, and the emphasis in medical economics, as its practitioners would readily concede, has been almost entirely on matters of policy. Admittedly, for the period before 1929 (the year for which the first national economic statistics on medical care are available for the United States), there is a paucity of data of the sort that economists could comfortably interpret. In such shadowy terrain, one is necessarily driven, as I will be, to hypothesize and speculate. But there are other reasons, besides scarcity of information and the reciprocal inattention of economists and historians, for the absence of an economic history of medicine. The subject itself is elusive. Before the 20th century, medical care was relatively unimportant as an economic activity. It did not constitute a major industry as it does today, nor did it absorb much of the resources of the state. Most care of the sick was not even part of the market economy; it took place within the household, or through quasi-familial relationships outside the realm of market exchange.

Insofar as care of the sick remained within the family and communal circle, it was not a commodity, in the sense that it had no price in money and was not "produced" for exchange, as were the trained skills and services of doctors. But as people in sickness and distress increasingly resorted to physicians, entered hospitals rather than be cared for at home, and bought patent medicines instead of preparing their own remedies, medicine passed from the household into the market. This steady drift is one of the main currents deep beneath the changing structure of medical institutions. The growth of the market thoroughly altered the social relations of illness, yet the rule of market forces could never be complete. There was resistance to treating medicine purely as a commodity and to giving free rein to commercial impulses. Consequently, the social history of medicine in the 19th century is a history both of the extension of the medical market, and of its restriction.

Nineteenth-century society, Karl Polanyi has written, was governed by just such a "double movement:" the market expanded continuously, reaching into almost every sphere of social life, but it was met by a countermovement restraining and resisting its expansion. On one side, the principal of economic liberalism called for the release of the market unchecked. On the other, the forces of what Polanyi calls "social protectionism" attempted to curb the devastating effects of the market on traditional institutions, nature and even the economic system itself.[1]

These two political responses had their counterparts in medicine. The advocates of economic liberalism believed that in the care of the sick, as in other activities, private choice should prevail — hence their support for the abolition of all medical licensing. People, they thought, should be able to contract for treatment with whomever they wished: the market, in other words, could best regulate itself. On the opposing side of the issue, seeking to protect themselves from the ravages of an unconstrained market, medical societies tried to establish restrictions on entry into practice and limits on commercial behavior, like price-cutting and advertising. The countermovement was also represented by public support for charity hospitals, medical aid to the indigent, and, around the turn of the century, regulation of the drug industry. In different but related ways, professionalism, the nonprofit structure of most medical institutuions, and government regulation were efforts to modify and soften the workings of the market, without abolishing it entirely.

Thus powerful normative considerations, embodied in law or in moral codes, continued to affect the social and economic relations between the sick and dependent and the rest of society. A market, in the pure, abstract sense of a web of relationships of exchange governed by nothing but independent transactions, was never fully realized in medical care. The economic structure of medicine could never be completely "disembedded" (the term is Polanyi's) from the cultural order: hence medicine has no purely economic history apart from its social and cultural development. And hence our concern here with the changing boundary between the economic and the social, the shifting balance between medicine as a commodity and medicine as a moral activity.

The Emerging Market Before the Civil War

In at least one respect, the commercial nature of professional practice was more forthrightly acknowledged in America than in Britain. English law, under an ancient legal fiction, regarded the services of physicians as wholly philanthropic. While surgeons and apothecaries could sue for their fees, physicians could not. Barristers, in contrast to the lower-ranking attorneys, were similarly presumed to be above material motives. These presumptions, like the gradations of status among practitioners, never successfully crossed the Atlantic.[2] The only doctors ever barred from suing for fees in the United States were unlicensed practitioners. To be placed outside the market was an honor in an aristocratic culture, but a penalty in a democratic and commercial one.

In the late 18th and early 19th centuries, the state relinquished control over the market in professional services in what was perhaps the most crucial area — the determination of professional fees. Before the 19th century and the rise of an ideology of laissez-faire, government played an active, explicit and direct role in economic life that included the regulation of prices. In 1633 in Massachusetts the charging of extortionate prices was made punishable by law, and in 1639 the Virginia Assembly passed the first of several medical practice acts specifically providing for judicial action against "griping and avaricious" doctors levying exorbitant charges.[3] In 1736, the Burgesses enacted a lengthy fee schedule for physicians. Whereas later schedules consisting of minimum fees would be issued by medical societies hoping to prevent price-cutting, the earliest consisted of maximum fees aimed at preventing price-gouging. Yet state determination of medical prices was short-lived. In 1766 the Chief Justice of Massachusetts ruled that "Travel for Physicians, their Drugs and Attendance had as fixed a Price as Goods sold by a Shopkeeper," but this decision was reversed four years later when a physician was permitted to sue in *quantum meruit* (for the reasonable value of his services).[4] State determination of lawyers' fees eroded more slowly, the last traces finally disappearing around 1850.[5] In professional practice there was a general movement in the determination of prices from statute to contract, restrained in some degree by the pressure of custom.

Thus the origins of the expansion of market forces in medicine lay in diminished state involvement as well as the attenuated role of the household in the treatment of the sick. In the mid-19th century, particularly after the decline of licensure in the 1830's and 40's, the state had almost nothing to do with the private transactions between medical practitioners and their patients, except insofar as it guaranteed the sanctity of contracts and provided a means for the determination and redress of negligence (malpractice). Some communities paid the cost of medical treatment of the poor and maintained hospitals and pesthouses for contagious disease; some states built mental asylums and gave small subsidies to medical schools. The federal government maintained a limited system of compulsory hospital insurance for merchant seamen. These essentially marginal functions were, up through the Civil War period, the extent of state intervention in the economics of medicine.

Medical societies assumed, or tried to assume, some functions the state had abandoned, as in the setting of fees. "The law no where settles the precise value of professional opinion or advice," noted an article in the *New England Journal of Medicine and Surgery* in 1825. "A fee table settles this...." "In the last resort, where individuals are not disposed to settle their differences, it is very convenient to possess such a standard for public reference."[6] Yet the fee bills often went unobserved and had, as one writer put it, "little importance as authorities." A Philadelphia journal, publishing a fee schedule of the local College of Physicians in 1861, noted that this would be the first time most practitioners in the city had ever seen it, as charges had "not been guided by any fee-bill" at all. "Like literary labor," the journal observed, "medical attendance is worth in the market what it will bring."[7]

Most physicians were paid by a fee per service or a fee per case. Some were retained for a fixed fee per annum to provide all needed care for that period to a family, a plantation or the indigent members of a community. Called "contract practice," this method — actually a primitive form of insurance — was generally resisted by doctors who believed they were exploited under the system because of the unlimited services they might be asked to provide. Indeed, such arrangements did place on the individual physician the entire burden of risk; their existence gives testimony to the weak bargaining position of many doctors. It should be noted, however, that "contract practice," despite its name, was no more or less contractual than other forms; the contract was just explicit, rather than implied. The legal system presumed a contract between doctor and patient (or someone acting on the patient's behalf) even where none was expressly made.[8]

Much medical care was provided on credit. Physicians tried to collect their fees quarterly or annually, but they usually lost a substantial portion of their income through unpaid bills. The "credit system," like contract practice, was a source of much irritation among doctors, but they were in no position to eliminate it. As probate records for New England doctors in the early 1800's indicate, many were enveloped in a tangled web of debtor and creditor relationships until their deaths. Practitioners in New England in the 1830's rarely received, more than $500 a year in gross income. Much of this was paid in kind rather than money.[9]

The supply of physicians in the early and mid-19th century was unrestricted by significant institutional barriers to entry. Because of the proliferation of medical schools, offering easy terms and quick degrees, the cost of medical education, in both money and time, was kept relatively low. Nor was an education beyond an apprenticeship always necessary. In five New England counties during the period 1790-1840, the proportion of medical school graduates among practicing physicians ranged from 20 to 35%.[10] In eastern Tennessee in 1850, according to a doctor of the era, there were 201 physicians, only 35 of whom (or 17%) were graduates of a school; 42 other practitioners claimed to have taken a course of lectures.[11] The total investment necessary to enter medical practice in 1850, including direct expenses and opportunity costs, probably ranged between $500 and $1300, depending on the degree of schooling.[12] By contrast, the cost of establishing a farm in the West during the same period was likely to be larger, in the range of $1,000 to $2,000.[13] In the 20th century the supply of physicians has been constrained by the limited number of places in medical schools and by licensing requirements, both of which have been influenced by medical societies desirous of limiting entry into the field. Neither of these barriers impeded access in the mid-1800's. It was relatively easy then to set oneself up in medical practice, and doctors complained endlessly about "overcrowding" in the profession.

As a result of the unrestricted entry into practice, doctors were apparently well distributed through rural areas. "Physicians, even in surplus quantity, were available to the most remote New England towns, but the competition was keen and not always amiable. The most common problems of new practice were the dearth of patients and lack of rapport with established doctors." [14] Had educational and licensing requirements for medicine been more rigorous, physicians would undoubtedly have been more scarce, especially in rural areas. The amount of money to be made in small towns and rural communities would have been too meager to recoup the investment in an extended education. The limited training of 19th century doctors was not so much an expression of ignorance and foolishness as it was a response to economic realities — in fact, to one reality in particular, the limits of effective demand.[15]

The Growth of Demand and Decline in Indirect Prices

The fundamental constraint on medicine in early American society was the relatively low demand for medical services, rather than any institutionalized restrictions on supply. Whether it was because of popular preference for domestic care and disbelief in the value of professional medicine, or the difficulty of obtaining and affording treatment, or the ease with which competitors entered the field, many physicians found it extremely difficult to support themselves solely from medical practice. A second occupation, usually farming, or a broadened conception of the doctor's role to include the making and selling of drugs, often proved necessary. Starting out in practice frequently meant protracted underemployment and hardship. "The fact is," stated the *Boston Medical and Surgical Journal* in 1836, "there are dozens of doctors in all great towns, who scarcely see a patient from christmas-time to christmas-coming."[16]

If the demand for physicians' services was relatively low, the demand for hospital services was still lower. Almost no one who had a choice sought hospital care; there was no market in it. Hospitals were regarded with dread, and rightly so. They were dangerous places; when sick, people were safer at home.[17] The few who became patients went into hospitals because of special circumstances, which generally had to do with isolation of one kind or another from the networks of familial assistance. They might be seamen in a strange port, travellers, homeless paupers, or the solitary aged — those who, travelling or destitute, were unlucky enough to fall sick without family, friends or servants to care for them. Isolation was also related, but in a converse fashion, to the kindred institutions of pesthouse and asylum. There, isolation (or respite) from the community was the intent rather than the occasion of removal to an institution.

The expansion of medical services and the growth of hospitals have been routinely ascribed to changes in science and technology (that is, to changes on the "supply side" of the market). However, advances in science, while formidable, did not immediately translate into advances in medical practice. Unquestionably, genuine and dramatic improvements in surgery followed the introduction of anesthesia and antisepsis. In other areas of medicine, the case is much more doubtful. Increased demand for medical services seems to have preceded significant improvement in the effectiveness of physicians. This may seem at odds with known improvements in health, but declining rates of mortality and morbidity were probably due to better nutrition, housing and other changes in the standard of living, and to public health measures, like improved sanitation, rather than higher rates of cure from therapeutic services.[18] Medical science did contribute to the development and refinement of public health methods, but it did not do much through the treatment of individual illness.

The objective effectiveness of medical services, however, is distinct from their perceived effectiveness, and there is good reason to believe that perceptions changed. Perhaps the most tangible sign was the restoration of medical licensing in the 1870's and 80's. The cultural status that science in general and medicine in particular acquired, partly through achievements unrelated to therapeutic care, lent prestige and authority to the medical profession. Socioeconomic changes may also have promoted demand for medical services. Greater education and income made more money available for professional care, and may have also strengthened the propensity to define physical symptoms as requiring the attention of physicians. In empirical studies in the 20th century, higher socioeconomic status has been associated with a greater tendency to interpret bodily symptoms as demanding professional examination.[19] The less "medicalized" lower social strata of recent decades may reflect beliefs, attitudes and necessities that were once far more widespread.

These various changes in the cultural authority of science, the income available for professional care, and the lay interpretation of illness may have contributed to a shift in preferences — that is, greater demand for medical care at a given price: in the economists' terms, a movement outward of the demand curve. But there also seems to have been movement along the demand curve as well, due to a secular decline in the total price of medical care.

The price of medical services consists not only of the direct price (i.e., the physician's fee, the charge for a hospital room, etc.) but also of the indirect price — the cost of transportation (if the patient travels to the doctor or sends another person to summon one) and the foregone value of the time taken to obtain medical care. In most discussions, only the direct price is taken into account, but this bias is unwarranted. Direct and indirect prices are "symmetrical" determinants of total price and "there is no analytical reason to stress one rather than the other." [20]

Toward the beginning of the 19th century, the indirect price of medical services from transportation and opportunity costs probably outweighed the direct price. Dispersed in a heavily rural society, lacking modern transportation, a large part of the population was effectively cut off from ordinary recourse to physicians because of the prohibitive cost of travel in both money and time. A trip of ten miles into town for a farmer could mean an entire day's lost work. Contemporary observers and historians have continually drawn attention to the isolation of rural life and most small communities before the 20th century. This was as much an economic as a psychological fact.

The self-sufficiency of the household in early American society was never complete, but it was quite extensive, particularly in frontier, back-country and rural communities, which had a large share of the population before the mid-1800's. [21] Families produced not only agricultural goods for their own consumption, but also many other necessities — clothes, furniture, household utensils, farm implements and building materials. After 1815, household manufacturers went into a steep decline; according to Rolla Tryon, the transition to shop- and factory-made goods was nearly accomplished by 1830, particularly in New England. Elsewhere it took longer; the presence of a large frontier population through mid-century meant that the transition was "always taking place but never quite completed" in the country as a whole. "As soon as manufactured goods could be supplied from the sale or barter of the products of the farm, the home gave up its system of manufacturing, which had been largely carried on more through necessity than desire. Generally speaking, by 1860 the factory, through the aid of improved means of transportation, was able to supply the needs of the people for manufactured commodities.[22]

A similar transition from the household to the market economy took place in the production of services. For non-urban families, the cost of procuring specialized services outside the household was greatly compounded by the value of the time it took to obtain them. The advent of modern means of transportation, the building of hard roads and increasing urbanization radically altered the structure of prices. By reducing the opportunity and transportation costs for services, urbanization and improved transportation generally promoted the substitution of paid, specialized labor for the unpaid, unspecialized labor of the household. Getting a haircut, visiting a prostitute, and consulting a doctor all became, on the average, less expensive because of reduced costs of time.

From data contained in 19th-century fee tables, we can make some estimates of the relative magnitude of direct and indirect prices. The fee bills published by medical societies are probably poor indicators of average charges, but they do give the ratio of prices between different procedures and, more importantly, the ratio of indirect prices (i.e., fees for travelling and lost time) to direct prices (i.e., fees for actual services). Almost all of the 19th century fee schedules list, in addition to a basic fee for a physician visit to a patient's home, a charge per mile if the doctor needed to travel out of town. The charge for mileage represents an estimate of the foregone value to the doctor of the time spent in travelling, plus the cost of maintaining a horse and gig. We may assume that time had roughly the same value for patients as for their physicians (an assumption that probably holds for the 19th century, though it would be untenable today because of the high median income of physicians, relative to the population at large). Thus the monetary value doctors assigned to travel may give us an estimate of the indirect prices faced by patients when they visited the doctor.

Nineteenth-century fee bills vary between regions, especially between urban and rural areas, but the importance of indirect prices is evident everywhere. A few examples will suffice to make the point. In Addison County, Vermont, in 1843, the fee for each visit by a doctor was 50 cents at less than half a mile; $1 between a half mile and two miles; $1.50 between two and four miles; $2.50 between four and six miles and so on. In Mississippi the same year, according to a report in a Boston journal, a visit cost $1, while the charge for travel was $1 per mile during the day ($2 at night).[23] These ratios between charges for service and mileage are typical. Even at relatively short distances, the share of the total price due to travelling and opportunity costs exceeded the physician's ordinary fee; at a distance of five or ten miles they typically amounted to four or five times the basic charge for a visit.[24]

The more major the service, the less significant the indirect price became; the fee for serious operations could overshadow the charge for mileage. Indirect prices were more of a factor in limiting demand for ordinary medical care than they were in limiting demand for major forms of treatment. In this way, they affected the character of medical practice; except in the most serious situations, many families would not think of calling in a doctor.

When patients were treated at home, before the advent of the telephone, the doctor had to be summoned in person, which meant the costs of travel were often doubled, as two people, the physician and an emissary, had to make the trip back and forth. Moreover, there was no guarantee that the doctor would be found when someone went in search of him, since he was often out on calls. A doctor from the District of Columbia, observing that no physician in Washington during the 1840's or 50's kept regular office hours, later recalled, "Patients and other persons wishing to consult [a doctor] waited at irregular times for indefinite periods, or went away and came back, or followed in pursuit in the direction last seen, and sometimes waited at houses to which it was known the doctor would come . . . The only certain time at which one could be found was when in bed and had not instructed the servant to deny the fact." [25]

The reduction of indirect prices from improvements in communication and transportation put medical care within the income range of more people; in this way, it had the same effect as cost reductions from new technology in manufacturing. Underlying the shift from household to market in manufactured goods were radical changes in productivity that drastically altered relative prices. In the production of textiles, for example, family manufacture was virtually eliminated in a remarkably short period. In 1815, the power loom was introduced in Massachusetts; by 1830, the price of ordinary brown shirting had fallen from 42 to 7½ cents a yard. A woman at home could weave four yards of the cloth in a day; one worker in a factory, tending several power looms, could turn out 90 to 160 yards daily. There was no way housewives could compete. [26]

In medicine, there was no radical or sudden change in technology that drastically cut the cost of producing physicians' services, only the gradual erosion of indirect prices that came from more rapid transportation and more concentrated urban life. Though difficult to measure, significant gains were almost certainly made in the "productivity" of physicians (measured as services to patients per day). The doctor of the early and mid-19th century passed a great deal of his time travelling; as one doctor put it, he spent "half of his life in the mud and the other half in the dust." [27] Underemployment in the early years of practice also cut into the physicians' average work load. In several 19th century fee schedules, a fee for an entire day's attendance by a doctor is given as $5 or $10. (The average daily income for doctors, depending on locality, probably fell within or below this range.) These same fee schedules list the charge for an office visit at $1 or $1.50. [28] It seems likely, therefore, that doctors in the 1800's were seeing no more than an average of 5-7 patients a day (in urban areas perhaps more, in rural less). In contrast, by the mid-20th century, the average load of general practitioners, rural and urban, was about 18-22 patients daily. [29] Such figures suggest a gain in productivity for practicing doctors on the order of 300%. For surgeons, the gains have probably been even larger, considering the danger and infrequency of surgery before antisepsis.

The invention and spread of the automobile and telephone at the turn of the century enormously advanced the productivity and income of the profession. Physicians who wrote to the *Journal of the American Medical Association,* which published several supplements on automobiles between 1906 and 1912, reported that an auto cut the time for house calls in half. "It is the same as if the day had forty-eight hours instead of twenty-four," a doctor from Iowa rejoiced. [30] "Besides making calls in one-half the time," wrote a physician from

Oklahoma, "there is something about the auto that is infatuating, and the more you ride the more you want to ride."[31] In a 1910 survey of readers that drew 324 replies concerning automobiles, three out of five doctors said they had increased their income; answering a slightly different question, four out of five agreed that it "pays to own a car." The survey asked physicians using either automobiles or horses to give their annual mileage and costs, including maintenance and depreciation. The 96 physicians still using horses reported costs that work out to thirteen cents a mile; for the 116 who owned low-priced cars (under $1,000), the cost per mile was 5.6 cents. It came to nine cents for 208 doctors who owned cars priced over $1,000. However, the initial investment in purchasing a car was greater than in buying a horse.[32] "To assert that it costs no more to run a car than to keep up a team is absurd," insisted one physician. "But if one considers the time saved on the road, and the consequent additional business made possible, to say nothing of the lessened discomfort, a busy practitioner will find a large balance on the side of the motor car."[33] In 1912, a Chicago physician noted that the residential mobility of patients required doctors to drive a car. "Chicago today is a city of flats [apartments], and people move so, that a patient living within a block to-day may be living five miles away next month. It is impossible to hold one's business unless one can answer calls quickly, and this is impossible without a motor car. I have not only held my own, but have increased my business by making distant calls promptly . . . [averaging] about 75 miles a day . . ."[34] One physician in central Illinois quite reasonably described hard roads as having been "the single greatest contribution toward the improvement of the practice of medicine" in his region.[35]

Just as automobiles and hard roads enabled physicians to cut down on travelling costs, so they enabled patients to do the same in visiting doctors' offices. Reduced travelling time in both directions cut the cost of medical care and raised the supply of physicians' services, by increasing the proportion of the doctors' time available for contact with patients.[36] In the same period, the telephone, which first became available in the late 1870's and spread rapidly after 1895, made it less costly to reach a physician, greatly reducing the old problem of tracking down the peripatetic practitioner on foot. Curiously, the first rudimentary telephone exchange on record, built in 1877, connected the Capital Avenue Drugstore in Hartford, Connecticut with 21 local doctors.[37] (Drugstores had often served as message centers for physicians.) Mechanized transportation and the telephone also improved the efficacy of treatment by making possible more rapid intervention in emergency situations. The ambulance was meant to accelerate that process. Reduced distances may also have had a psychological effect: increasingly, one came to expect the doctor's intervention. Improved access ultimately brought greater dependency.

The Evolution of the Medical Workplace

Once medical practitioners are called in to help care for the sick, they can provide services in the homes of their patients, at their own offices, or in a hospital or some other institution. Wherever medical care takes place, the relationship between practitioner and patient is quite different from the ties between members of a family when they care for each other. The responsibilities as well, as the skills of the physician are specialized. But the setting is important in that it affects the relative power of the patient, the doctor and other parties, as well as the balance of costs and perhaps the effectiveness of the treatment itself. In the 19th century, the different settings of medical care had different moral connotations. The families in the "better" classes of society received physicians in their homes when someone was ill; they generally did not go to the doctor's office or to a hospital. Treatment in those settings was generally regarded as a mark of lower status. One of the great changes occurring in the last century was that the office and the hospital lost their traditional moral taint, and the home gradually declined in importance as a place for physicians' services.

The shift in the locus of medical care out of the household bears comparison with the same transition as took place in the production of industrial goods. The two developments share some similarities, but their nature and causes were somewhat different. In her study of the evolution of household into factory production in America, Tryon identified what seemed to her five "well-marked" stages: (1) family manufacture, in which the producer and consumer were virtually identical; (2) itinerant-supplementary production, in which the family either hired an outsider (e.g., a tailor) to come in to do part of the work, or sent out raw materials or semi-finished products to establishments that supplemented household labor; (3) shop manufacture, where the shopkeeper owned his business and provided labor, raw materials and tools; (4) mill and small-factory production; and (5) large-factory production.[38]

While there are forms of medical care analogous to these stages (i.e., domestic medicine, itinerant healers, office practitioners, small clinics and hospitals, large medical centers), medical practice did not pass through them in simple historical succession. Once past the most rudimentary stages of settlement, medicine moved from household self-sufficiency into the "itinerant-supplementary" phase: that is, physicians or other practitioners were called in by a family to provide advice or services, but most of the care was still given by the family itself. Much medical care remains in this and the "shop" (office) phase even today. What seems to have happened in medicine is not so much a clear, well-marked series of stages as a differentiation of sectors. Solo practitioners in the "shop" stage, clinics in the "small-factory" stage, and hospital medical centers in the "large-factory" stage developed side by side, acquiring different functions, rather than succeeding one another. (In psychiatric treatment, the sequence was even reversed: the "factory" came before the "shop," in that large mental hospitals existed before psychiatrists had regular office practices. But this is an exceptional case. The general drift in the development of medicine was from the household to entrepreneurial professional practice, with bureaucratic organization and state intervention increasing in the 20th century.) The medical "workplace," once the patient's bedside in the patient's own home, switched to the doctor's office for minor problems and to the hospital for more serious ones. All three settings – home, office and institution – have been in use since the first hospitals were built, but the proportion and nature of medical work taking place in each have shifted.

Home to Office. The movement from the patient's home to the doctor's office as the setting for professional advice and routine medical services probably began in the 19th century, though it became virtually complete only recently.[39] The telephone made it much easier for patients to see a physician at his office at a prearranged time, reducing the risk of dropping in while he was out on call; it also made office practice more attractive to the doctor, who could now make orderly appointment hours and see more patients than when relying on an uneven stream, or trickle, to his door. Moreover, as physicians' incomes have risen relative to the population at large, patients have had an increased incentive to substitute their own time for that of the doctor's by travelling to his office instead of paying him to visit their homes. The nature of medical practice has also changed; patients increasingly come to physicians for chronic diseases, minor complaints and regular examinations, which permit them to travel. The shift from home to office has also been encouraged by the growing use of clinical equipment and ancillary personnel. Finally, beyond the material changes, there seems to have been a shift in the expectations of doctor and patient. The doctor is no longer a body servant to the upper classes as he quite frequently used to be; his social position has risen and he expects the patient not to waste any of his time beyond that required for his service. It is a measure of the relative position of the two parties that the inconvenience of travel is no longer borne by the doctor, and that care of sick patients takes place in his sphere of action rather than theirs.[40]

Home to Hospital. Somewhat different, though related, forces seem to have been at work in the shift from the home to the hospital as the setting for major medical treatment and care of the acutely ill. The rise of hospitals occurred in a relatively brief time. In 1873, a government survey counted fewer than two hundred hospitals; by 1910, there were over four thousand, and by 1920 more than six thousand.[41] The number has not greatly increased since then, though their size and ownership have altered. Changes in both the nature of the hospital and the structure of the family affected their relative capacity to provide and manage treatment of the sick. The developments in hospitals are well-known: they ceased to be repositories of filth and infection and became desirable as places for medical care. Whether this was due to progress in science and technology or to changes in cultural beliefs and practices is not entirely clear. The movement to improve hygienic conditions in hospitals and professionalize nursing received much of its inspiration from people, like Florence Nightingale, who refused to believe in the "germ" theory of disease. Like many of her contemporaries in public health, Nightingale thought disease was communicated by vague miasmas — a theory now known to be scientifically incorrect. Yet while wrong as a theory, it was still effective as a motive of action. As an influence in the improvement of hospital hygiene and nursing, cultural attitudes toward dirt and contagion may have preceded scientific discovery. In any event, the two were quickly integrated and reinforced one another. One might point to the discovery of ether and antiseptic surgery as scientific advances that precipitated the rise of hospitals. But both ether and antisepsis were used in surgery in the home; they did not require recourse to a hospital. However, they did make hospitals safer and less forbidding, and consequently softened their image in society. In the long run, the growth of medical technology has ruled out a complete reversion to treatment in the home. But it does not account for the initial rise of hospitals at the end of the 19th century, when the technological aspects of hospital care were still undeveloped.

While hospitals improved both their objective and perceived capacity to manage serious illness, changes in the family and its relationship to society made it less able to care for the sick. The separation of work from residence that came with the growth of the market economy and factory system made it more difficult to attend the sick at home during the day. With industrialization and high geographic mobility in America, the conjugal family also became more isolated from the larger network of kinship, so fewer relatives were available to call on for assistance in case of illness. We need not argue here that there was a shift from an "extended" to a "nuclear" family; such terms may exaggerate the degree of change.[42] At least in terms of household size, the decline in the 19th century was not that striking. In 1790, households averaged 5.7 members in the United States; in 1900, 4.8.[43] On the whole, family structure in America seems to have had a "modern" shape before industrialization.[44] But significant change did take place during the 19th century in the size of upper-strata households. In 1790 in Salem, Massachusetts, merchants averaged 9.8 persons per family, master carpenters 6.7, and laborers 5.4.[45] By the end of the 19th century, families in different classes were equally small.[46] Upper-strata households diminished in size because of declines both in fertility and in the number of domestic servants. Also, urban growth led to higher property values, forcing many families to abandon single dwellings for apartment houses: this too affected the size of families they could afford to have; more particularly, it limited their ability to set aside rooms for sickness or childbirth. Finally, industrialization and urban life brought an increase in the number of unattached individuals living alone in cities; in a sense, they represented the extreme case of the attenuation of the household. In Boston between 1880 and 1900, boarding and lodging house keepers rose in number from 601 to 1,570, almost double the rate of population growth for the city. An array of new establishments—laundries, eating places, tailors — sprung up to meet the needs of this class. The hospital, as Morris Vogel points out, was one of these "corollary" institutions.[47] Both in England and America many of the first hospitals to care for private patients were built with lodgers and apartment house dwellers especially in mind.[48]

All these changes deprived the household of labor-power and physical space to handle the acutely ill. Adults increasingly had to go out of the home to work; there were fewer children, kin or servants around to help; space in the home became more precious; more isolated individuals had no one to take care of them. Talcott Parsons and Renée Fox have further speculated that in the modern urban family, there has been a loss of emotional and motivational capacity to deal with illness. They argue that the small size and increased isolation of the conjugal family have made it peculiarly vulnerable to strains created by illness: one member of the family cannot be attended at home without draining emotional support and attention from the others. The relations of the family, they maintain, have also become more emotionally intense, so when one person becomes ill, others are often likely to be overly indulgent, inviting perpetuation of sickness, or possibly overly severe, disrupting recovery. Moreover, in their view, illness has become an increasingly attractive response to a variety of pressures as a "semi-legitimate channel" of withdrawal from daily obligations and routines. To counter these tendencies, the doctor and hospital provide institutionalized mechanisms, in some respects "functionally alternative" to those of the family for handling the motivational problems of illness. The lack of emotional involvement in the professional setting encourages neither indulgence nor impatience; the status of patients is legitimized as long, and only as long, as they make an effort to get well. The physician's task is to make conformity with his advice more rewarding than the "secondary gain" of the "sick role" (i.e., the pleasures of dependency and respite from obligation). Thus for Parsons and Fox, care outside the family is "positively functional" in three respects: It shields the family from the disruptive effects of illness; it directs the passive deviance of sickness into supervised arenas where it can be contained; and it facilitates the therapeutic process.[49]

Working-class households do not seem to have undergone the changes in size and structure that this line of argument presumes. They were small even before the 19th century because of high infant mortality and the early departure of children into the labor force. The Parsons-Fox hypothesis seems more plausible if restricted to the upper social strata. At the time the shift to hospital care was taking place, there definitely were allusions to its effects on the family. One newspaper account in 1900, headlined "The New York Hospitals: A Boon Not Only to the Poor But to the Well-to-do," describes hospitals as affording "great relief to the family from physical as well as mental strain" and quotes a hospital director as saying, "It can be put down as one of the advantages of a hospital that the relatives and friends do not take care of the patients. It is much better for them not to be under the care of anyone who is overconcerned for them." The article concludes, "Many people who have had the experience of being ill in and out of the hospital are greatly in favor of the former, especially where, as in many cases [of illness at home], the breaking down of some member of the family from overwork and anxiety follows . . ."[50]

While the growth of hospitals occurred principally at the end of the 19th century, there were two distinct waves of innovation. About a half century separated the initial spread of mental hospitals in the 1830's and 40's and that of general hospitals in the 1880's and 90's. While the mental asylum began to receive patients from the middle classes in the earlier part of the century, the general hospital waited until after the Civil War. This disjunction in the evolution of their clientele seems related to the difference in the timing of their growth. From the beginning of the industrial era, changes in work and family structure probably created a growing disposition in favor of extra-familial care, but because of the dangers of cross-infection in general hospitals, families that could possibly manage treatment of the physically ill at home did so. The reforms in hospital hygiene and the acceptance of antiseptic surgery, both of which date from the period after the Civil War, precipitated the proliferation of the general hospital, but only because a prior demand for extra-familial care already existed.

The abbreviation of distances is also relevant here. In a society with primitive transportation, not yet heavily urbanized, the general hospital is accessible to relatively few people; on the other hand, a mental hospital is less dependent on quick access and can still serve important functions. Because of its relation to the system of social control and broad cultural concerns over the stability of the social order, the mental asylum has, sociologically, been a quite different institution from the general hospital. In its functions, its financing and its organization, it has had a more thoroughly public stamp. In the 19th century, the effective demand for psychiatric treatment came first of all from the society and only secondarily from individual patients. This difference in the nature of the demand for its services may account for the reversed sequence of institutional development that put the bureaucratic stage ahead of the entrepreneurial (that is, the hospital ahead of private office practice). The hospital could more appropriately serve the public functions of the control and confinement of disorder.

Each of these various transfers in the medical workplace — from the home to the mental asylum for treatment of serious psychological disorder, to the general hospital for major medical procedures and care of the acutely ill, and to the doctor's office for routine medical services — involved somewhat disparate sociological considerations and took place on a different historical "schedule." But they were also clearly part of a single larger transition in social life. The family lost its economic function as a unit of production, first with the passing of household manufactures, and then of family capitalism. With the rise of schooling, it ceased to play the central part in educating the young; with the rise of social insurance, its role in supporting the aged, disabled and dependent diminished. Day-care centers for pre-school children have advanced the process in one direction, nursing homes in another. And as the recent growth od day-care and nursing homes well illustrates, specialized services often relieve the household of obligations that interfere with employment in the market economy.[51] Hospitals have also served that function. The segregation of sickness and insanity, childbirth and death, has been part of a rationalization of everyday life — the exclusion from daily experience of disturbances and strains that make difficult participation in the routine of industrial society. In this sense, the rationalization of personal disorder has been complementary to the rationalization of economic life.

Yet, in comparison with industrial goods, personal services like medical care have passed out of the family into specialized institutions under somewhat less commercial conditions. The state has played a much greater role in setting up and running many of the new institutions, explicit profit-making has been less common, and the normal rules of the market (e.g., caveat emptor) have less often applied. While there are exceptions, the pattern has been unmistakable. The restriction of the market has been much more pronounced in the sphere of personal services than in the industrial sector of the economy.

Part of the explanation probably resides in the nature of personal services, which, as some economists have emphasized, are often simultaneously vital and difficult for consumers to assess.[52] Going outside the family for medical care entails a distinctive loss of privacy. It places the patient and the family in a vulnerable and exposed position. The physician vouchsafes their security through his professionalism. This is not merely a matter of ideology; to some extent, it is also a matter of law. Physicians are in a position of trust; they cannot abuse their patients' confidence or abandon treatment whenever it suits them. The relationship between doctor and patient is a market relationship, but because of the vulnerability of the sick, it is fiduciary as well as contractual.

The operation of the market in medicine has been limited in other ways, and these have specific historical origins. By the late 19th century, medical licensing had been restored and strengthened, and changes were under way in medical education that would culminate in the rapid decline of the proprietary medical school after 1906. The structure of the medical market by the end of the Progressive ear was vastly different from what it had been before. Where entry into the market had once been easy and relatively inexpensive, now it was difficult and costly. Shortages of physicians began to appear in rural areas.[53] If the market for medical services in the mid-19th century had been characterized by a relative insufficiency of demand, the chief characteristic in the mid-20th century became a relative insufficiency of supply. The continued growth of demand, while the supply of physicians was relatively inelastic, drastically altered the structure of the medical market and the position of the medical profession. The market grew under a distinctive kind of constraint, and we live with the consequences today.

Harvard University   Paul Starr

FOOTNOTES

1. Karl Polanyi, *The Great Transformation* (Boston, 1957). Though Polanyi never mentions medicine, I have been much influenced by his general theoretical views. For a survey and critique of Polanyi and his followers, see S. C. Humphreys, "History, Economics and Anthropology: The Work of Karl Polanyi," *History and Theory* 8 (1969), 165-212.

2. Judah v. M'Namee, 3 Blackf. 269 (Indiana, 1833).

3. Wyndham B. Blanton, *Medicine in Virginia in the Seventeenth Century* (Richmond, 1930), 250-259; Wilhelm Moll, "Medical Fee Bills," *Virginia Medical Monthly* 93 (1966), 657-664.

4. Pynchon v. Brewster, Quincy 224 (Mass. 1776); Glover v. Le Testue, Quincy 225 (Mass. 1770).

5. Ruth E. Peters, "Statutory Regulation of Lawyers' Fees in Massachusetts, New York, Pennsylvania, South Carolina, Tennessee, and Virginia from the mid-Seventeenth Century to the mid-Nineteenth Century," unpublished paper, (Harvard Law School, May 1975).

6. *New England Journal of Medicine and Surgery* 14 (1825), 50-51; cited in George Rosen, *Fees and Fee Bills: Some Economic Aspects of Medical Practice in 19th-Century America* (Baltimore, 1946), 6.

7. "Fees and Fee Bills," *Medical and Surgical Reporter* 7 (Dec. 7, 1861), 231-2.

8. Pray v. Stinson, 21 Me. (8 Shep) 402; Peck v. Hutchinson, 88 Iowa 320, 55 N.W. 511.

9. Barnes Riznik, "Medicine in New England, 1790-1840," unpublished manuscript, Old Sturbridge Village, 1963, 78-81. A gross income of $500 would probably mean about $350 net, assuming the costs of general practice were relatively as large in the early 1800's as in

the early 1900's. In ascertaining debts, Riznik examined the probate records for 34 "typical" physicians from Worcester County, Massachusetts; 26 had unsettled debts when they died and more than half owed between $2,500 and $10,000.

10. Idem, "Medicine in New England, 1790-1840," Old Sturbridge Village, 1965, 24. (This pamphlet is a shorter version of Riznik's 1963 manuscript.)

11. Richard H. Shryock, *Medical Licensing in America, 1650-1965* (Baltimore, 1967), 31-2.

12. Estimating the necessary investment for medical practice is difficult because so many of the costs are uncertain. Many doctors never attended medical school or, if they attended, remained for only one term or even part of a term; apprenticeships varied in length. Accordingly, we have given a range of costs rather than a single average. The elements are as follows:

(1) the fee for three years of apprenticeship or office study;
(2) tuition and living costs for two terms (about 26 weeks) of medical school;
(3) the cost of a horse and buggy;
(4) the cost of books, medicines and equipment;
(5) the opportunity cost of time invested in an apprenticeship and medical education;
(6) the opportunity cost of money invested, assuming a normal rate of return of ten percent.

Our rough estimates of these are as follows: (1) 3x$50-100 per year; (2) $150-300, depending on whether the school was rural or urban; (3) $200-300; (4) $25-100; (5) $150; (6) $35-125. The low estimate assumes three years of apprenticeship at the lowest fee, no formal medical education and minimal expenditures for books and medicines (total $560). The high estimate assumes three years of apprenticeship at the higher fee, an urban medical education, and larger expenditures for a library and medicines (total $1275). Obviously, if one were to include the cost of a house and the need to support a family through the lean early years of practice, the costs would go higher.

The data for apprenticeship and medical school costs come directly from William F. Norwood, *Medical Education in the United States Before the Civil War* (Philadelphia, 1944), 393-5. The estimate of the opportunity cost of time assume that an unskilled 20-year-old male would be able to earn no more than $50 a year more than he might receive in kind as an apprentice, or during his weeks in medical school.

13. See Clarence H. Danhof, "Farm-making Costs and the 'Safety Valve': 1850-1860," *Journal of Political Economy,* 49 (1941), 317-359.

14. Riznik, "Medicine in New England," (1965), 15.

15. Technically, there was another factor – the "indivisibility" of physicians' services due to the limits of contemporary transportation. While a poor rural area might not have been able to support one well-trained doctor, it conceivably could have supported one-eighth, if the physician could have covered eight such areas with the help of modern cars and roads. But because transportation was primitive, communities did not have the opportunity to choose a fraction of a well-trained and more highly priced physician over the full services of a less trained and lower-priced doctor.

16. *Boston Medical and Surgical Journal* 15 (Nov. 30, 1836), 273.

17. See John E. Erichsen, *On Hospitalism and the Causes of Death After Operations* (London, 1874).

18. Edward Meeker, "The Improving Health of the United States, 1850-1915," *Explorations in Economic History* 9 (1972), 353-373.

19. Earl L. Koos, *The Health of Regionville* (New York, 1954), 30-39.

20. Gary Becker, "A Theory of the Allocation of Time," *The Economic Journal* 75 (Sept. 1965), 26-31.

21. Stewart Bruchey, *The Roots of American Economic Growth 1607-1861* (New York, 1965), 493-517.

22. Rolla M. Tryon, *Household Manufactures in the United States 1640-1860* (Chicago, 1917), 243, 11.

23. These data have been culled from Rosen, *Fees and Fee Bills,* 15-16, which contains numerous other fee tables that would make the point equally well.

24. Direct estimates of transportation and opportunity costs yield roughly the same result. The cost of transportation by horse and buggy to a doctor in 1850 was about 9 cents per mile; the opportunity cost of time probably came to about 8 cents a mile. Going in both directions to and from the patient, therefore, travelling costs should have been about 34 cents for each mile the patient lay distant. Since the fee for a visit to the doctor was typically about 50 or 75 cents, the charge for mileage should have exceeded the ordinary fee at about two miles. This is roughly what the fee schedules indicate.

My estimates for transportation costs and the opportunity cost of time are based on the following calculations:

Cost of transportation by horse. In 1910, the *Journal of the American Medical Association* (JAMA), questioning readers of costs of cars versus horses, received 96 replies regarding the cost of horses. The average annual cost of a horse (maintenance plus depreciation) was $356.85. Average annual mileage totalled 2,680. (*JAMA* 54 [April 9, 1910] 1274). Deflating to 1850 price levels, according to the relative cost of farm products, yields a cost per mile of 9 cents. This however, should be seen as a high estimate since the 1910 figures include "some" instances where "more than one horse was used," as in a team-driven buggy. By horseback alone the cost of travel may have been somewhat lower than 9 cents.

Opportunity cost of time. Doctors probably covered about five or six miles per hour (see Riznik [1963] 84). Assume that they earned an average of $4 in gross income a day (probably a little high) and worked a daily average of 10 hours (perhaps a little low). With earnings of forty cents an hour and travelling at a speed of .2 hours per mile, the opportunity cost of time for travel should have been about 8 cents per mile.

This suggests a simple formula. Let P be the total price of physician visit, p_1 the fee of the doctor, p_2 the price of transportation per mile, and wt the opportunity cost of time. Then

$$P = p_1 + 2p_2d + w\left(\frac{2d}{s}\right) \qquad (1)$$

where 2d is the distance back and forth between doctor and patient and s is the average speed. Substituting the values indicated above, we have

$$P = .50 + 2(.09)d + .40\left(\frac{2d}{s}\right) \qquad (2)$$

$$P = .50 + .34d \qquad (3)$$

This agrees fairly well with actual fee tables.

We can elaborate the analysis by breaking time into three components: travelling time $(t_1 = \frac{2d}{s})$, waiting time (t_2) and time taken for the actual service (t_3):

$$P = p_1 + 2p_2d + w\left(\frac{2d}{s} + t_2 + t_3\right) \qquad (4)$$

$$P = p_1 + 2d\left(p_2 + \frac{w}{s}\right) + w(t_2 + t_3) \qquad (5)$$

In (5), the second term, $2d(p_2 + \frac{w}{s})$, represents the full cost of travel; the last term, w

$w(t_2 + t_3)$, represents the cost of time spent at the doctor's office. The history of indirect prices in medicine, I would argue, has seen the second term greatly diminish in significance, especially during the late 19th and early 20th centuries, as distances (d) and transportation prices (p_2) declined, while the speed of transportation (s) increased. The result, as I've indicated, may have been a declining total price in the late 1800's, and consequently an expanded market.

I should add one caveat. There is no continuous series for medical fees in the 19th century, but fragmentary evidence from fee tables suggests that there were increases during wartime periods of inflation that seem to have persisted even when the general level of prices declined. This does not necessarily conflict with the point being made here. For a decline in indirect prices to have significantly expanded the market for medical services, the total price need have declined only for that part of the population that shifted from low-density rural areas to cities. This it almost certainly did. For the part of the population that resided in high-density areas from the beginning of the century, prices for medical care may have remained the same, or increased.

25. Samuel C. Busey, *Personal Reminiscences and Recollections . . .* (Washington D.C., 1895), 157-158.

26. Tryon, *Household Manufactures*, 275-6; 291-3.

27. Thomas N. Bonner, *Medicine in Chicago, 1850-1950* (Madison, Wis., 1957), 200.

28. Rosen, *Fees and Fee Bills*, 30; 41.

29. Antonio Ciocco and Isidore Altman, "The Patient Load of Physicians in Private Practice, A Comparative Statistical Study of Three Areas," *Public Health Reports*, 58 (Sept. 3, 1943), 1329-1351.

30. George Kessel, "Would Not Practice Without an Auto," *Journal of the American Medical Association* 50 (March 7, 1908), 814.

31. J. A. Bowling, "Testimony from the Southwest," *JAMA* 46 (April 21, 1906), 1179.

32. "A Compilation of Automobile Statistics," *JAMA* 54 (April 9, 1910), 1273-74.

33. H. A. Stalker, "The Automobile as a Physician's Vehicle," *JAMA* 52 (March 7, 1908), 812.

34. C. A. Hibbert, "Transient Flat Life Requires Physician to Cover Wide Territory," *JAMA* 58 (April 6, 1912), 1080..

35. C. E. Black, "Medical Practice in Illinois before Hard Roads," *Bulletin of the Society of Medical History of Chicago* 5 (1946), 401-423.

36. Thus when professional leaders went on a campaign after 1900 to curb what they saw as an oversupply of doctors, they were responding not only to the growth of medical colleges, but also to the increase in supply that resulted from the automobile.

37. John Brooks, *Telephone: The First Hundred Years* (New York, 1976), 65; Marion May Dilts, *The Telephone in a Changing World* (New York, 1941), 9. A financial guide for doctors commented in 1923 that the telephone had become "of equal importance in practice as the stethoscope." Verlin C. Thomas, *The Successful Physician* (Philadelphia, 1923), 146.

38. Tryon, *Household Manufactures*, 242-248.

39. There are, so far as I know, no systematic data on the distribution of home versus office visits in the 1800's, and even for this century the statistics are fragmentary. My assumption

is that the decline of home visits has been fairly steady since the advent of the telephone, but this may be wrong. The first national survey of visits by general practitioners was made by the Committee on the Costs of Medical Care for the period 1928-31. Of the total number of calls made by general practitioners then, half were office and half were home calls. The major variation on this pattern was for children under ten, for whom about two thirds of the calls were at home. [See Selwyn D. Collins, "Frequency and Volume of Doctors' Calls Among Males and Females in 9000 Families, Based on Nation-Wide Periodic Canvasses, 1928-31," *Public Health Reports,* 55 (Nov. 1, 1940), 1983.] In 1932, a survey of 500 physicians, all recent graduates of medical schools practicing in communities of 50,000 people or less, reported that 55% of their calls were office visits; 35% home visits; and 10% hospital visits. [See the *Final Report of the Commission on Medical Education* (New York, 1932) 73.] In 1942, a survey of general practitioners in three areas of the country showed no significant differences between rural and urban counties, but did find that doctors over 65 years of age were making many more home visits than their younger colleagues under 35. The younger men made about 25% as many home as office visits; the older practitioners from about a third to half as many home visits. [See Antonio Ciocco and Isidore Altman, "The Patient Load of Physicians in Private Practice, a Comparative Statistical Study of Three Areas," *Public Health Reports,* 58 (Sept. 3, 1943), 1329-1351.] The first nation-wide data based on household interviews were collected by the federal government for the period July 1957 to June 1958; at that time, home visits represented 10.2% of all physician visits. By 1963-64, they were down to 5.4% and in 1971 to 1.7%. This merely confirms what everyone knows from experience – the house call is a thing of the past. [See U.S. Dept. of Health, Education and Welfare, "Physician Visits, Volume and Interval Since Last Visit, United States – 1971," Public Health Service Series 10, No. 97, 9.]

40. The decline of home calls has clearly gone beyond any purely economic considerations since it is now virtually impossible to find physicians who offer to make calls even at inflated prices. I think the physicians' preference to work in his own territory is as much a matter of status and power as it is the result of the relative cost of his time or the technological advantages of the office or hospital.

41. For 1873, see J. M. Toner, "Statistics of Regular Medical Associations and Hospitals of the United States," *Transactions of the American Medical Association* 24 (1873), 314-33; for the later dates, U.S. Bureau of the Census, *Historical Statistics of the United States, Colonial Times to 1957* (Washington, D.C., 1960), 35; for a state-by-state survey for this period, "Twenty-five Years' Growth of the Hospital Field," *National Hospital Record* (Sept. 1903), 23-27.

42. William J. Goode, *World Revolution and Family Patterns* (New York, 1963), 70-76.

43. *Historical Statistics,* 16. The data do show a steady decline in household size from 5.55 members in 1850 to 5.09 in 1870, 4.93 in 1890, 3.52 in 1950.

44. See Frank Furstenberg, "Industrialization and the American Family: A Look Backward," *American Sociological Review* 31 (June 1966), 326-337 and Edward Shorter, *The Making of the Modern Family* (New York, 1975).

45. Bernard Farber, *Guardians of Virtue: Salem Families in 1800* (New York, 1972), 46.

46. Richard Sennett, *Families Against the City: Middle Class Homes of Industrial Chicago, 1872-1890.* (Cambridge, Mass., 1970), 79.

47. Morris Vogel, "Boston's Hospitals, 1870-1930: A Social History," Ph.D. dissertation, University of Chicago, 1974, 188-199. See also John Modell and Tamara K. Hareven, "Urbanization and the Malleable Household: An Examination of Boarding and Lodging in American Families," *Journal of Marriage and the Family* 35 (1973), 467-479. Modell and Hareven point out that one-person households have gone from 3.7 to 20% of total households between 1790 and 1970.

48. For the English case, see Brian Abel-Smith, *The Hospitals, 1800-1948: A Study in Social Administration in England and Wales* (Cambridge, Mass., 1967), 141.

49. Talcott Parsons and Renée Fox, "Illness, Therapy and the Modern Urban Family," *Journal of Social Issues* 8 (1952), 31-44. The article by Parsons and Fox was written at a point in history that, in retrospect, appears to have been the high water point of hospital medicine. In the next two decades, mental hospitals underwent a drastic decline, and increasing attention began to be paid to unnecessary hospitalization in the general medical system. While correctly identifying the positive functions of hospitals, Parsons and Fox had neglected its dysfunctional aspects – that patients learn sickness behavior from each other, that prolonged isolation from the world makes it difficult for patients to function on return, and that hospitals impose an enormous cost on society. This last point especially has begun to tell in recent years. Parsons and Fox failed to see that much hospitalization was produced by the insurance system and the professional interests of physicians. They gave only two alternative explanations – family structure and technology – and missed entirely the structure of economic incentives.

50. *The New York Times,* (Dec. 31, 1900). Another account of the period cites "the trend toward the city" and "the necessity in many instances that women should engage in wage-earning occupations" as having "done away in great measure with home care of the sick."

> Home conditions are also changed. Fewer families occupy a single dwelling, and the tiny flat or contracted apartment no longer is sufficient to accommodate sick members of the family. Economic conditions are no longer favorable to home care, and recourse to the hospital has become necessary. It is not strange that the hospital has flourished . . . The sick are better cared for with less waste of energy, and their presence in the home does not interrupt the occupations and exhaust the means of wage earners . . . The day of the general home care of the sick can never return."

Henry Hurd, "The Hospital as a Factor in Modern Society," *The Modern Hospital* (Sept. 1913).

51. For an analysis of the causes of the growth of day-care, see Richard R. Nelson and Michael Krashinsky, "Public Control and Economic Organization of Day Care for Young Children," *Public Policy* 22 (Winter, 1974), esp. 54-60.

52. Kenneth J. Arrow, "Uncertainty and the Welfare Economics of Medical Care," *American Economic Review* 53 (1963), 941-967.

53. On the barriers to entry to the market, see Milton Friedman and Simon Kuznets, *Income from Independent Professional Practice* (New York, 1945), 8-21; 89-94; on the rural shortages, see Lewis Mayers and Leonard V. Harrison, *The Distribution of Physicians in the United States* (New York, 1924).

Edward Shorter

MATERNAL SENTIMENT AND DEATH IN CHILDBIRTH: A NEW AGENDA FOR PSYCHO-MEDICAL HISTORY

The forgotten person in psychohistory is the mother. A scad of studies speculate about changes in the father's relationship to the infant as a source of psychic trauma.[1] The socializing of the children themselves, normally in the period from weaning until kindergarten, has been carefully examined, although, usually from the viewpoint of how the child experienced the world rather than how the mother experienced the child.[2] And a large number of psychobiographies have traced the upward bounding of various famous individual children, J.S. Mill, Hitler, Luther, etcetera, emphasizing of course the *father's* role, and finding heavy torpedo damage down there in those libidinal bulkheads because the father had been too oppressive, too harsh, too overpowering, too remote, or too affectionless.

But childrearing from the mother's viewpoint has been underplayed in these accounts. I am not carping at the authors for "sexism." Women appear less prominently than men do in much of the basic source material, and so there's less to say about how Bismarck's mother cuddled him. But if the first twelve months or so are in fact crucial in the molding of personality, and if it is indeed the mother who fills the child's horizon for most of this time, some under-standing of how mothers interacted with tiny infants will clearly be central in understanding psychogenic changes in history.

The assumption that the "maternal instinct" is somehow "universal" doubt-lessly explains why the question has been so neglected up to now. If we can assume that mothers have always acted more or less the same way towards their infants, we could be confident that infant socializing regimes in 1620 were roughly the same as in 1920, and thus free ourselves to address other factors in personality formation likely to have been more variable over the years. Within cultural anthropology one school argues that, in fact, some kind of basic, radiant maternal love for infants is a constant to be found in all cultures, and if a historian seems to have found something different, then the fault lies with that historian rather than with the mothers of the time.[3] He has simply been blinded by his (bourgeois) (twentieth-century) (romantic) worldview to the fact that mothers always behave in roughly the same ways in all times and places. And a number of historians have taken this lead in their own analyses of the history of childhood.

Thus Christopher Lasch has recently argued that if by-gone mothers appeared to be unfeeling or indifferent towards their infants, it could only be because a harsh surrounding world had *forced* them to be so, that grim material conditions obliged them wilfully to subdue whatever stirrings of empathy they may have felt within their breasts and instead to affect placidity as their children sickened and died. According to this view, the rigors of poverty forced mothers to give time to chores more economically essential than infant care, and the high mortality resulting from externally-introduced infection made infant life so precarious that individual parents had forcibly to curtail their emotional investment in childrearing.[4]

If this view is correct, the main key to changes in the relationship between mothers and infants would lie in understanding poverty, for it was destitution that tugged individual mothers away from the cribside, where otherwise they would like to have dallied. And it was squalor that exposed infants to such deadly diseases as diptheria and smallpox, resulting in the loss of one in every two children before adulthood.

If in fact these variables are crucial, and if the maternal instinct lies just beneath the surface of all historical peoples, ready to blossom forth as soon as the kiss of prosperity descends, a history of "mothering" as such would be relatively uninteresting. What counts is the history of oppression and misery, and how the working classes have managed to lift themselves from this valley of despair. Writing this sort of history, of course, is what social historians have always more or less done. So their new contribution to psychohistory will be: just a bit more of the same. Keep up the good work, boys.

Recently, however, a second view of the history of mothering has appeared. For this hesitant little band of scholars, the "maternal instinct" has nothing universal or constant about it at all, and to say that mothers have always wanted to beam upon their babies would be historically as inexact as saying "People have always wanted to be happy." This view sees, rather, an articulate sense of maternal sentiment evolving over the years in response to a specific, though as yet imperfectly understood, set of historical changes. According to this school, maternal sentiment is as culturally-enhanced as are such other kinds of sentiment as romantic love, or love for dogs, or love of standing alone in the forest at night.[5] Which means that some cultures in some centuries will promote it, others in other times and places won't.

Several circumstances work against the notion that mothers who didn't seem to love their babies were prevented only by misery from doing so. The misery argument normally emphasizes infection as the cause of death, pathogens contracted from spoiled, contaminated food or from unhygienic surroundings. But keep in mind that one quarter to one third of the astoundingly high infant mortality of traditional society occurred in the first month of life, indeed as much as a quarter within the first week.[6] Now, the significance of this pattern of infant mortality is that neonatal deaths are rarely caused by externally-induced infections. They are rather the result of prematurity, birth trauma, improper feeding, or congenital weaknesses acquired during gestation.[7] "Misery" of course is ultimately responsible for some of those pathologies as well, but the role of human volition in overcoming them is much more significant than in fighting germ-born diseases, as we shall see later.

The second circumstance frequently overlooked by the "misery" historians is that not everyone ever to have lived in past times was desperately poor. While here is not the place to descend into discussions of "just how many people did starve?" or when did the proletariat's immiseration actually commence? I should nonetheless like to point out that in the villages and small towns where Europeans and North Americans lived in past centuries a sizeable "middle class" did exist. By "middle class" we should understand not so much the bourgeois merchants and bankers who constitute the *bourgeoisie,* but the group which Marx labelled the "lower middle classes," the millions of shopkeepers, independent peasants, and master artisans who hired one journeyman and had an apprentice living in as well.[8] These people, though rarely so well off that a bad year wouldn't shroud them in hardship, had nonetheless in normal times (which, by definition, is most of the time) a modest surplus, about which we know because we see them buying land, or financing big weddings, or paying daughters' dowries, or buying militia uniforms with it.

The point is that this village middle class, the backbone of traditional society, treated their children in exactly the same way as did the genuinely wretched of the earth, the landless laborers, and eternal journeymen. Evidence abounds of "middle-class" families abandoning unwanted infants, affecting indifference in the face of infant death, or neglecting to breast-feed their children and handing them instead pap or cow's milk from wooden baby bottles. Peasants' wives who hung their infants, bound tightly in swaddling clothes, from tree limbs for long periods or who permitted by neglect the pig to wander in and devour the child weren't absolutely compelled by poverty to be out there working in those fields; they could have made alternate baby-sitting arrangements when they left the farm house – had they cared enough to do so.[9] The point was they didn't care, because their entire culture was indifferent. They had not internalized rules of the social game which commanded: "Preserve infant life about all else," and so went about their days guided by different priorities, prepared to accept the mortality risks they knew their actions entitled.

The "new agenda for psycho-medical history" mentioned in the title of this paper will not be, therefore, a grand scheme to study the impact of poverty upon mother-infant relations in the traditional family. Though ultimately important in the way that all resource questions matter, "poverty" played only a secondary role in shaping maternal attitudes towards infants.

What did matter? Here the new school of historians of childhood has given us two options to choose from. One is Lloyd deMause's "psychogenic theory of childhood."[10] The other represents a loose group of historians we might call the "great transformation" school.

DeMause argues that the basic motor that drives relations between parents and infants is the parents' desire to regress subconsciously "to the psychic age of their children and work through the anxieties of that age in a better manner the second time they encounter them than they did during their own childhood."[11] Psychoanalysts recognize this sort of "regression" as a therapeutic aid. DeMause is suggesting that it becomes the fundamental socializing mechanism of entire cultures. Parents who are raised lovingly will have relatively few psychic traumas to work through, and so behave lovingly towards their children. But parents who themselves were the victims of unfeeling brutality as children will have a much more ambivalent response to their own children, accouding to deMause. Their own recollections of childhood beatings will rustle through their unconscious and they may tend to use their own children as a sounding board upon which to project their anxieties. Or they may use their children as substitutes for adult figures of their own pasts, actually seeing them unconsciously as their own parents and reversing upon them the rage they felt towards their parents. DeMause calls this second possible response the "reversal reaction." The third possible response to children is for parents to "empathize with the child's needs and satisfy them," which is, in deMause's view, the humane solution towards which contemporary society is now groping.

So we have a theory that outlines three possible responses to children as ways of reliving and working through the traumas of one's own childhood: the first two, projection and reversal, occur in tandem as part of a "double image" that traditional parents had of children: you beat them to show "that the child is both very bad (projective reaction) and very loving (reversal reaction)."[12] These first two dominate most of the history of childhood. In deMause's view the essential story in this history is that of projection-reversal giving way to empathy, the third response, over the last two millenia.

For convenience, deMause subdivides this long history of childhood into five separate "modes:"[13]

The "infanticidal" mode (Antiquity to Fourth Century A.D.) This mode makes of childhood a horror story: "parents routinely resolved their anxieties about taking care of children by killing them. . . " And many of those who were not killed were sodomized, according to deMause.

The "abandonment" mode (Fourth to Thirteenth Century A.D.) Parents continue to project all the anger and fear they themselves felt about growing up upon their children, but because the Church has made killing and sodomizing rather outré behavior, parents content themselves with merely beating their progeny often, or abandoning them "to the wetnurse, to the monastery or nunnery, to foster families, to the homes of other nobles as servants or hostages, or by severe emotional abandonment at home."

The "ambivalent" mode (Fourteenth to Seventeenth Centuries) To contain what they still perceive as their children's dangerousness, parents now try to mold them rather than just flailing away. DeMause notes the emergence of child instruction manuals in the fourteenth century and comments on the frequency in art of the "close-mother" image.

The "intrusive" mode (Eighteenth Century) Now we're reaching the origins of our own times. For unexplained reasons many parents start to feel "true empathy" with their children, and even those still bent upon molding their kids do so in more psychological rather than physical ways, which means controlling children by making them feel guilt rather than pain. The storybook replaces the enema.

The "socialization" mode (Nineteenth to Mid-twentieth Centuries) is basically a continuation of the intrusive mode, with more gentleness and understanding. Fathers, however, now involve themselves a bit in the picture. DeMause observes perceptively that "the socializing mode is still thought of by most people as the only model within which discussion of child care can proceed, and it has been the source of all twentieth-century psychological models, from Freud's 'channeling of impulses' to Skinner's behaviorism."

The "helping" mode (begins Mid-twentieth Century) This is the A.S. Neill "Summerhill" approach, based upon "the proposition that the child knows better than the parent what it needs at each stage of its life. . . . There is no attempt at all to discipline or form 'habits'." Etcetera. Thus far, this historic "mode" seems to have been adopted only by a handful of upper-middle-class intellectuals, but I mention it here for the sake of indicating what is, in deMause's view, the termination stage of this essentially teleological progression, a progression from bestialness and violence to love and understanding. Much as we once thought governments progressed inevitably from autocracy to liberalism, and religions from orthodoxy to toleration, now we have a historical scheme in which parents march just as inevitably across the ages from anxiety and resentment to the ability to put themselves in their children's shoes and thus to let their children form their own happy little lives.

Please note the "inevitability" with which these changes take place. DeMause has enunciated the Iron Laws of Childrearing, recalling Marx, who evolved similar set of Iron Laws. Yet whereas for Marx all changes which take place in social behavior have their origin in external shifts in the mode of production, for deMause nothing from the outside impinges at all upon this inner dynamic between parents and children: it evolves for autonomous reasons, at its own pace, and is undeflected by structural changes raging about the nursery.

An alternative to the psychogenic theory is the "great transformation" theory, used by several historians who see a crucial change in the experience of childhood occurring in the eighteenth and nineteenth centuries, at the time as other elements in the mentalite´ domain change as well.[14] Although the great transformation people agree with deMause that the basic direction of change is towards more loving child-care, and away from the affectionless indifference — with its hideous infant mortality — of the old regime, they differ on two essential points:

1. The great transformation school sees modernization occurring in one fell swoop, rather than slowly jerking away at popular mentalities across the ages. Whereas for deMause childrearing modes have been in constant evolution since the Greeks and Romans, for the "modernizers" a relative stability in patterns of popular life prevailed from the high middle ages (what happened before that time in childrearing no one knows) until the 18th century. Thereafter this stable "traditional society" is hammered by a number of blows that transform its sentimental life completely within a century and a half. So if deMause has five modes that extend over two millenia, the modernization people have just two main prototypes: "before" and "after," traditional "village" childrearing vs. the "modern" sentimental family.

2. The great transformation school sees changes occurring within the family, especially between mother and infant, as a consequence of external changes in the social structures which encadre sentimental life. At some level, greater attachment to children must be associated with changes in how people make their living, or whether they live in cities, or whether they have acquired a feeling of personal autonomy, or whether they feel their fellow citizen are, fundamentally, competitors or *communards*. As I have observed, deMause militantly rejects any possibility that shifts from one mode to another were brought

about by outside factors: "Not only is this 'generational pressure' for psychic change . . . spontaneous, originating in the adult's need to regress and in the child's striving for relationship, but it also occurs independent of social and technological change. It therefore can be found even in periods of social and technological stagnation."[15] Thus for deMause the history of childhood marches to the beat of an internal drummer, not at the command of outside forces in the substructure of society. Just as intellectual historians, for example, often believe that ideas change as a result of some internal dynamic quite independent of changes in the surrounding society, so deMause feels that parents' historic transition from anxiety to love is accomplished quite independently of the gut-wrenching changes of the great transformation.

The disagreement is quite fundamental. For deMause, childrearing itself is the prime mover of social life, and all that transpires in the economy or the intellectual life of a civilization will reflect the way in which children are socialized. For the great transformation people, childhood is another of many "dependent" variables, factors which shift as a result of massive, subterranean structural changes in the modes of production, the organization of communities, or the level of technology. Just another tail, in other words, wagged by the giant dog of modernization.

Where the great transformation school has fallen down is in specifying the psychodynamics of change in childhood. DeMause has a clear schema: projection, reversal, empathy. Among the great transformation people, Weinstein and Platt have probably come closest to spelling out the psychic mechanisms through their analysis of authority patterns in "the father's leaving the home," a consequence of the growing subdivision of labor.[16]

My own work has pointed to changes in the relationship between the family and surrounding community as the key to the shift. I have suggested that the family's desire for privacy and isolation, to permit its individual members to develop a rich sentimental life, put down a base for the crystallizing of maternal sentiment towards infants. But these are "sociological" variables rather than "psychological:" they permit us to account for the rise of the privatized nuclear family, and for the destruction of the traditional community, with arguments that owe nothing to Freud, Erikson, or any of the other masters. So if we have mothers suddenly bathing affection upon their nurslings, it's not because they've started to work through their own anxieties about their own childhoods in any different way but rather because, for external structural reasons: (a) they feel more "sentimental" in every aspect of their intimate relations and (b) they find themselves in a family environment that supports mothering and cherishes infant life.

If pressed to elaborate a psychoschema of change, I would probably suggest that in traditional communities the boundary line between the individual ego and the surrounding social world was much less distinct than it would later be. Individuals were much less attuned to their personal gratification, to "happiness" and the whole bagful of tricks that later would associate with western individualism. They were accordingly more prepared to subordinate their ego-related demands to the needs of the surrounding community for stability and the maintenance of custom. Once, however, a strong sense of individual self-identification starts becoming elaborated, allegiance to the old, confining rules falls by the wayside and people start asking themselves: "What can I do to be happy?"[17] Among the answers that women, at least, receive echoing back from the new culture is: "Love your babies." This is the crystallization of maternal sentiment.

Where the "misery" and the "great transformation" schools both have an advantage over deMause, however, is in permitting verification of their arguments, in specifying the evidence whereby they may be proved right or disproved, and in laying out quantitative procedures for tracing the diffusion of various "mentalities" among the millions of anonymous people whose behavior we all, ultimately, are trying to account for. Verification has always been the achilles heel of psychohistory, and of psychoanalysis in general, isolating it from such relatively "hard" social sciences as sociology or economics. DeMause is no exception. Let us take, for example, the transition from the ambivalent to the intrusive modes, which evidently occurred around the beginning of the great transformation, in England starting doubtlessly at some point during the seventeenth century, in France during the eighteenth, in Germany during the nineteenth. DeMause gives us no indication whether this major historical change began first in the cities or the countryside among the aristocracy, the *grande bourgeoisie* or the peasants in the villages. Did it parallel the diffusion of the "popular enlightenment," or instead follow the spreading wake of the free marketplace? Did this major historical transition have, in short, *any* social dimensions at all? Or did it progress among all those millions of people simultaneously and at the same pace.

DeMause's argument has no *handles* on it, no social characteristics for us to get hold of and shout, "Yes, by God, here it is, happening among the barrelmakers of Dijon! They've started breast-feeding their kids!" Nor are we able to cry "Aha! He's wrong. Here are *newly* infanticidal parents among the factory workers of Sheffield, eight centuries after deMause has assured us that child-murder ceased to be the leading edge of pyschochange."

The great transformation school makes, at least, certain "predictions" about what happened: that we find first involved in newstyle mothering the upper-middle classes, the movement then spreading downwards from that group, through not necessarily as the result of some kind of *gesunkenes Kulturgut* or social diffusion process. This school predicts we'll encounter new-style tenderness first in the great cities, last in the isolated hinterland, first among the office workers, last among the Breton or Upper Bavarian peasantries.[18] And if these predictions are proven wrong, then we shall ruefully declare ourselves licked, and return to the drawing boards to devise some new arguments.

The bulk of recent historical scholarship has suggested that these predicted differentials actually exist. In Yves Castan's recent work on Languedoc, for example, we see mothers among the provincial bourgeoisie ignoring their younger, non-inheriting sons in favor of the eldest.[19] These cadets, unlike their older brothers, were then sent out to rural wetnurses, where infants generally experienced a harrowing chance of dying.[20] Meanwhile in England, as J.H. Plumb has pointed out, mothers among a comparable social group were lavishing affection upon all their children, dressing them up as little soldiers and sailors or "wasting" their money on "useless toys."[21] Randolph Trumbach's forthcoming book shows that by mid-18th century maternal sentiment had already crystallized among most of England's great aristocratic families.[22] So in that century of supposed universal pivoting from ambivalent-to-intrusive-to-socializing modes, we note unmistakable social and national differentials: while the German peasants still resolutely swaddled and handfed their infants, maternal breastfeeding and free movement of infant limbs was making progress among the Parisian middle classes; while the hidebound French provincials were still practicing the traditional politics of favoritism, the English middle and upper classes were rushing headlong into modern patterns of tenderness and impartiality.

Enormous social differentials in childrearing have recently become visible in the 19th century too. Patricia Branca, in her study of middle-class and lower-middle-class Victorian women, argues for an "evolution toward increasingly intimate and loving bonds between mother and child." By the end of the century parental treatment of children had, according to her, "altered significantly." The child was beginning to be viewed as an "individual with very particular needs which only a loving mother could fulfill."[23] Now, let us contrast these adoring Victorians with the working-class Lyon mothers who, around the same time, were still sending their children out to wetnurses, so that among Lyon's textile population infant mortality was in 1903 still 23%.[24] We could range back and forth across Europe like this, spotting variations at any given time in the way mothers of different countries, social classes and city-sizes treated their infants. The presence of these gulches practically screams at us that those mothers who in some places *did* become more loving were animated by certain social, economic or cultural forces which were absent in those places where the mothers *didn't.*

The point of all this talk about differences from mother to mother is merely to establish that (a) at some point in time virtually everywhere this dramatic, historic change in the quality of mothering which I have called "The crystallization of maternal sentiment" does in fact take place, and (b) that deMause's argument about its unrelatedness to the major social transformations of modernization is not to be taken seriously.

The evidence available now does not let us pin down the subterranean structrual forces behind this change. A number of people, including myself, have speculated about the root causes, but it's as with a sailor trying to navigate in a thunderstorm who sees only the occasional star. We need to spread out the whole horizon in front of us in some systematic way.

That is the second point. We should start thinking about a research agenda that will, by a study of group-to-group variation, help determine what lies behind the great transformation in mothering.

II

The agenda must have some minimum ground rules:

(a) We should focus primarily upon women because it has been upon women that the burden of infant care has fallen until very recently.

(b) We should focus upon domains of life and death amenable to some extent to human control, and slide by those dark reaches where famine, war and pestilence carry people away despite their best individual efforts.

(c) We should aim at "measuring" behavior with readily standardized yardsticks, so we can be sure we're comparing the same trait among mothers in places as apparently disparate as Scotland and Swabia.

To this end I propose the study of death in childbirth.

Pregnancy, labor and childbed may claim as victims both mother and infant. We are accustomed today to thinking of delivery as a "normal" biological process. And of course it is. But at the same time, at no moment in their lives are women usually so close to death as when they give birth. And no other mammalian infant so close to perishing as is the human child in the weeks and months immediately following birth. Childbirth is a crossroads where life, death and affection intersect along roads that otherwise almost never meet. And I think that, historically, the behavior of women at that crossroads has undergone some major changes.

Virtually nothing is now known about how women have responded in past times to pregnancy and parturition, to sickness in the lying-in period and to early-infant death. This must be noted at the outset. So the first step in observing the woman at that crossroads is not to ask what emotions dance across her face, but what were in reality her objective chances of dying in labor or of contracting postpartum sepsis? What in fact was the risk of losing her infant, either during pregnancy, in labor or in the neonatal period? And what might she have undertaken, through her own initiative, to minimize that loss?

Suddenly we spring from psychohistory to medical history. Let me first develop a rationale for focussing upon obstetric and perinatal mortality (to call things by their technical names), and then point out the possible psychohistorical implications of this knowledge.

The maternal mortality of childbirth is important not as an index of how mothers behaved, but rather of the risks to which they might have suspected their infants would subject them. Remember that we are talking about women who might be pregnant ten or twelve times over their fertile years and give birth six or eight times, about a 2-4% chance that each time the infant would be stillborn (to say nothing of miscarriages), and about a 2% chance that each time the woman herself would actually succumb during or shortly after delivery. When in 1908 Gustav Zinke, a Cincinnati obstetrician, called childbirth a "conflict unto death between mother and child," he was describing a situation that had already improved enormously since the middle of the nineteenth century.[25] In normal births, of course, a "conflict" between the interests of the parturient mother and of the infant, who is about to descend the birth canal, wouldn't be anticipated. A speedy delivery free of obstetric intervention serves equally the interest of both. It is when complications of pregnancy or labor develop that the survival of the infant can become diametrically opposed to the survival of the mother.

Consider, among the many possible complications, the problem of "dystocia." All of a sudden, labor stops. The contractions subside. The fetal head ceases to advance. Nowadays we have a quick solution in the form of caesarian section, but only around 1900 did the caesarian become a relatively risk-free operation. And its ghastly mortality made it, for all practical purposes, quite unavailable before 1880. So what did people do in those pre-antiseptic, pre-anaesthetic times in case of dystocia? The three available options placed maternal and fetal interests directly at loggerheads:

(1) A "high forceps" delivery, which means reaching directly into the uterus with the tongs, grasping the presenting part, and tugging it out. Forceps left something of a chance that the infant's life would be saved, but only at the cost of terrible lacerations to the mother, such as cervical tears or fistulae that might not necessarily be fatal but which would subject the woman to agony, and then leave her an invalid for long periods.[26]

(2) An operation called "version and extraction," which meant the accoucheur or midwife's reaching their hand into the uterus to grasp the fetal feet, in order to turn the infant foot-down (hence "podalic" version); then pulling the child out of the womb by its feet (extraction). Again, this procedure offered a chance of saving the child, but at the risk of introducing infection into the mother's uterus, or of tearing her perhaps only partially-dilated cervix.[27]

(3) Embryotomy, essentially, the perforating of the fetal head with a hook or a pair of scissors, then letting the woman herself deliver the rest of the child's body once the large, obstructing head had been collapsed.[28]

In all three of these operations the life of the infant might be sacrificed to save the life of the mother. If no operation were done, then the mother's life might trickle away as the accoucheur waited for her to deliver herself naturally, a decision that would, of course, favor the infant over the mother.

A similar choice between mother and infant presents itself in numerous other complications of pregnancy, such as "placenta praevia" (the placenta implanting itself across the entrance to the cervix), the premature separation of the placenta, or the various toxemias of pregnancy. In each, the interests of mother and infant may be opposed.

How frequent were such complications? If they occurred only rarely, we have little more than a curiosity of medical history. If they occurred, on the other hand, quite often, we have the makings of an intriguing explicandum in psychohistory: what did average mothers, pregnant for the n-th time, think about their fetuses and newborn children whose uterine existence placed their own lives so much at stake?

That women often risked death in childbirth goes without saying. Whereas women generally had a lower mortality than men at most ages (then as now), only in their twenties and thirties was the reverse true: that women died more often. In Norway, for example, between 1889 and 1932 married women at ages 20-24, 25-29 and 30-34 (before 1922, 35-44 as well) died much more frequently than the men in those age groups. After 1932 the difference is reversed, and women start to outlive men even in those age groups as a result of better obstetric care. We know it was something about marriage, probably childbearing, that imposed this excess mortality upon women because *single* women at those ages had a lower mortality than single men. This surplus female childbirth mortality shows up in a number of other studies as well.[29]

Much of the mortality of childbirth is associated with complications, rather than with infection that just happens to drift in. Labor is protracted; the tissue that has started to die along the birth canal becomes infected with bacteria from the vagina; sepsis begins. Or the accoucheur introduces some deadly pathogen from the outside in trying to intervene. So the pressing research problem becomes to establish just how often were women confronted with the grim realization that their survival might be incompatible with the survival of their child? How often did labor stretch out to two and three days, with the relatives hysterical, the midwife in tears and horsemen riding frantically into town to fetch the doctor with his decapitation hook?

If the architecture and physiology of the pelvis were some immutable fact of nature, we could compute the incidence of complications merely by looking at the obstetric statistics of our own time. But here the story acquires nuances: what happens to the female pelvis has changed over the years.

Consider, for example, the problem of the contracted pelvis. Pelvic deformities are quite unusual in modern obstetrics (about 5% of all deliveries) because most women today have been well nourished as babies, received sufficient vitamin D, avoid rickets, and experience adequate physical development.[30] But even around the middle of the 19th century many women suffered from rickets as infants, and so grew up with pelves too narrow to permit a normal delivery.[31] Ultimately many of them would deliver anyway through natural means, after a long, painful labor, but for many others some kind of dystocia would accur, placing their accoucheur before the terrible dilemma mentioned above: which to favor, the mother's interests or the infant's?

If we are to get at the psychodynamics of the mother's relationship to infant child, we must develop at least an approximate notion of the incidence of rickets, dystocia, and operative intervention in labor. But at present, outside the statistics of a few lying-in hospitals — untypical because they served mainly young, unmarried primiparous women and because the people who ran them were quite keen to intervene surgically at every opportunity — we know nothing about the typical risks that an average parturient mother would run in the usual situation: delivering at home in the hands of a midwife.

We do have a few shards of data on obstetric mortality. Consider the statistics in table 1, the death rate in childbirth for selected places over some longer period of time. No general trends at all emerge. In some places the risk of dying in childbed seems to have risen during the late-18th and 19th centuries, such as in England, Wales and Scotland, the Marseille Lying In Hospital (!), and those two Austrian villages. In others it apparently declined, such as in that Scottish private practice and in the state of Mecklenourg. These data, the only published series I have been able to locate, must be taken with about nine grains of salt because (a) the tendancy of doctors to conceal mortality from sepsis during the lying-in period may have changed, and thus the death certificates, on which national morbidity statistics are based, may underreport puerperal deaths more severely at some times than at others; (b) these maternal death statistics combine indiscriminately the mortality from induced late-term abortions and from full-term pregnancies.[32] At some point during the nineteenth century the mortality from abortions begins a deadly rise, simply because so many more abortions were being performed, but without data which separate full-term pregnancies from "miscarriages" we won't be able to tell how much a genuine decline in obstetric mortality may have been obscured by rises in abortion deaths.[33]

Enough technical data. The main point is that without further archival research based upon the midwives' and doctors' casebooks themselves, we won't be able to discern how the mother's real risk of dying in childbirth actually did change during the crucial period in which maternal sentiment was coming alive. Nor will we know the extent to which "normal" labor was disrupted by these terrible complications of pregnancy.

A second index promises to cast light more directly upon the mother's attitude to her young infant: "perinatal mortality," to use the current medical jargon.

Perinatal mortality means simply the number of miscarriages and stillbirths that occur after 28 weeks of pregnancy, plus the number of newborn who die in the first week, or first month, of life. These deaths of live children are called "neonatal" mortality. So noramlly adding together the stillbirth rate and the neonatal death rate will give us "perinatal mortality."

Why would psychohistorians want to know such a thing?

Of all the points in life at which the infant is at risk of death, the few weeks before and after delivery are those when the mother is most able to influence its survival. Intrauterine fetal loss is significantly affected by whether the mother does hard field or shop work in the final weeks of her pregnancy and by how well she eats. Women who toil at the hoe and stick to their traditional bowls of porridge seem to have suffered more premature labors and macerated fetuses than those who rested up at the end and who ate those extra eggs and chunks of meat.[34]

The stillbirth rate is probably influenced — though to what extent is unclear — by the quality of medical help the family is able to afford: by whether they let the husband deliver her himself, bring in a "granny" or helping neighbor, or pay the fees of a competent midwife.[35] Calling in a male physician was, in the epochs that interest us, essentially the decision of the midwife, not of the mother herself or of her family. A resource decision, the engaging of a midwife can be taken as a mirror of the valuation which the mother, or her family, places upon having a live birth.

We find a third point at which maternal attitudes affect perinatal loss in the weeks just after confinement: how the mother feeds the infant, whether the house (or hut) is kept warm, and quite probably the amount of attention she lavishes upon it as a stimulus for it to remain in life. Today we take all three of these circumstances for granted, and virtually all newborn are fed digestible food, kept in warm quarters and showered with attention. So the causes of neonatal death today (aside from prematurity) boil down to a handful of obscure diseases of early infancy plus some cases of birth trauma and deformity.[36] But in the 18th century, when routinely 2 or 3 % of all infants were stillborn, and another goodly share, as indicated above, died in the first week or two of life, the components of perinatal death were much more subject to external influence.[37]

Thus I am arguing that mothers could improve their infants' chances of survival at three distinct moments: late in pregnancy through diet and work regime, during labor by hiring a good midwife, and in the puerperium by further abstaining from work in order to care for the newborn and feed it at the breast, rather than with goat's milk out of a wooden bottle or with pap.

Two possible objections might be offered to this analysis. How many of these decisions did the woman herself actually control? Surely her diet, for example, would be determined by the sheer availability of food, and by the willingness of others to let her eat more than her normal share of meat or eggs? And in part, of course, this objection would be true, for traditional society generally was chronically undernourished simply because calories were scarce. But even within the family differential allocation of food took place, the men, for example, customarily getting more meat than the women.[38] Peasants usually sent their beef and dairy products away to the urban bourgeois, and themselves ate only occasionally a bit of pork, from the one pig slaughtered every year. A society hellbent upon nourishing its womenfolk adequately in pregnancy could simply have decided that more of these customary exports would be consumed at home. As for working till the end of term, then resuming the grinding routine as speedily as possible after parturition, who can say right now how much of this labor was essential in economic terms, how much merely "traditional"?[39] We need more information about the options available to normal women in typical peasant, sub-peasant, artisanal and small-merchant households. At some level these labor inputs were all subject to human allocation.

The second objection is, did people really know how much these factors mattered in pregnancy wastage and in early-infant death? How much reliable information was available to the village and smalltown culture of traditional Europe? In some places, for example, it was customary to give newborn babies biscuits or cow's milk as their first food, mother's milk only later, as a test of survival. Lily Weiser-Aall, who has studied this practice in detail for Norway and Iceland, suspects it may have been a sort of *Kraftprobe* to ensure that only the fittest would grow up.[40] Obviously these mothers realized the potential consequences of their infants' diets. European mothers in general would have come increasingly within earshot of sensible medical advice about breast-feeding as time progressed, for doctors all over began a huge propaganda campaign. How many women picked up these messages, and continued traditional practices anyway? We need research on these questions.

The final question is the one psychohistorians should try most urgently to answer: if the women knew that certain practices were bad for the health of their infants, did they really care? We have accumulated over the past ten years a considerable amount of evidence to the effect that they did not care, that infanticide was used routinely as a means of birth control, that infant-abandonment came as casually to parents from the popular classes as going to market, and that divorcing parents were quite unconcerned about the kinds of child custody questions that would later put mothers and fathers at each other's throats.[41] All these data, unfortunately, are difficult to standardize for comparative purposes. The mortality data offer us a new avenue to plumbing the real attitudes of parents towards children, and to understanding why those attitudes changed in the long pull over the mountains that we call "modernization."

An indirect way of establishing the sensitivity of perinatal death to material conditions in the mother's world is to compute year-to-year correlations between the cost of living and mortality. If this variety of mortality really is sensitive to such factors as diet, the parents' ability to pay a midwife, afford fuel to superheat their dwelling and so forth, it should decrease in years of prosperity, increase in years of dearth.

I performed this sample test upon perinatal mortality data from Italy, the only large country to have published both stillbirths and neonatal deaths in uniform series over long periods of time. Both living standards and infant mortality are subject to powerful trends over the years. So to measure reliably the effect of year-to-year changes in one variable upon the other, without picking up the false correlation that two simultaneous trends might produce, I have "de-trended" the data. The coefficients in the bottom half of table 2 are therefore most important, and more or less confirm the initial hypothesis.

Before 1908 the correlation is minimal (and has moreover a positive sign!), which means, basically, no relationship. Traditional practices maintain their heavy sway regardless of the possibly ameliorating influences of higher wages. After 1908 a powerful inverse correlation emerges, demonstrating the sensitivity of infant death to living conditions: the better off people become, the fewer infants that die *in utero* and in the first week of life. These numbers should not be taken too seriously. Many conflicting patterns can show up in a country as diverse as Italy, making national-level data the sum of a number of vastly different apples and oranges. But we get some hint that quantitative regression analyses of this nature may offer a promising avenue of research.

Can we relate these exercises in numerology to John Demos's call for greater use of "developmental" models of childhood?[42] Demos encourages historians to employ "horizontal" models, which relate various aspects of the child's existence one to another, or "vertical" models such as that of Erik Erikson, which specify psychogenic stages through which the individual passes on the way to adulthood. Demos's own work, for example, has leaned heavily on Erikson's "eight stages of man" model. He finds the first stage in Puritan communities full of love and tenderness for the tiny infants: they're breastfed, clad in light, warm clothing, sleep in their parents' beds, and enjoy surroundings that are "animated, warm and intimate." The personality types this early-infant experience produces are, according to Demos, balanced ambivalently between a tropism towards "harmony, unity, and concord," on the one hand, and "contentiousness" or "outright conflict" on the other.

Now, consider the neonatal experience of most European babies in the years before 1850. Rather than being coddled by doting parents in warm environments, they are swaddled tightly and cast aside by exhausted, resentful mothers, fed only intermittently, and permitted to stew for hours in their own ordure. In view of the statistics we have just rehearsed, is it any wonder that these high-parity mothers might have not greeted joyously their newborn? That they might have seen infants as a curse of God rather than a blessing? What kinds of adult personalities ultimately emerged from this sort of perinatal crucible? *That* is a compelling new item on the agenda for psychohistory.

University of Toronto   Edward Shorter

Table 1: Maternal Mortality, Selected Time Series

Area	*Author*	*Social Group*	*Maternal deaths per 1000 confinements*	
Unterinntal (Austria)	Fliri[1]	peasants	1700-1749	3
			1750-1799	10
			1800-1849	15
			1850-1899	13
			1900-1939	2
Martelltal (Austria)	Winkler[2]	full peasants	1634-1650	3
		and half-peasants	1651-1700	1
			1701-1750	7
			1751-1800	7
			1801-1850	8
			1851-1900	9
			1901-1950	12
			1951-1968	7
Mecklenburg	Prinzing[3]	whole pop.	1777-1800	11
			1801-1815	10
			1816-1875	9
			1886-1900	7
			1901-1909	4
Sweden	Henriks[4]	whole pop.	1776-1780	8.9
			1781-1785	8.3
			1786-1790	9.3
			1791-1795	10.1
			1796-1800	8.5
			1801-1805	7.8
			1806-1810	8.9
			1811-1815	7.9
			1816-1820	7.4
			1821-1825	6.7
			1826-1830	6.6
			1831-1835	5.7
			1836-1840	5.1
			1841-1845	4.5
			1846-1850	4.4
			1851-1855	4.4
London Lying in Hospital	Fox[5]		1790-1810	5
			1855-1875	13
Rotunda Hospital Dublin	Fox[5]		1786-1793	12
			1792-1800	8
			1800-1807	11
			1807-1814	12

Area	Author	Social Group	Maternal deaths per 1000 confinements	
British Lying-In Hospital, London	Buer[6]	married women	1749-1758	24
			1779-1788	17
			1789-1798	4
			1799-1808	5
Scotland	Watson[7]	whole pop.	1855-1864	4.9
			1865-1874	5.1
			1875-1884	5.2
			1885-1894	5.3
			1895-1904	4.6
			1905-1914	5.6
			1915-1922	6.2
small town in Scotland	Watson[7]	a "mixed town and country" private practice	1847-1864	17.0
			1880-1891	7.2
			1891-1923	1.7
England and Wales	Boxall[8]	whole pop.	1847-1849	6.0
			1850-1854	5.2
			1855-1859	4.6
			1860-1864	4.7
			1865-1869	4.6
			1870-1874	5.3
			1875-1879	4.4
			1880-1884	4.7
			1885-1889	4.6
			1890-1891	5.1
Marseille Lying-in Hospital	Queirel[9]	mainly unwed mothers and poor married women	1695-1720	2
			1735-1739	4
			1740-1749	8
			1750-1759	2
			1760-1769	4
			1770-1779	1
			1780-1789	1
			1815-1826	9
			1827-1867	56
Labriboisiere	Siredey[10]		1882-1886	32

			From all causes	"puerperal" causes
Hospital (Paris)		unwed mothers, poor married women		
			1855-1859 73	67
			1860-1869 33	28
			1870-1879 28	22
			1880-1881 25	18

Notes to Table 1:

1. Franz Fliri, *Bevölkerungsgeographische Untersuchungen im Uterinntal* (Innsbruck: Universitäts-Verlag Wagner, 1948), p. 56. Deaths within 4 weeks of parturition.

2. Gisela Winkler, *Bevölkerungsgeographische Untersuchungen in Martelltal* (Innsbruck: Universitäts-Verlag Wagner, 1973), pp. 70-71. Deaths within 4 weeks of parturition.

3. Friedrich Prinzing, *Handbuch der medizinischen Statistik,* 2nd ed. (Jena, 1931), p. 106.

4. Freidrich Hendriks, "On the Vital Statistics of Sweden from 1749-1855," *Journal of the Statistical Society of London,* 25 (1862), p. 167. N confinements taken from Gustav Sundbarg, *Bevölkerungsstatistik Schwedens, 1750-1900* (reprint Stockholm: Statistiska Centralbyran, 1970), p. 127.

5. Claire E. Fox, *Pregnancy, Childbirth and Early Infancy in Anglo-American Culture, 1675-1830* (American civ. diss., University of Pennsylvania, 1966), pp. 361-363. London Lying-In data per 1000 confinements, Dublin data per 1000 live births.

6. M.C. Buer, *Health, Wealth, and Population in the Early Days of the Industrial Revolution* (London, 1926), p. 145.

7. B.P. Watson, "The Responsibility of the Obstetric Teacher in Relation to Maternal Mortality and Morbidity," *American Journal of Obstetrics and Gynecology,* 14 (1927), 278. Private practice deaths are from "sepsis."

8. Robert Boxall, "The Mortality of Childbirth," *The Lancet,* 1 July 1893, p. 9.

9. Dr. Queirel, *Histoire de la maternité de Marseille* (Marseille, 1889), pp. 7, 14, 31, 43, 91.

10. F. Siredey, *Les Maladies peurpérales: étude clinique* (Paris, 1884), pp. 89, 91. 92.

Table 2.: Correlations in Year-to-Year Fluctuation between
Perinatal-Neonatal Mortality and the Standard
of Living in Italy, 1871-1939

Zero-order correlation coefficients between:
Perinatal mortality and standard of living:
    1871-1890 r = -.61
    1907-1939 r = -.68

Neonatal mortality and standard of living:
1871-1890 r = -.81
1907-1939 r = -.74

First-order correlation coefficients (partialling for trends) between:
Perinatal mortality and standard of living:
    1872-1890 r = +.21
    1908-1939 r = -.47

Neonatal mortality and standard of living:
    1872-1890 r = +.20
    1908-1939r = -.46

Notes to table 2.:

Standard of living data for Italy taken from Vannutelli Cesare, "Occupazione et Salari dal 1861 al 1961," in *L'Economia italiana dal 1861 al 1961* (Milan: Giuffrè, 1961), pp. 568-571. Data from 1871 to 1903 represent the "ore di lavoro necessarie per comperare un q. le di fremento." To make of these cost-of-living data a standard-of-living time series, I took the inverse of the index number given in the source. Data for 1901-1939 provide an index of "retribuzioni reali."

Data on infant deaths in the first month are from Stefano Somogyi, *La Mortalita nei primi cinque anni di età in Italia, 1863-1962* (Palermo: S. Consentino, 1967), p. 145 for 1863-93, p. 147 for 1926-62, p. 153 for 1890, 1907-1925. Note the gap in neonatal deaths from 1891 to 1906.

Data on total live and stillbirths are from *Annali di statistica,* ser. VIII, vol. 17 (1965), p. 688 ff.

Detrending done with the formula $[X_i - X_i - 1] = X_i^{dt}$

I am grateful to David Keane for having undertaken the computer work involved in these computations.

FOOTNOTES

1. What kind of book would Alexander Mitscherlich have written, for example, had he entitled it "Society Without the Mother"? Erikson himself, in organizing the chapter subheadings of his Gandhi book, appears to give mother and father equal billing, but the evidence in the mother section is skimpy and rushed, in the father section lovingly delected, which section is concluded by Erikson agreeing with Gandhi's observation that, "in order to make sexuality amenable to mastery . . . a man must . . . above all give an account of his conflicts with his father." *Gandhi's Truth: On the Origins of Militant Nonviolence* (New York, 1969), 123.

2. The mother disappears from John Demos's informative chapter on "Infancy and Childhood" among the Puritans after the second paragraph. *A Little Commonwealth: Family Life in Plymouth Colony* (New York, 1970), 131-132.

3. One noted anthropologist, Professor Beatrice Whiting, has suggested to me that a minimum level of maternal nurture is to be found in all societies, else the species would not perpetuate itself. Professor Whiting argued that high infant mortality rates, which do ultimately threaten the continuation of the species, are the result of external conditions over which the mother has no control rather than owing to deficient "mothering" as such. Recent cross-cultural studies have, however, observed significant variation in the quality of maternal care, maternal warmth and such. Ronald P. Rohner, for example, writes that "the more children are wanted before they are born, the more they are loved after parturition." *They Love Me, They Love Me Not: A Worldwide Study of the Effects of Parental Acceptance and Rejections* (N.p.: HRAF Press, 1975), 170. Leigh Minturn and William W. Lambert speculate that "the degree of warmth expressed by mothers is related to the privacy of living arrangements," and to "the presence of other people in the household." *Mothers of Six Cultures: Antecedents of Child Rearing* (New York, 1964), 282, 289. The maternal remoteness which both Rohner and Minturn-Lambert observe, however, could be ascribable to the poverty in which their subjects live.

4. "What the Doctor Ordered," *New York Review of Books,* 11 December 1975, 50. Lasch asks rhetorically, "Did 'premodern' parents abandon children because they were indifferent to their welfare or because they could not bear to see them starve?"

5. Several feminist scholars who have traced the origins of the 19th-century "cult of motherhood" fit into this camp, as for example Linda Gordon, *Woman's Body, Woman's Right: A Social History of Birth Control in America* (New York, 1976). See also Shorter, *Making of the Modern Family* (New York, 1975), ch. 5.

6. In one Swiss village, for example, one half of the infant mortality in 1790-1799 occurred within the first month, and of that over one half within the first *day*. Silvio Bucher, *Bevölkerung und Wirtschaft des Amtes Entlebuch im 18. Jahrhundert* (Lucerne, 1974), 80. The concentration of infant deaths in the first few days of life was even more overwhelming around the same time in the French town of Meulan, Marcel Lachiver, *La Population de Meulan du XVIIe au XIXe siècle* (Paris, 1969), 196-197. These statistics are merely meant, however, to establish the importance of neonatal mortality in the general pattern of death. Over the last hundred years neonatal deaths have occupied an ever *greater* share of total infant deaths because post-neonatal mortality, heavily influenced by infection, recedes much more quickly than does the mortality of the first week.

7. In the United States in 1959-61, for example, the death rate for diseases of the respiratory system – most of which like bronchitis and influenza are infective – was 28/10,000 live births for infants aged 1-11 months. For infants less than 1 month the rate was 0.8/10,000. For infants older than 1 month the death rate from gastritis, duodenitis, enteritis and colitis was 5.8; for infants less than 1 month the death rate from those diseases was zero, and the death rate from "diarrhea of newborn" was only 1.0. See Sam Shapiro, *et al., Infant, Perinatal, Maternal and Childhood Mortality in the United States* (Cambridge, Mass., 1968), 284.

8. Mack Walker illuminated this "middle-class" nature of smalltown life in, *German Home Towns: Community, State, and General Estate, 1648-1871* (Ithaca, 1971), esp. chs. 3 and 4.

9. These examples are documented in Shorter, *Making of Modern Family,* ch. 5.

10. For a succinct statement of deMause's theories see his article "The Evolution of Childhood" in deMause, ed., *The History of Childhood* (New York, 1974), 1-74.

11. *Ibid.,* 3.

12. *Ibid.* 8.

13. *Ibid.,* 51-52.

14. Three disparate works in this school are Eugen Weber, *Peasants into Frenchmen: The Modernization of Rural France, 1870-1914* (Stanford, 1976), ch. 11, which seems to put the grand divide around 1900 – a little late from my viewpoint; Fred Weinstein and Gerald M. Platt, *The Wish to be Free* (Berkeley, 1969), 14-15 and *passim,* and Shorter, *The Making of the Modern Family,* esp. ch. 7.

Philippe Ariès, the great pioneer of the history of childhood, argued of course that the change begins first around the time of the Reformation among the aristocracy and *haute bourgeoisie.* See the Eng. trans. of his book, *Centuries of Childhood: A Social History of Family Life* (New York, 1965). Among the "popular classes" who interest us here however – the butcher, baker and candlestickmakers who lived in towns like Memmingen and Agen – the change commences only during the eighteenth century.

15. "Evolution of Childhood," 3.

16. *Wish to be Free, passim.*

17. I have found several of the recent articles by Philippe Aries most instructive in this regard. "L'Amour dans le mariage et en dehors," in *La Maison-Dieu,* 127 (1976), 139-145, "Les Rituels de mariage," *Ibid.,* 121 (1975), 143-150, and "La Famille hier et aujourd'hui," *Contre-Point, 1974, 89-98.*

18. These are, at least, some of the differentials I observed in *Making of the Modern Family,* ch. 5.

19. *Honnetete et relations sociales en Languedoc, 1715-1780* (Paris, 1974), 212. .

20. Castan, "Pères et fils en Languedoc à l'époque classique," *XVIIe siecle,* nos. 102-103 (1974), 39.

21. J.H. Plumb, "The New World of Children in Eighteenth-Century England," *Past and Present, no. 67 (May, 1975), 90-91* and *passim.*

22. Trumbach's study "The Rise of the Egalitarian Family: Kinship, Childhood and Aristocracy in Enlightenment England" will be forthcoming from Academic Press in 1977.

23. *Silent Sisterhood: Middle Class Women in the Victorian Home* (Pittsburgh, 1975), quotes from 102, 108-109.

24. A. Vitrey, *Contribution a l'étude de la mortalité infantile* (Paris, 1907), 14.

25. "Solving the Problem of Obstetrics," *American Journal of Obstetrics*, 58 (1908), 736.

26. Early nineteenth-century maternal mortality in forceps operations for England, France and Germany was about 7%, fetal mortality around 20 percent. Fleetwood Churchill, *On the Theory and Practice of Midwifery*, 3rd American edition (Philadelphia, 1848), 327.

27. In Kurhessen during 1836-38, for instance, around 10 percent of all podalic versions ended fatally for the mother, 40 percent for the fetus. K. Schreiber, "Ein Beitrag zur Statistik der Gebrutshülfe mit besonderer Beziehung auf Kurhessen," *Neue Zeitschrift für Geburtskunde*, 11 (1842), 195, 200.

28. According to the statistics which John S. Parry reviewed, over a third of all mothers with contracted pelves who underwent craniotomies died. "The Comparative Merits of Craniotomy and the Caesarean Section in Pelves with a Conjugate Diameter of Two and Half Inches or Less," *American Journal of Obstetrics*, 5 (1872-73), 672, Churchill put craniotomy mortality at about 20%, *Theory of Midwifery*, p. 354.

29. *Dødeligheten og dens arsaker i Norge, 1856-1955* (Oslo, 1961), p. 188. See also G. Arbellot, *Cinq paroisses du Vallage (XVIIe-XVIIIe)* (Paris: Microeditions Hachette, 1973), p. 68, who speculates that childbed mortality is the cause of a huge tear in the age pyramid for women 30-34. Gilbert Garrier shows how many marriages among vinters were ended by maternal deaths during the first or second pregnancies during the 19th century. *Paysans du Beaujolais et du Lyonnais, 1800-1970* (Grenoble, 1973), I, 73.

30. Of 47,700 cases in the U.S. Obstetrical Statistical Cooperative, only 5 percent of the deliveries were complicated by a contracted pelvis. Louis M. Hellman, *et. al., Williams Obstetrics*, 14th ed. (New York, 1971), 897.

31. Exactly how many women had contracted pelves in past times is an important question for research. Although Jean-Louis Baudelocque invented the pelvimeter in 1789, only in 1861 was the first classification of pelves by both form and size published. In 1897 George Dobbin found 11% of his Baltimore patients to have contracted pelves, a figure which was probably higher than the U.S. average because of Baltimore's large black population. Reported contractions in Europe around that time ranged from 5 to 24 percent. "The Frequency of Contracted Pelves," *American Journal of Obstetrics*, 36 (1897), 147, 150.
   The literature on the prevalence of rickets is mentioned in Max Hirsch, *Fruchtabtreibung und Praventivverkehr im Zusammenhang mit dem Geburtenruckgang* (Würzburg, 1914), 228. Hirsch believes rickets increased in Germany during the 19th century. See also August Hirsch, *Handbuch der historisch-geographischen Pathologie*, vol. II: *Die Organkrankheiten*, 2nd ed. (Stuttgart, 1886), 514-521. By way of example, among those working on the social sources of perinatality, G.F.D. Smith discovered that malnutrition among working-class women in London and Dublin resulted in frequent prematurity and a high incidence of perinatal mortality in general. "An Investigation into Some of the Effects of the State of Nutrition of the Mother During Pregnancy and Labour on the Condition of the Child at Birth and for the First Few Days of Life," *The Lancet*, 191 (1916), 54-56.

32. Several researchers interrogated the doctors who signed the death certificates to determine how often cases of peurperal mortality lay behind such diagnoses as "pneumonia." In 1896, for example, the number of peurperal deaths (minus abortion deaths) discovered by checking back to doctors through the death certificates was 47% higher than the number which the city's statistical office officially published. Over three times as many abortion deaths took place as officially reported. Philipp Ehlers, *Die Sterblichkeit "Im Kindbett" in Berlin und Preussen, 1877-1896* (Stuttgart, 1900), 30.

33. On the masking of full-term obstetric deaths by induced-abortion deaths, see Walter Sigwart, "Die Pathologie des Wochenbetts," in Josef Halban and Ludwig Seitz, *Biologie und Pathologie des Weibes: Ein Handbuch der Frauenheilkunde und Geburtshilfe*, vol. 8, pt. 1 (Berlin, 1927), p. 465, which shows that in Switzerland from 1901 to 1914, full-term pregnancy mortality was cut by 40 percent, whereas – because of a trippling in the number of deaths from "Fehlgeburt" – the overall maternal mortality rate dropped by only 16%. In the second edition of that work, edited by Seitz and Alfred Amreich, Sigwart's article on "Das Wochenbettfieber" demonstrated that the almost three-fold increase in general maternal mortality which occurred in Berlin from 1910 to 1922 was exclusively a result of a rise in abortion mortality: the death rate for full-term births occupied almost the same level at the end of the period as at the beginning, 10.

34. Sigismund Peller supplied some important data on Viennese women who had rested up in Lying-In Hospital before their delivery vs. those who had not, to give one example of a flood of clinical pre-World War II data on this matter. *Der Geburstod (Mutter und Kind)* (Leipzig, 1936), 49 ff.

35. Reports abound of the horrors wrought by untrained obstetric helpers, all of whom were by no means female. One mother perished of gangrene at the hands of an incompetent male accoucheur after he, together with the woman's husband, had both tugged mightily with a pair of forceps upon a fetal head, causing a huge perineal tear and killing the infant as its brow emerged "with a loud pop." F. Haugk, "Gutachten . . . uber den fraglichen Kunstfehler einer Medicinal-person," *Zeitschrift für Staatsarzneikunde*, 34 Ergänzungsheft (1845), 82-113. The mother had suffered from rickets as an infant. We observe village incompetents violating the rules of sensible obstetric practice – even in the terms of the medicine of the time – in literally hundreds of such accounts. That this malfeasance could have not influenced overall maternal mortality is unlikely. *Trained* midwives, however, do not seem to have had a significantly higher mortality than physicians in home deliveries, if we may go by the few systematic comparisons, such as the New York Academy of Medicine's Committee on Public Health Relations' survey, *Maternal Mortality in New York City: A Study of all Puerperal Deaths, 1930-1932* (New York, 1933), which found 2.9 deaths per 1000 live births in all those cases where a midwife had made some contact with the mother (however brief); the physicians' death rate in home delivery was only 1.8/1000 (196, table 83). If those cases whom physicians saw first at home and then were taken to hospital are added in, the physicians' death rate rises to 2.2, leading the Academy of Medicine to conclude that "no great disparity" existed between the work of the two groups (198).

A 1904 survey of birth lists in Mecklenburg found that, for breech presentations, doctors had a fetal mortality of 21%, midwives of only 14%. The author speculated that this difference was due to the doctors' greater tendency to intervene in the labor of *multiparas* (rather than of primiparas, as is commonly assumed), killing the fetus through their efforts. Otto Büttner, "Mecklenburg-Schwerins Gueburtshilfe im Jahre 1904," *Zeitschrift für Guburtshilfe und Gynäkologie*, 61 (1908), 188-189.

36. Shapiro, *Maternal, Perinatal . . . Mortality*, ch. 1.

37. Dr. Kessler's and A. Laube's study of the decline in infant mortality shows the declining share of factors amenable to maternal volition, such as digestive diseases and rickets (which would depend also upon how well the mother herself has been treated as an

infant). The small *rise* in neonatal deaths in Germany after the First World War appears due to the greater percentage of first births among births in general, and to a rise in the number of elderly primiparas, rather than to a decline in the quality of care. "Totgeburten und Sauglingsfruhsterblichkeit, ihre Ursachen und Bekampfung ... 1923-1928," *Zeitschrift für Geburtshülfe,* 98 (1930), 426-444, esp. 429-430.

38. Numerous accounts show that men would routinely get the largest share of food at the table, and that pregnant women received nothing extra to eat. For Norway, as an example, see Lily Weiser-Aall, "Die Speise des Neugeborenen," in Edith Ennen and Günter Wiegelmann, eds., *Festschrift Matthias Zender* (Bonn: Röhrscheid, 1972), I, 542-544. In at least one German village around 1900 mothers received nothing special to eat during the peurperium. Gertrud Herrig, *Ländliche Nahrung im Strukturwandel des 20. Jahrhunderts: Untersuchungen im Westeifeler Relikgebiet am Beispiel der Gemeinde Wolsfeld* (Meisenheim am Glan, 1974), 97.

39. Hard labor until the very end of term seems to have been typical of peasants. See for example Weiser-Aall, "Speise des Neugeborenen," p. 544. Robert Debré, *et al., La Mortalite infantile et la mortinatalité: Résultats de l'enquete poursuivie en France et dans cinq pays d'Europe sous les auspices du comité d'hygiene de la Société des Nations* (Paris, 1933), reports of "surmenage des femmes enceintes" in various rural districts, pp. 264 ff.

40. "Speise des Neugeborenen," 539.

41. For recent illustrations of these assertions, see Alain Lottin, *La Desunion du couple sous l'ancien régime: L'Example du Nord* (Paris:, 1975), 158-159; Lloyd deMause, "On the Demography of Filicide," *History of Childhood Quarterly,* 4 (1976), 16-30.

42. "Development Perspectives on the History of Childhood," *Journal of Interdisciplinary History,* 11 (1971), 315-328.

Patricia Branca

TOWARDS A SOCIAL HISTORY OF MEDICINE

Medicine is a social activity embracing increasing interest and time on the part of more and more people. The importance of medical developments as they slowly emerged in the late 18th century and burgeoned in the 20th century is undeniable. The aura of medicine extends further and further into our daily existence affecting, not only, our physical state, but, our psychic condition, as well. While the impact of medicine is undisputable, the progress by which this phenomenon which must been seen as a health revolution in that it changed people's lives, the way they think, eat, sleep, work, play, procreate, even die, is not at all clear. How the physician became omnipresent partaking of joyous events such as the birth of a child to those emotional pressure points when sickness and death draw the doctor and patient closer together is a topic open for discussion. Obviously, this close relationship has not always existed. Did the doctor force himself on the individual, the family, the community, making all its members — particularly the presumed weakest women and children — totally dependent upon him as he monopolized all aspects of health care by regulating the sale of drugs, by banning charlatans through legislation requiring medical certification for all those purporting to deal with the sick? Did the monopolization come about by doctors keeping their art, like their hand-writing, unintelligible to the lay person — their white coats symbolizing their sacrosanct mystic — if their technical jargon and control over health facilities, such as hospitals did not do the trick?

The health revolution is as worthy of socio-historical inquiry as are the political and economic revolutions which marked and shaped modern Europe and America from the late 18th century into the present. The health revolution was most pervasive — it has touched us all directly. There has been little in the way of outright protest against the workings of the health revolution. Few voices are heard longing for the "good old days" when medicine was restricted to the realm of black or white magic. On the contrary the vanguard of the health revolution is still marching strongly.

Research into the relationships that define the dynamics of the health revolution; for example, the development of health care institutions from dens of poverty and deprivation to highly specialized institutions with budgets and staff to rival the major economic potentates in both private enterprise and government; the rise of the physician from stumbling country bumpkin, a jack of all trades to super specialist; the advances in the field of medical tech-nology from leeches to pacemakers; and, the establishment of the modern drug industry from home grown herb gardens to pill factories — serves several functions. Primarily from a scholarly standpoint it explains a keynote to the development of modern society useful to both the professional social scientist and the student. Little effort has been made to educate the non-specialist student in the field of medicine. Criticism has been made of the short comings of the history of medicine that is presented even to medical students. Medicine alone among the major professions has guarded its secrets from undergraduate instruction. Preachers pine for undergraduate attention; engineers and scientists take training at this level as a matter of course; lawyers have condenscended even to offering, at least, a course in first principles. One is not proposing to desanctify formal medicine by teaching it in an undergraduate classroom. Yet, there are many topics to be pursued in understanding the development of the health revolution as it has interacted with actual people. History as a social science is an appropriate vehicle for this kind of introduction if it is informed by proper medical and related scientific knowledge.

At the practical level research into the working of the health revolution as it developed in the 19th and 20th centuries provides essential data for policy makers concerned with the welfare of society be it at the micro level, the family, or the macro level, the state.

Medical histories are not new of course. But one need only look at the typical table of contents to see that they have been written largely from an antiquarian vantagepoint often by retired physicians; as such they are either unintelligible to laymen or so confident that a list of medical discoveries and great men in medicine is *ipso facto* illuminating. A narrative description of the great pioneers in medicine and their discoveries is not sufficient. The underlying implication in the traditional medical history approach is that since the discoveries were designed for society they automatically had positive social effects. How many of the actual medical breakthroughs were designed to improve health be it physical or mental? The story of Alexander Graham Bell's attempt to devise a hearing aid and instead inventing a telephone which the deaf cannot use at all is one example, here in the reverse, of the problem of assuming automatic cause and effect. Obviously we need to know the discoveries but this is the merest beginning; the larger task is to find out what happened next.

One of the more promising attempts to go beyond conventional medical history is the historical suvey of public health. This was the first approach to show the broad scope and implications of health care through detailed discussions of the history of sanitary commissions and their reports; laws regulating health facilities and safety standards for factories and housing, sewage, and other urban developments antedating a clear germ theory; and, public innoculation against various epidemic diseases. The new work in the field of public health demonstrated, also, the close relationship between government bureaucracy and public health care.

The history of public health was a step in the right direction to opening new vistas. It is of vital concern for the scholar of the health revolution but it shares a certain weakness with the conventional medical history narrative. It tends to leave people out – the people who actually get sick and therefore are patients or potential patients. It is necessary to describe the many laws and commissions created to deal with the conditions of public health, but we need to know, also, how these reacted on people — how they actually improved health and changed expectations about the treatment of disease. The social history of medicine must embrace the common everyday practices of health care which include the interaction between doctor and patient and, relatedly, the development of supportive institutions along with a study of the healthy population. The last subject is most important for the history of *modern* medicine. There seems to be among those who write medical history a penchant for the macabre. Blood, pus and pain, however, are not the whole of medical history. For preventive medicine is as important to the health revolution as is therapeutic medicine.

More recently, efforts have been made to explore the interrelationship between doctor and patient. The major focus at this time has been on the general state of women's health in the 19th century particularly in England and America. The new work has opened up exciting vistas and much controversy. Leaving aside the political interpretations of a number of the newer studies, one cannot fail to recognize that for the first time important questions are being posed. How were women treated as patients from the 19th century into the present? How did they respond? What laid behind the soaring interest in women's health in the 19th century? These are critical issues for the social historian which will be addressed directly in this paper. The difficulties involved in finding answers to these questions are enormous as will become apparent as we proceed further. One of the more pressing problems is trying to determine what was in fact "common" practice. Too much attention has been given to the atypical, the medical craze. The work on women's health in the 19th century illustrates the potential pitfalls in this type of concentration. References are made often to the "neurasthenic" women as being the typical female health problem of the 19th century. The patient diagnosed as suffering from "neurasthenia" (which covered a wide variety of symptoms from being over active to listlessness) was subjected to an assortment of cures: water cures; electric shock treatment; rest cures with special diets and exercise programs. Equally important and certainly more dramatic was the so-called "uterine" craze, wherein all female disorders were believed to be a result of a malfunction of the uterus. Treatment here was more severe starting with cauterization to clitoraldectomies and ovariotomies. While it is true that all of the above treatments were practiced it is not clear how widespread they were. It is very difficult to generalize about the social history of women's health through a study of a few individual doctors. Ovariotomies, for example, often cited because doctors specializing in gynecology discussed the importance of the surgical procedures, were rarely performed in the 19th century. A study of 117 hospitals in England in 1867 showed that a total of 22 were performed. It was not until anesthesia, plus the application of the germ theory, along with an understanding of blood transfusions, were known that the operation was conducted with a feeling of safety. In the few cases where ovaraiotomies were necessary they were performed generally as the last possible measure for the suffering woman. There was certainly by no means a crusade to sterilize women as has been implied in recent studies on women's health in the 19th century.

How does one make medical history not only intelligible to the lay reader but also relevant? The purpose of this paper is to present a research agenda that would expand the parameters of the paradigm which for too long has governed the research and interpretation of the working of medicine in modern society. The proposed research design is by no means complete and thus subject to further modification, even total revision, if future work proves this necessary. The research model is set up to deemphasize the macabre and help ameliorate some of the grosser problems of the history of public health, as well as the history of the medical craze by focusing on the patient.

A few preliminaries by way of setting the background for the research design. The model is based on research in the history of family medicine, i.e. obstetrics and pediatrics. Principle examples for this paper will be drawn from the field of obstetrics in England and France. The comparative framework proved most valuable in the formulation of the model. With this in mind let me sketch the construct in very simple terms with complexities to be added in large dosages. The social history of medicine involves three layers: great men and women at the top (the Pasteurs, the Marie Curies); patients or prospective patients at the bottom (you and me); and the ordinary practitioner or intermediate specialist in the middle. Developments at the top follow their own rhythm, related to general developments in science and institutional support though not untouched by the other layers. A social history of the top spectrum, perfectly feasible, would be largely in terms of the sociology of knowledge and a history of the relationship between grantsmanship and scientific development.

As implied earlier, the crux of the social history of medicine, taking the top layer as backdrop, lies with the relationship between the two lower layers and their role in the development and application of medicine. With the development of the modern industrial network, the bottom layer became increasingly important as modern men and women strove for control over their personal well being. This growing interest played a prominent role in determining what the middle level − the ordinary practitioner − did. This trinitarian approach would not please doctors probably, though they do note increasingly the demands patients place upon them. The model so ordered implicitly suggests that given God the Father and God the Son their due, the social history of medicine must pay particular attention to the Holy Ghost, a particularly apt if haunting image for the medical profession. It is necessary to look to the hopes and expectations of the patient, and to what doctors had to do to attract patients in order to grasp the development of actual medical practice, with the top level researcher a necessary precondition for but not always an active cause of change.

With the construct neatly ordered the complexities need to be added. First the model suggests obvious division, or gaps. In medicine, as is true for most scientific and technological developments, there is a time lag between actual breakthrough by those at the top and its application at the bottom. The time lag is not surprising, it needs mention primarily because most formal medical histories ignore it in the blithe assumption that discovery equals practice equals massive improvements in human health. But the classic problem of dissemination of new knowledge is particularly important in the history of modern medicine because most gaps involved human suffering, indeed human lives, when time was lost between discovery and practice. Also, the very fact of discovery, plus more general attitudes associated with modern life styles, conditioned key groups of patients to expect improvements which their doctors would not provide.

The implications for the gap go further. Let us assume a breakthrough at the top to be dealt with particularly by the social historian of science. The assumption behind many of our present social policies based on the paradigm of traditional medical history insists that the process of dissemination is automatic. Pour money into the top layer and its magic fruits will fall, perhaps through some blend of Newton and Johnny Appleseed, to the doctor who will in turn transmit them to the patient. The patient is seen, of course, as passive, open to anything poured into his or her mouth or any other portion of one's anatomy; hence the word *patient*. Without meaning to play upon the implication of the last medical recourse, if one looks at medical developments from the bottom up, from the vantagepoint of social history, that is from the viewpoint of patients or potential patients, the process is far from automatic and relies in great part on the pressures applied by the patient. Practicing doctors, the middle layer, may have had a less autonomous role than has been traditionally assumed. In other words, the construct suggest that what the patient deems his or her particular needs and concerns will play a major role in determining whether a new technique or wonder drug will be successfully implemented and what the timing of this implementation will be. If the patient is not ready for change, the change will not occur or it will have to be enforced by legislative action, ranging from educational programs to innoculation requirements. The legislative avenue historically has provoked not only hostility and resentment but evasion. However, if the patient is primed for change, he or she will jump at innovation, sometimes even initiating it (in so far as this is within range) forcing the intermediary level — the ordinary doctor — to innovate against his will.

By placing the patient in a prominent position in the history of medical developments in modern society we hit upon inevitiably the most complex ingredient to the model and a necessary digression. Who are the patients? The definition of a patient depends upon society's definition of sickness. A very telling point in the history of medicine which is worthy of investigation is the ever expanding definition of sickness in modern society. Despite the fact that medical advances have played an important role in combating sickness, we find that sickness, the trauma of sickness concerns us all. Perhaps within the historical framework the concern today is not comparable to the fears of the patient in premodern society. Presumably one major difference was that sickness and death were more closely related, indeed corollaries in premodern society: One got sick, one died. At the same time, the expectations of the premodern patient were rather limited compared to the modern patient. It is crucial in pursuing the social history of medicine to understand that sickness is not an absolute: it is relative to the individual. Sickness is very much a function of society's expectations.

An integral aspect of modern living is that it has challenged successfully the traditional corollary that sickness is the first throe of death. In order to do this it was necessary to grapple with the concept that death was beyond the province of human control. By the 19th century, in Western Europe and America, the acceptance of death as inevitable for key sectors of society was denied, starting with the crusade against the futility of infant and maternal mortality. By the 20th century, the age at which one could expect to die was progressively delayed. We are at the point today wherein the very concept that death should be allowed to pursue its own course is definitely anathema to modern living. The spectrum that death colors has been significantly curtailed.

At the same time, the whole concept of what constitutes sickness has been steadily redefined. As death was found to be unacceptable in modern society, so too was sickness. The social history of medicine starting in the 19th century but especially in the 20th century is more and more the history of people's refusal to endure sickness. It could be said that the modern man and woman are by definition healthy. In very simple terms the progression can be seen from the individual's standpoint as: I do not want to die; I do not want to be sick; I do not want to endure physical discomfort; I do not want to endure mental stress. Achieving these goals was heavily dependent obviously upon innovations from the top level of the model — the researcher/scientist — in addition to the adaptation of the middle level — the doctor. The point to be argued here is that the patient's expectations played as central a role in determining the course of medical history. The patient as an intermediary, at times even a catalyst to medical advances, has not been fully credited and needs to be investigated.

In pursuing the social history of medicine from this vantagepoint the nature of the patient population under study is significantly different from the more conventional studies of medicine. The focus here is not so much on the sickly, the hospital patient, the victims of epidemics or diseases in general, but those who wished not to get sick. The modern doctor/patient relationship has expanded considerably. In traditional society the doctor saw *only* the sick, of this sector only those who were upon the door of death. Starting in the 19th century not only did more sick people seek the services of the medical profession but also, and more importantly, more healthy people used, directly and indirectly the resources of the medical community; doctors, nurses, clinics and hospitals.

The expectations of patients are heavily dependent on social position — class. To the present, the patient-as-innovator, the healthy patient who wishes to maintain good health, has derived primarily from the middle class. The rise in health consciousness began first among the middle class. The new middle class outlook toward life as it has developed from the late 18th century into the present pivots around the desire for personal control, comfort and predictability. It saw no reason to maintain traditional passivity toward pain or needless deaths. Investigations into the study of changes over time in the threshold of pain are being conducted now. It would appear that the middle class' threshold to pain decreased faster than the working class'. If this is the case (admittedly only impressionistic evidence is available at this point) one would need to know why this developed.

The middle-class patient has been largely ignored by most medical studies. Public health studies, particularly of the 19th century, are essentially descriptions of state actions to improve the health condition of the working class (while noting middle-class initiative as a means of self-protection). One is often left with the impression that the class had no health problems at all or at least none serious enough to investigate; if mentioned at all they were the ultra-clean and physically fit who at best wish to spread their ways to the less fortunate. The fact of the matter is that they were subject to serious health problems which prompted them to develop a new outlook on the whole issue of sickness and death. We know that the middle class was open particularly to the idea of scientific innovation: Thus more receptive to new procedures, in some instances even before the middle layer — the general practitioner — was comfortable in applying them. Obviously differences in economic resources played a vital role in the development of different attitudes, as in actual health conditions. Economic determinism must be given its due. The middle class had the economic surplus to indulge in speculation for improved health. Yet cast of mind, expectations, have a way of hanging on well beyond the dictates of economic necessities.

Also to be considered is the fact the most doctors in the 19th and 20th centuries came from the middle class. Therefore, there was no direct cultural conflict in the middle-class doctor/patient relationship. It is possible that the slower acceptance of doctors by the working class went beyond economics and attitudes toward sickness and death and was related to a communication gap between the doctor and patient. The middle-class doctor dressed differently and talked differently. Eventually he would live and see his patients only in his terrain.

Beyond class, sex marked a distinction, in the definition of patient-as-innovator. Within the middle class women were quicker than men to attune themselves to medical science and insist on change. Desire for better physical health was fundamental to women's advancement in modern society. Women's charge for the care of children prompted also a more intense interest in medicine. Women's use of doctors and hospitals demonstrably increased at a faster rate than men's. The course of the health revolution in modern society involves relationships between multi-dimension levels.

Now to illustrate the model. Obstetrical and gynecological developments are a vital part of the social history of medicine because they formed one of the earliest medical specializations, obviously based on the problems of a major, identifiable segment of the population, women. It should be understood that both specialties developed before there was a great deal of new knowledge to purvey, which suggests three related points: first, doctors sought extra income or, in France, even bare subsistence by trying to define themselves in special ways — on a more modest basis psychiatric practice developed similarly during the same period in the United States: second, this premature specialization might serve as the basis for creation of new knowledge — level two affecting level one; and third, in this specific instance, women may have demonstrated the kind of new concern with health that made this specialization particularly logical. Toward this last point the rising tide of indignation of maternal mortality and other women's ailments in women's magazines, particularly in Britain, by mid-century, long before massive medical advance, suggests that this is a plausible instance of potential patients influencing the course of medical practice.

French and English obstetrics originated essentially in the late 18th century — we'll start with a dose of conventional medical history, to be sure we get some names in. The French claim Dr. J.L. Baudeloque as the founder of modern obstetrics. England can offer Dr. Charles Gordon for the title. But, as most medical histories note, it was in the 19th century that the most important milestones in midwifery were launched. The list of innovations is indeed impressive: the development of sophisticated forceps; the vaginal speculum (over 400 different designs were introduced); the dilator; the uterine sound, and anethesia. One of the most important 19th century obstetrical improvements involved the discovery of the spread of "puerperal fever," a septic poisoning, which killed thousands of parturient women yearly. The new medical procedure developed to prevent the spread of the infection was simple — requiring the sterilization of all instruments that came into contact with the patient and the careful cleansing of all persons who touched the parturient patient.

Equally dramatic was the transition of power held for centuries by the female midwife to the male physician. This transition, or usurpation of power, was more complete in England than in France. Explaining the process whereby the advances in medical obstetrics were implemented beyond the laboratory and became common practices exposes the intricacies of pursuing the social history of medicine.

Our focus here is on the nature and relationship of levels two and three- the doctor/patient relationship for at level one — the level of scientific knowledge in the field of obstetrics in England and France was progressing at the same rate. And impact of the new advances of obstetrics was slow as reflected in the continuing high rates of maternal mortality which plagued 19th century England and France: maternal mortality hovered about the 4-5% mark per total births from 1800 into the 1920's. How many of these lives would have been spared if proper examination of the uterus was made early in the pregnancy thereby alerting the doctor of possible pelvic disorders complicating the delivery? How many women's strength was so weakened because they had to endure a long delivery without the relief offered from anesthetics? And how many as a result were left an easy prey for infection? How many women suffered the pains and died from puerperal fever because few doctors, or for that matter midwives, believed in the need to cleanse themselves carefully before attending the woman in labor?

Fundamental changes had to occur at levels two and three before the scientific breakthroughs of level one became part of everyday practice. These changes had to be reciprocal, i.e. the recognition had to reflect mutual self-interest. This process moved more quickly in England than in France.

By mid-19th century England, middle-class women had set clear goals for themselves: to improve their own personal lot and that of their children. This new desire for control was articulated in the many articles in women's magazines of the day. In their efforts to improve upon the ills of nature women in England turned to science whose spokeman was the doctor. Numerous health care manuals and journals were produced instructing women in the details of managing pregnancy and child birth, topics that were not discussed openly before this time. Dr. Bull's *Hints to Mothers,* first published in 1833, ran through fifteen editions to 1877, illustrates the popularity of this new literature. A survey of the manuals and periodical literature gives one an indirect measure of the patient's concerns during this time. It would appear that women were most anxious to determine their pregnancy as soon as possible. Next they were anxious to know what care should be taken to insure a full term pregnancy and an easy delivery. This last concern was most important. Many expressed their fears of the pains of childbirth and thus were quick to sieze upon the news that anesthesia would help ameliorate the worst pains of delivery.

However, even for the English woman, there was a significant lag between rising expectations and rewards. On the whole doctors were slow, sometimes obstinately opposed to the new directions being taken in obstetrics, particularly in the case of application of anesthesia. The controversy that erupted over the use of ether and chloroform is interesting because it demonstrates that the process of medical developments is by no means automatic. In this particular instance the process of acceptance ran from researcher to patient who in turn put pressure on the general practitioner.

While stressing the lag it is important not to lose sight of the fact that English doctors were changing in the direction of their patients' needs. As noted above the numerous mass publications on women's concerns during pregnancy and child birth were penned by physicians and are examples of the growing reciprocal relationship. By mid-19th century, British doctors were required to have some training in midwifery before they could practice medicine. A part of this recognition of the growing importance of women's medical care was the founding of the British Obstetrical and Gynecological Society in the 1850's. Relatedly British doctors launched a savage attack against the traditional purveyor of child delivery, the midwife, coming close to eliminating her by the end of the century. Doctors sought government intervention in the form of legislation requiring the licensing of all who attended lying-in women. Their argument centered around their worries for the health of the woman and the new born. So while there were gaps — points of controversy between the doctor and the pregnant woman — they were both determined to alter the ways of childbirth for the good of the patient.

The situation in France was ironically different. At the top level the French could claim a slight edge over the English in such matters as pre-natal exam, for example. French obstetricians were urging early internal examination in order to determine probable date of conception in case induced birth was needed. Hence the word *toucher* to describe the tactile examination which was eventually adopted into English medical parlance. French researchers were more advanced in their efforts to determine the state of pregnancy. Early in the 19th century Dr. Frassines noted that the urine of a pregnant woman was discernibly different from that of a non-pregnant woman. In 1836 Dr. Jacquiemier noted that the interior of the vagina assumed a bluish discoloration in a pregnant woman. French researchers were coming to terms with means to determine as soon as possible the state of pregnancy. Yet none of the practices were used at the patient/doctor level. The expectations of French patients, plus the interest of the French general practitioners, made for a significantly different relationship between the two lower levels of the model.

In France there was no counterpart to the English "medical philosophes," the manual writers, the health column advisers who sought to explain in common language the mysteries of childbirth. French doctors wrote; they had every reason to seek this kind of income. But there was no comparable consumer market in 19th century France as there was in England. To be sure, more French manuals retained a religious influence, resisting the scientific clamor that adorned the new press in England. The manuals that were sophisticated in terms of medical knowledge simply did not find a wide readership.

A clearer indication that the doctor/patient relationship in childbirth was significantly lagging behind in France was the continual preference for midwives over doctors. Not only throughout the 19th century but into the mid-20th century, the majority of French women chose to deliver their babies at home with the assistance of only a midwife. Whereas in England, by the end of the 19th century the switch from midwives to doctors was almost complete, as was the move to the supportive medical facilities – maternity wards and hospitals.

General health statistics reflect the difference between the two countries. Female mortality, as well as infant mortality, was higher in France than in England. French female mortality rates ranged almost 13% higher than in England during the second half of the 19th century. As female health in England began a marked improvement during the early years of the 20th century the rate soared to 43%. The gap narrowed only after WWII, when among other things French women began to make the switch to doctors and hospitals.

Explanation here is complicated. France was of course a more rural country. Rural populations after 1850 tend to have higher mortality rates and are obviously more prone to stick to traditions such as the use of midwives. French doctors through the 19th century were content apparently to let midwives care for childbirth on conditions that they be trained under their supervision, examined, and certified. The contrast with England has already been suggested, for here doctors opposed midwives as lacking in training and knowledge and responsible through their carelessness for the high rate of infant mortality; and English midwives resisted training and licensing. Can this aspect be explained simply by a greater selfish professionalism on the part of the English doctor? French doctors were in such sorry straits that they surely would have seized upon this specialization were they able. Midwife opposition would have been strong, but the effort was not even made.

There were fewer births in France than in England, so the market was less obvious, particularly at those social levels that had the money to afford private medical treatment and were the first to limit family size. But this cannot take us too far since French and English birth rates per marriage were quite comparable – in fact England had a lower fecundity rate per marriage until the 1870s when a marked difference did appear, but this was well after English obstetrics was launched on its distinctive course – so that only by noting that the French marriage rate was considerable lower than the English (by about 21%) can this be considered as a causal factor.

The urbanization factor evoked above must also be handled with care. That England developed more advanced obstetrics earlier than France follows from earlier urbanization, and relatedly a larger, progressive middle class. Yet by 1920

France was an urban country, and still obstetrical practice remained very traditional. A persistent culture, developed in the 19th century remained long after any necessity, and defined patients' expectations.

The French midwife, thanks to some training and licensing, had a certain panache. She combined traditional care, women taking care of women, with perhaps sufficient marks of science to make her acceptable to a modernizing society. The French were, however, also open longer than the English to outright charlatanism, although here too claims to scientific reliability proved increasingly useful. This approach long seemed acceptable to expectant mothers (and to others in the population needing medical care). This can hardly exhaust the reasons for the greater traditionalism of the French with regard to medicine in general. It is clear, however, that a distinctive culture existed which discouraged the use of doctors. Undoubtedly this helped maintain doctors in their traditional ways, whatever the research advances in the great schools; and to this extent, having nothing new to offer, they in turn maintained their patients' desire to stick to relatively traditional methods now gaining a new scientific or pseudo-scientific gloss.

There is yet another reason for the persistent French pattern. French doctors were not as receptive to the changes occuring at the top level and the needs of the lower level. In general, the contact between doctor and patient was more remote in France. In the 1870's the English ratio was one doctor per 1500 patients while the French was one per 3300. To this one must add that French doctors were often unemployed – up to 25% sometimes – a problem unheard of in England. French women may have been exercising very good sense, not sheer traditionalism in staying away from them. As late as 1911-1924 French doctors were averaging 2 dead babies to 1 live in deliveries; the midwives scored .71 dead to 1 live. Of course doctors were called in mainly in the more complicated cases, which helps explain their bad track record. But explanations were not terribly useful to women who could logically associate the doctor with death and combine the track record with other common practices. Well into the later 19th century French doctors bled pregnant women for very minor ailments; it was widely believed, despite some challenges from researchers, that women should be bled automatically in their fourth month. But here again patients were not always patient. We have direct statements from doctors of the horror women expressed at the prospect of the application of leeches and the refusal, in many cases, to subject themselves to a doctor's care as a result. Leeches were fairly well gone from the French doctor's armamentarium by 1900, although pharmacists still sold them and individual French doctors remained capable of recommending almost anything. But a culture in this case on the part of the patient, had been established and would long persist. Doctors were simply not seen as specially scientific, innovative, or advantageous.

From the patient's standpoint which experience, the English or the French, was more beneficial? Higher mortality rates observed earlier (while admitting that a host of factors, from housing through medical care enter into these) would suggest a conclusion that the English relationship though marked by anxiety was in the long run more beneficial. In addition women in contact even with conservative doctors benefited by learning that a number of traditional beliefs related to childbirth were erroneous; for example, English doctors began to urge women after delivery to sit up and move about within 24 hours of delivery thereby stimulating circulation and combatting infection. In France, doctors continued to insist that the parturient woman remain in a dorsal position for two weeks. This stagnation was an ideal place for infection to take its ugly course.

More important still, precisely because of their inability to wipe out completely the horrors of maternal mortality English doctors from the mid-19th century onward actively advocated birth control, through the use primarily of new contraceptive devices. By the turn of the century a few French doctors realized the benefits to be derived from limiting the number of pregnancies a woman endured. But overall interaction was not there. Hence the high probability of a greater French reliance on abortion, as well as, outright abstinence, to accomplish goals that the English achieved largely by contraceptives. In England the alliance of women and doctors helped bring about a lead in the democratization of birth control information and eventual liberalization of abortion laws. In France – again as one among many factors, but a vital one – the absence of a strong doctor/patient is no doubt related to the slowness to modernize birth control and abortion legislation.

Another consequence of the development of the obstetrician doctor/patient relationship to benefit English women sooner than French, was that it accustomed women to the *modern* medical process in general. While fear of death and pain were strong motivators in the seeking of medical relief in the case of childbirth, the fact is that this was the first time that medical services were sought as a means of preventive medicine (an insurance for the continuation of good health) as opposed to the traditional doctor/patient relationship which was found only in the advanced stages of sickness. The impact of preventive medicine on the health revolution, particularly in the 20th century, has not been fully realized. In the new relationship, wherein the patient is healthy and desires to remain so, the chances that demands will be dictated to the doctor from the patient are significantly greater.

From this initial relationship others grew. Women as mothers and wives sought medical consultation for other health problems. The concern and pressure for improvements in children's health among middle-class women in England (more so than in France) was intense throughout the nineteenth century. As a result pediatric medicine, as a specialized field, developed quickly upon the heels of obstetrics, well before there were significant breakthroughs at the top levels.

With the three-tier model one sees that medical developments depended upon a variety of responses and inputs. Medical developments in obstetrics did not follow a one way street. The three-tier approach provides another dimension in that it pursues the interrelationships between the levels, the network of motion that ran both ways among all three sectors. How much influence each sector had in a particular area of reform would vary.

The implications of the three-tier construct (however much it must be modified for different kinds of medical problems and specialities) for medical policy today is considerable as noted from the start. Contemporary medical policy based on the medical funnel idea — pour money into research and it will run down into general practice and eventually change patients' attitudes is too simple and consequently misses many problem areas. The situation as seen from the application here is far more complex. One need only look to the controversy in America today over the drug laetrile as a cancer cure — to find that patients are indeed impatient and will apply heavy pressures. What patients want, what they will accept how they will relate to medical personnel all have as much to do with the development and advancement of medicine and the actual levels of health as formal medicine itself. Class, ethnic, sex and age factors need careful social-scientific as well as medical investigation. Where, as is very often the case, the culture of patients and or of doctors was formed in the past, this investigation must include a serious historical component. From the application of the model here, it can be seen that the middle class played an important role in fostering and maintaining new attitudes toward health care. Thus one tentative conclusion that can be drawn and tested for further reforms is that it is necessary or advantageous in terms of application to have middle-class support for a particular health reform. If the middle class does not identify with a particular cause this could result in a serious lag between the implementation of a breakthrough at the top and its acceptance into general practice. Thus policy makers would be wise to direct their efforts towards the middle class for economic support and moral consent, especially in areas which involve a cultural conflict.

At the same time, it is important to recognize that there are different cultures which need to be addressed in their own particular milieu. If a health reform effort is to be geared to the working class, specifically, it is important for the policy maker to understand the cultural bases of this sector if the reform is to be adopted. As suggested earlier it is possible that the working-class lag was a result in part of the inability of the class to identify with the reformers who represented themselves as better than thou- more educated- ultra clean etc. Efforts to recruit medical personnel from the working class should be more vigorously supported not only to democratize the system but also in order to meet the demands of the patient population.

For the historian the task of pursuing the social implication and application of medicine be it at the top theoretical level — the discovery of a new virus or drug or scientific procedure; or, at the intermediary level — the paramedics, the hospital staffs; or at the most complex level, the patients expectations, requires an interdisciplinary approach relying heavily upon social scientific methodology but also informed medical expertise. With this process the complexities of the health revolution as it developed over time, as it is pursued in the present, and its future course are better understood.

Carnegie-Mellon University   Patricia Branca

Regina Markell Morantz

MAKING WOMEN MODERN:
MIDDLE CLASS WOMEN AND HEALTH
REFORM IN 19TH CENTURY AMERICA

I

Social historians have yet to explore adequately either the connection between health reform and advances in 19th-century medicine or the role of women in the active promotion and adoption of rationalistic health practices. As life expectancy increased and infant mortality declined, sickness gradually ceased to be endemic. More important, fatalistic attitudes toward death and disease gave way to the conviction that good health was within the reach of each and every citizen. The nature and impact of these changes cannot be explained merely by recounting the heroic strides made by medical scientists during these years. While the work of Pasteur, Koch, and others was vitally important, advances in bacteriology and medical therapeutics do not tell the whole story. The 19th-century revolution in health was far more pervasive; its advocates were not only great men of science, but ordinary men and women who promulgated and implemented new attitudes toward public and personal cleanliness.

Beginning in the ante-bellum period, self-help in health matters, public hygiene, dietary reform, temperance, hydro-therapy and physiological instruction merged as ingredients in a coherent and articulate campaign to save the nation by combating the ill-health of its citizenry. Although such attention to personal health and hygiene was not wholly original, never before had the regard for good health given rise to such widespread public activity.[1]

In the modernizing world of the 19th century, health reformers played a critical role in transforming traditional attitudes toward sickness and death. They promoted the active assumption by men and women of the responsibility for their own health, the health of their families, and the health of society at large. Itinerant speakers lecturing to enthusiastic audiences and dedicated to furthering common knowledge of health and hygiene traversed the cities and towns of the North and West. Hundreds of heuristic tracts instructed eager readers in the "laws of life." A handful of journals kept men and women informed of new developments. The popular *Water Cure Journal,* for example, boasted 10,000 subscribers in 1849, the second year of its publication.[2]

Although the movement held attractions for both men and women, and, as we shall see, the contributions of male spokesmen were vital, middle-class women, by virtue of their new roles in an increasingly complex society, became the health reformers' primary constituency. Because the changing structure of the 19th-century family increasingly required women to school their children in "modern" values, they welcomed with relief the practical solutions to bewildering problems offered in health reform journals and tracts.

The concern with hygiene was an integral part of the ante-bellum reformist world view. Indeed, the health crusade converged with several better known radical concerns. Historians have been quick to point out this identity of ideas and personnel. No study of ante-bellum reform can ignore the fundamental role of hygienic and physiologic concepts. Abolitionist speakers, for example, lodged at health reform boarding houses, and a large number of women's rights advocates followed some form of Sylvester Graham's vegetarian diet. Oberlin College, familiar as a breeding ground for abolitionism and women's rights, adopted strict vegetarianism in its dining room in 1835. Asa Mahan, the college's president, put a "reformation in food, drink, and dress" high on the list of important causes.[3]

Moreover, a cursory glance at the men and women who actively promoted the health revolution suggests that, like other reformers, they came from the Northeastern, predominantly middle-class sectors of the American population. Sylvester Graham began his career in New Jersey as a Presbyterian minister and temperance lecturer. William A. Alcott, cousin of Bronson, was a thoughtful, Yale-trained physician. Joel Shew and Russell Trall graduated from regular medical schools in New York. James Caleb Jackson, a self-made man, was the son of a yeoman farmer in upstate New York. Mary Gove Nichols became a teacher in Maine. Rachel Brooks Gleason graduated from New York's Central Eclectic School of Medicine and ran a water cure establishment with her physician husband. Paulina Wright Davis and Elizabeth Oakes Smith both hailed from prominent New York landholding families. Harriot Hunt's father, a skilled navigator, invested his small capital in Boston's commerical shipping industry. Lydia Folger Fowler, wife of the phrenologist publisher Lorenzo, was the second woman to receive a medical degree in the United States. A descendant of the Puritan settlers of Nantucket Island and distant cousin of the astronomer Maria Mitchell, Lydia's father was a manufacturer, a shipowner, and a selectman of his native town. Recently, an intensive study of the rank and file of the Boston Ladies Physiological Society found that the large majority were predominantly the wives and mothers of Boston's middle class.[4]

Previous students of the health reform movement have offered us a number of useful insights. We know, for example, that health crusaders shared with other reformers of the period a fundamental Enlightenment rationalism. Implicit in their theory of sickness was a concept of self-help and a conviction that disease could be prevented by teaching people the "laws" of physiology and hygiene. Other scholars suggest that the rationalistic impulse in health reform rhetoric was overshadowed by heavy doses of Christian perfectionism. Preaching the interconnectedness of the moral and physical life, health reformers agreed that man could not achieve success in the one without total control over the other. Medical historians, in contrast, have emphasized a causal relationship between the rise of health reform and the decline of heroic medical therapeutics. Health crusaders stood united in their criticism of the bleeding, purging and dosing of the professional practice of the day. Finally, a few scholars attribute the rise of the movement to the pervasive anti-elitism characteristic of the ante-bellum period, an atmosphere which fueled the public animus against established medical practice.[5]

While earlier work has been informative, two crucial questions remain virtually unexplored in the historiographical literature. The first concerns the relationship of health reform to modernization; the second relates to the connection between women's interest in health reform and changes in their status.[6] Although this essay will make some brief and admittedly speculative observations concerning the first of these problems, its primary focus will be to suggest a tentative framework for explaining women's role in the health reform movement. It is hoped that such a framework will aid others in further explorations of the subject.

Former accounts have only briefly acknowledged and never analyzed women's participation. We know a great deal about Sylvester Graham, William A. Alcott, and James Harvey Kellogg, but our information about the many women who preached, implemented and occasionally elaborated on the ideas of these more prominent health reformers remains sketchy.[7] Yet a number of the most outspoken of the health crusaders were female, and women swelled the ranks of the new movement.

In 1837 the American Physiological Society was founded in Boston to foster health by teaching physiology. Almost a third of its members were women and at its second annual meeting the new organization acknowledged women's central role in promoting good health in the following resolution:

> *Resolved,* That woman in her character as wife and mother is only second to the Deity in the influence that she exerts on the physical, the intellectual, and the moral interests of the human race, and that her education should be adapted to qualify her in the highest degree to cherish those interests in the wisest and best manner. [8]

Women took to the field as lecturers. Ladies' Physiological Societies appeared throughout the Northeast. The names of Mary Gove Nichols, Harriot Hunt, and Lydia Folger Fowler are only the most familiar of the dozens of women who taught enthusiastic female audiences the "laws of life."

Profound changes in women's roles underlay their active interest in health reform. The social transformation touched off by industrialization and urbanization gradually forced them to redefine their responsibilities in an altered family setting. Since colonial times traditional verities had suggested that woman's place was in the home. But women had experienced family, home and work as an integrated, stable whole. The heavy burden of household production and the immediate concern with economic subsistence left them little time and less inclination to question their duties. Moreover, social roles for women in the 17th and 18th centuries in reality remained quite fluid and imperfectly defined. It was left to the 19th century to institutionalize the concept of "woman's sphere."

As productive labor shifted from the home to the factory, men, acting on premodern conceptions of men's and women's responsibilities, increasingly sought outside employment. Masculine and feminine spheres became more rigidly separated. This development quickly colored 19th-century cultural expectations.

Economic changes suddenly made it possible for the first time for large numbers of women to become primarily wives and mothers. No longer did playing a vital role in the family economy compete for their time and attentiom. The ideal of the modern family — small in size, emotionally intense, and woman supervised — made its appearance as a distinctive emblem of middle-class culture.

Contemporaries noted these changes with satisfaction. In a letter to the *Water Cure Journal* in 1854, the reformer Frances Dana Gage observed:

> Steam power suggested steam power, [sic] and one invention gave leisure for another; mind was released from physical labor, and gained time and leisure for higher and nobler development; woman was obliged to keep sight of the age. She was a help-meet, suggesting, striving, planning, and executing; thinking for the young, and leading them to the depots of usefulness.... Woman ... thirty years ago seldom went from the home, because she *could not be spared,* now that spinning-jennies and patent looms do the spinning and weaving, and sewing machines are doing the needle-work, steam-power does the knitting, and garments are made so cheap... it seems an idle waste of time to use 'Her needle'...[9]

Paralleling these economic developments was the desire to educate women to their duties as mothers which sparked the spread of female education in the first half of the 19th century. Enlightenment theorists had been the first to propose that, within the home, women should have primary responsibility for rearing the nation's young. Only an astute mother, they argued, could raise her sons to be proper citizens of the Republic. Health reformers merely eleaborated on this theme. "Now who," asked a typical contributor to the *Practical Educator and Journal of Health* in 1847, "is the best qualified to supervise a household? She who has been thoroughly trained... or she who knows practically nothing about it.... Let woman be intellectually educated as highly as possible."[10]

Educational opportunity brought middle-class women into contact with Enlightenment ideas about progress and individual freedom. Such concepts colored their adjustments to underlying social changes and helped produce a talented minority with rising status expectations who came to feel frustration, distate, anger, even desperation at the severe limitations imposed on them by the growing popularity of the "cult of the lady." Trained in a more ascetic Protestant tradition of usefulness, strength, duty, and good works, many middle-class women rejected the fashionable, indolent life of the leisured wife. Gradually two competing images of the ideal 19th-century woman emerged. On the one hand, woman was described as weak, sickly, dependent and ornamental. On the other she was exalted as highly spiritual and morally superior — confined to the home, yet invested with genuine power and responsibility within her sphere. Both health reformers and women's rights advocates would reject the first and seize on the second ideal — that of woman's moral power — using it effectively in this century to explore significant and divergent outlets for female energies. These women would practice domesticity, not as a cult, but as a science. Responding to changes in women's traditional role which left them devoid of adequate models and established forms of behavior, they sought to elevate and professionalize the domestic sphere as a means of seeking an effective and practical role for women in a new and unpredictable social setting.[11]

The middle-class woman's new domestic orientation required a single-minded concern with the problems of health and hygiene. Her own good health became a matter of conscious choice. She took an assiduous interest in questions concerning marriage, childbearing and childrearing, family health, sexuality and family limitation. Health reformers, both men and women, shared these interests and attempted to provide practical solutions to unsettling problems. Indeed, health reformers gave to the majority of their female constituents a justification for devoting their fulltime efforts to woman's traditional role of homemaking, recast, it is important to note, in a modern and scientific setting.

For the ordinary woman, the health revolution became a fundamental ingredient in women's modernization, allowing her to cope with the problems created by industrial and urban living and easing her transition into a more complex and modern world. Yet the movement also produced a smaller number of female activists who linked their concern with health problems to a more aggressive feminism. The health reform movement thus touched the average woman and the feminist in slightly different ways. Ironically, even as health reformers aided in readjusting female roles to coincide with traditional values concerning woman's place, they helped, sometimes unwittingly, to lay the groundwork for the eventual erosion of ancient pieties. To the female leaders of the campaign health reform offered a path out of the home and a more active role in social change.

II

Because woman's procreative role often made her health more precarious than man's, it seemed natural for the health reformers to begin their efforts with an aggressive concern for the state of female health. "If a plan for *destroying female health,* in all the ways in which it could be most effectively done, were drawn up," announced Catherine Beecher, "it would be exactly the course which is now pursued by a large portion of this nation, especially in the more wealthy classes." Dr. James C. Jackson, founder of the Danville water cure agreed. "American girls," he lamented, "are all sickly." "You are sick," wrote Mrs. S.M. Estee to the feminine readers of the *Water Cure Journal,* "and have been for months, years, and some of you your whole lives."[12]

We cannot know for sure whether or not this generation of women was sicker than their grandmothers. What is certain, however, is that they *thought* they were. Indeed, they well may have been. Fashionable dress took its toll on female health; the corset and tight lacing did much to damage female anatomy. Increased urbanization brought crowded and unsanitary living conditions. More and more middle-class women denied themselves the fresh air and exercise experienced by the rural housewife out of necessity rather than by choice. And the psychological strains of dislocation may have prompted some women to opt for ill-health, rather than stand and face changes which they could still barely comprehend.[13]

It soon became apparent that only healthy vigorous women could meet the challenges thrust upon them by a society in transition. Health reformers believed that woman was in the process of creating a new role for herself. "Woman ... is a new element in society," wrote Dr. James Jackson to his associate Dr. Harriet A. Judd, "just emerging from her hybernation... and so much better fitted to take to herself *new* ideas, and develop them...."[14] Good health was essential to woman's new self-expression and improved status. "Let mothers be educated in all that concerns life and health...." insisted Mrs. Eliza de La Vergue, M.D. "Let them learn that *knowledge gives the highest order of power.*"[15]

Good health became a prerequisite to woman's new place in the world. "Woman was neither made a toy nor a slave, but a help-meet to man," wrote "A Bloomer to Her Sisters," "and as such devolves upon her very many important duties and obligations which cannot be met so long as she is the puny, sickly, aching, weakly, dying creature that we find her to be; and woman must, to a very considerable extent, redeem herself — she must throw off the shackles that have hitherto bound both body and mind, and rise into the newness of life."[16]

Women could achieve none of these goals until they learned to dress properly. Health reformers made dress reform a symbol of women's new aspirations. Impractical clothes immobilized women and kept them from their responsibilities. Some regular physicians had linked fashionable dress to female ill health, but health reformers succeeded in making dress reform a moral imperative. Good health was doomed, they argued, as long as women clung to the dictates of French fashion. They called upon women to liberate their sould by freeing their bodies from the harmful effects of tight lacing and long, heavy unhygienic skirts. "How... glorious, "mused Rachel Brooks Gleason, M.D. "would it be to see every woman free from *every* fetter that fashion has imposed! Such a day of 'universal emancipation' of the sex would worthy of a celebration through all coming time." "We can expect but small achievement from women," warned Mary Gove Nichols, "so long as it is the labor of their lives to carry about their clothes." "How in the name of common sense," asked Edith Denner, "is a woman with long, full skirts, ever to become a practical Ornithologist, Geologist, or Bontanist. . .?"[17]

Health reform journals pressed the issue. Lengthy technical descriptions of the damage wrought on female anatomy by the corset appeared, complete with diagrams. Pictures entitled the "Allopathic Lady, or Pure Cod Liver Oil Female, Who Patronizes a Fashionable Doctor, And Considers It Decidedly Vulgar to Enjoy Good Health," were published side by side with those of women in reformed dress. A typical caption read "A Water-Cure Bloomer, Who Believes In The Equal Rights Of Men And Women To Help Themselves And Each Other, And Who Thinks It Respectable, If Not Genteel, To Be Well." Not content merely to admonish their readers, some journals printed sewing instructions. For a modest sum, the *Laws of Life* sold patterns to its subscribers.[18]

In a society where women were expected to play an increasingly complex role in the nurture of children and the organization of family life, health crusaders brought to the bewildered housewife, not just sympathy and compassion, but a structured regimen and way of life. William A. Alcott, as early as 1839, took for granted the mother's primary responsibility in childrearing and the father's extended absence from the home. "All, or nearly all," he wrote in his book *The Young Mother,* "must devolve on the mother. The father has not time to attend to his children."[19]

Burdened by this reorientation toward their family responsibilities, many ordinary women found in the health reform movement a means of coping with an imprecise, undependable and often hostile environment. Lectures, journals and domestic tracts provided friendly advice and companionship in an era characterized by weakening ties between relatives and neighbors. Women found a means to end their isolation and make contact with others of their sex. In study groups and through letters to the various journals, they shared their common experiences with other women. No longer must woman bear her burden alone. This collective sensitivity to the community among women was symbolized by the frequent references to "sisterhood" in health reform literature.[20]

"I wish," wrote Mary Gove Nichols of her motives in becoming a health reformer, "to teach mothers how to cure their own diseases, and those of their children; and to increase health, purity, and happiness in the family and the home."[21] For some women, Mrs. Nichols and her fellow reformers achieved these goals.[22] Numerous articles on Cookery, Bathing, Teething, Care of Infants, Childhood Sexuality, Cleanliness, and Domestic Economy carefully taught women how to manage their households properly. Itinerant physiological lecturers assaulted women's widespread ignorance of their bodies. Nichols relied heavily on discussion of anatomy and physiology in her lectures. She instructed her listeners in the formation of bone structure, the role of respiration and circulation, the anatomy and physiology of the stomach. The process of digestion was described in detail. The remainder of her course involved information on dietetics and the importance of physical education. The evils of "tight lacing," and dire warnings against the harmful effects of the "solitary vice" also proved popular topics for discussion.[23]

Advice on the supervision of pregnancy and childbirth was strikingly prophetic of today's feminist critique of professional obstetrical practice. Health reformers questioned regular physicians' very approach to the process of parturition, calling their treatment "unnatural and often outrageous." "Here," observed Thomas Low Nichols,

> where august nature should reign supreme, her laws are too often violated, and all her teachings set at naught. Instead of preparing a woman to go through the process of labor with all the energy of her vitality, she is weakened by medication and blood-letting. Instead of being put upon a proper regimen, and a diet suited to her condition, she is more than ever pampered and indulged. And when labor comes on, the chances are that it will be interfered with in the most mistaken, the most unjustifiable ... manner. The uterus will be stimulated into excessive and spasmodic action by the deadly ergot; the mother, at this most interesting and sacred hour of life, will be made dead drunk with ether or chloroform ...and if a weakened and deranged system does not act as promptly as the doctor wishes, he proceeds to deliver with instruments, with the risk, often the certainty of destroying the child, and very often inflicting upon the mother irreparable injury.

"Under the popular medical orders of the day," agreed Russell Trall, "pregnant females are regarded as invalids, and are bled, paregoric'd, magnesia'd, stimulated, mineralized and poisoned, just as though they were going through a regular course of fever."[24] In contrast, health reformers viewed conception, gestation, and parturition as natural functions. They rejected the notion that pain in childbirth was inevitable, labeling such a belief "an insult to Providence." They urged exercise, fresh air, proper diet, and cleanliness. Daily bathing was advised for infants, who were to be dressed in loose-fitting, comfortable garments to give plenty of opportunity for movement. No drugs were allowed for mother or child. Such attention to hygiene and diet probably improved the health of many, if we can believe the numerous testimonials from satisfied individuals to be found in the back pages of health reform journals.[25]

When the middle-class woman took possession of her life and the lives of those around her in the area of health, she also provided herself with a platform from which to effect other changes, both within the family constellation and in society at large. One doubts if this process was always conscious. Yet it seems equally clear that her psychological acceptance of various domestic responsibilities often led to subtle shifts in the power relationship between the sexes, giving rise to new attitudes toward what was, and what was not acceptable in marriage. Nowhere was this process more apparent than in the health reformers' attitudes toward sexual intercourse.[26]

Health reformers were among the first 19th-century thinkers to prescribe restraint in sexual matters. Believing that good health required constant control, vigilant self-discipline, and vigorous dominion over man's animal nature, they warned that of all the sensual passions, "the sexual element" was the most difficult to subdue. "No other element in our own nature," wrote Henry C. Wright, "has so much to do in ... forming our character and shaping our destiny ... But what is done ... to bring the sexual element under the control of an enlightened reason and a tender conscience?"[27]

Reformers clearly intended sexual restraint to benefit women and urged them to assert their rights in the sexual sphere. Much of female ill-health and infant mortality, they argued, could be attributed to husbands' sexual abuse of their wives. Believing that the male's passion for copulation far outdistanced his wife's, thinkers and educators urged men to follow the sexual rhythms of their more delicate spouses.[28]

Excessive childbearing endangered female health while it drained most women of the energy needed to perform the duties of scientific motherhood. Hence, health reformers linked their insistence on sexual restraint to family limitation. They were among the first to advocate birth control publicly. Children, they argued, must never be the result "of chance, of mere reckless, selfish passion." When, they asked "will men and women show a rational, conscientious, loving forethought, in giving existence to their children as they do in commerce, politics, and religion?" Every child should be a welcome child. "Welcome" became a code word for "planned." The "great object" of sexual intercourse, declared Henry C. Wright, was the *"perpetuation and perfection of the race."* Couples not ready to have children should remain sexually continent.[29]

In an era still largely ignorant of mechanical means of contraception, women benefitted from such cautious attitudes in numerous ways. Historians have already documented women's profound fears of pregnancy in this period. Less frequent childbearing did improve female health. Furthermore, the desire to avoid conception probably colored women's enjoyment of coitus. Some undoubtedly followed the common belief that failure to achieve orgasm would prevent pregnancy. Moreover, lovemaking techniques were often brutal and aggressive.[30] Even 19th-century physicians, although aware of female orgasm, knew very little else about the intricate nature of female sexual response. One suspects that middle-class women instructed their husbands and sons in the laws of sexual continence with a degree of enthusiasm and a measure of self-defense.[31]

While exalting the rewards of parenthood and elevating the motherly role, health reformers enjoined couples to limit their offspring. The contradiction in such views remains more apparent than real. The ideal of educated motherhood eventually proved antithetical to large families. Women were simply incapable of achieving either the emotional intensity or the domestic expertise required of them when caring for a large brood. Margaret Sanger's injunction that parents should have "fewer and better babies" had its origins in the antebellum period, among these "enlightened" sections of the middle class.[32]

III

Rarely in any century have human beings been content to view health and disease as matters of mere chance. The health reformers' approach, however, was distinctly novel. To the Puritans and other colonials, sickness had been primarily a moral and spiritual dilemma which called for introspection and soul searching. But the 19th-century health reformers insisted that it resulted from a violation of God's and Nature's laws. Such laws were eminently sensible, and the individual could, indeed, he *must,* keep himself well. No longer was sickness and death to be tolerated with the stoicism and resignation that contrasted the limited moral choices of man with the all-powerful inscrutability of God. "Many people," observed Mary Gove Nichols, "seem to think that all diseases are immediate visitations from the Almighty, arising from no cause but his *immediate* dispensation . . . Many seem to have no idea that there are established laws with respect to life and health, and that the transgression of these laws is followed by disease." Man, agreed Marie Louise Shew, was designed to live in good health to a ripe old age. Disease was man's doing, not God's. The prevention of disease and premature death was indeed within the control of mankind.[33]

The emergence of health reform as a coherent crusade cannot be understood apart from the gradual appearance of a novel set of assumptions about the world — an attitude which historians, for want of a more precise theoretical model, have attributed to the modernization process. Health reformers insisted upon the efficacy of individual action. They were certain that human beings could affect the future by manipulating the environment and controlling themselves. This was a conviction that they shared with all other reformers of the ante-bellum period. Yet this common outlook was itself a reflection of a more fundamental change in thought and feeling.

Even many critics of the concept of modernization agree that if used carefully it can serve as a helpful organizing principle for studying the social, political, and cultural fragmentation which accompanied industrialization.[34] The modernization model can be of aid in relating changes in individual and family dynamics to other aspects of social history.

Although we may differ as to the cause, most of us would agree that modern men and women behave differently from their ancestors: they exhibit high occupational and educational goals, they value mobility, personal freedom, and self-improvement, and their fundamental belief in progress leads to an implicit abandonment of passivity in the face of life's difficulties.[35] Health reformers filled their literature with such themes. Indeed, one could argue that health reform facilitated the adjustment of men and women in the 19th century to industrialization and urbanization.

Occasionally health tracts revealed the reformers' profound ambivalence toward social and economic change, and such equivocation was itself significant. By no means did all health crusaders welcome the new order with unbridled enthusiasm.[36] As other historians have shown, many individuals looked nostalgically backward to an idealized "republic of virtue" where the mutual interdependency of family members and society at large promoted "good health" in the form of physical and spiritual unity.[37] While they desired "progress," health reformers did not always realize that it would lead inevitably to changes in values. Arguing, on the one hand, that an excessive application to business led to insanity in men, while luxury and idleness produced nervousness in women, they simultaneously sought the creation of a personality type remarkably well-suited to the competitive atmosphere of the industrial order.[38] Preaching moderation and self-control, reformers strove to provide men and women with a coherent mode of adjustment to the physical and psychological demands of an urbanizing environment. By helping, willy-nilly, to effect a transformation of personality which equipped individuals to deal with other aspects of modernization, health reform itself became a part

By the end of the 19th century, reform ideas about personal cleanliness, public health, and family hygiene had become familiar axioms of middle-class American culture − a badge of distinction by which members set themselves off from "illegitimate" immigrant groups, many of whom retained distinctly premodern daily habits and attitudes toward disease. Indeed, those health reformers primarily concerned with public health had long been aware of the relationship between ignorance, immoral habits, poverty and sickness. The allegedly "filthy" and "depraved" customs attributed to the immigrant poor proved particularly vexing. Health reformers of all persuasions believed that they worked to make good health a measure of middle-class respectability.[39]

To the middle-class women, troubled by the contradictory demands of urbanization and industrialization, health reform offered both physical and psychological relief. Holding out to confused wives and mothers the prospect of improving the quality of life, not merely by changing the environment, but by gaining control of themselves, health reformers promised women that they could raise their children healthy in mind and clean in body. Reformers offered wives the possibility of keeping their husbands moral by cooking the right foods. Preaching sexual continence and physiological knowledge, they helped to legitimate female rights in the bedroom at a time when sexual contact need not universally have been a positive experience. Indeed, health reform manuals supported women's right to limit the number of their children and control their own bodies, though they accepted only sexual continence as a moral means of birth control. Nevertheless, the idea that fertility should, or even could be consistently tampered with was distinctly modern, and neatly complemented other social and economic developments.[40]

For a minority of brave, ambitious and talented women health reform also provided an outlet and an escape from an intolerably narrow and confining role. Health reformers shared with other 19th-century Americans the belief that woman's role was invested with cosmic moral significance. But unlike many of their contemporaries, female health activists subscribed to the widest possible definition of woman's sphere. They understood that to purify society, women would indeed have to enter it. Admitting women into the masculine sphere, even in a limited way, would eventually have profound effects on future definitions of sex roles.

Most middle-class women, however, were not feminists. Health reform gave them a coherent program to ease their adjustment to a society in transition. Over and over again the reformers identified poor female health with underemployment and idleness. This familiar refrain suggests a lack of integration in the lives of middle-class women, a tenuousness and uncertainty about their role. Female health reformers especially addressed themselves to this problem. Elevating the art of domesticity to a science, they restored to their followers a sense of purpose and direction, while they preserved in a new form traditional assumptions about woman's role which were deeply imbedded in the culture. The health reform regimen established new standards by which ordinary women could measure their own respectability and worth.[41]

Reformers underscored woman's importance by emphasizing her central role in the task of human betterment. Improvement of female health, they argued, would lead to social regeneration. Woman was invested with awesome responsibilities. "There are no duties on earth so nearly angelic as those which devolve upon woman. . . ." declared Alcott. "If all wives loved and delighted in their homes as Solomon would have them, few husbands would go down to a premature grave through the avenues of intemperance and lust, and their kindred vices." *The Lily,* a feminist and temperance journal, emphasized woman's moral power. "Woman's influence is truly kingly [sic] in general society. It is powerful in a daughter and a sister; but it is the mother who weaves the garlands that flourish in eternity." The gravity of woman's influence went even beyond her own family, for health reformers shared a contemporary belief in the inheritance of acquired characteristics. "For the sake of the race," explained Mary Gove Nichols, "I ask that all be done for woman that can be done, for it is an awful truth that fools are the mothers of fools." James C. Jackson was even more blunt: "God punishes as well as rewards mankind *through woman.* . . . She is appointed to dispense divine retributions as well as divine blessings. . . through her does God visit the iniquities of the father on the children to the third and fourth generations."[42]

Though such attitudes gave women genuine responsibility and power, they also exacted a large measure of anxiety and even guilt. "Women are answerable, in a very large degree," admonished Paulina Wright Davis, "for the imbecilities of disease, mental and bodily, and for the premature deaths prevailing throughout society — for the weakness, wretchedness, and shortness of life — and no remedy will be radical till reformation of life and practice obtains among our sex. . . ."[43] Such a psychological burden might well have been unbearable had not health reformers given to women fellowship, moral support, and practical information.

The health reformers' emphasis on educated motherhood and scientific domesticity in a sense helped make middle-class women modern. But being modern did not necessarily mean being equal. If the concept of female moral superiority was a source of *power* for women in the 19th century, it cannot be confused with *liberation*.[44] Indeed, it may have merely guaranteed the perpetuation and elaboration of traditional assumptions about mothering and housekeeping in an altered social setting. Full equality for women continued to be undermined by a single-minded concern with woman's maternal role. Even the most feminist of health reformers failed to realize that women would never be equal as long as they remained confined to a sphere — no matter how expansively that sphere was defined.

University of Kansas   Regina Markell Morantz

FOOTNOTES

This article grew out of a paper presented at a symposium on "Medicine Without Doctors: Home Health Care in American History," sponsored by the Department of the History of Medicine, University of Wisconsin, Madison, April 14, 1975. The author is grateful to Ellen Chesler, Rita Napier, Cliff Griffin, Eric Foner, John Clark and Martin Pernick for reading and criticizing the manuscript.

1. The most recent treatments of the health reform movement include William B. Walker, "The Health Reform Movement in the United States, 1830-1870" (Ph.D. Thesis, John Hopkins, 1955); Richard Shryock, "Sylvester Graham and the Popular Health Movement, 1830-1870," in *Medicine in America, Historical Essays* (Baltimore, 1966), 111-125; John Blake, "Health Reform," in E.S. Gaustad, ed., *The Rise of Adventism: Religion and Society in Mid-Nineteenth Century America* (New York, 1974), 30-49; H.E. Hoff and J. Fulton, "The Centenary of the First American Physiological Society Founded at Boston by William A. Alcott and Sylvester Graham," *Bull. Hist. Med.,* 5, (Oct., 1937) 687-734; Stephen Wilner Nissenbaum, "Careful Love: Sylvester Graham and the Emergence of Victorian Sexual Theory in America, 1830-1840" (Ph.D. Thesis, University of Wisconsin, 1968); James C. Whorton, "Christian Physiology: William Alcott's Prescription for the Millenium," *Bull. Hist. Med.,* 49, (Winter, 1975) 466-481. Two lively popular works are James H. Young, *The Toadstool Millionaires: A Social History of Patent Medicines in America Before Federal Regulation* (Princeton, 1961) and Gerald Carson, *Cornflake Crusade* (New York, 1967). The public health movement is dealt with in Charles and Carroll Smith-Rosenberg, "Pietism and the Origins of the American Public Health Movement: A Note on John H. Griscom and Robert W. Hartley," *Jour. Hist. Med.* 23 (1968) 16-35; Richard H. Shryock, "The Early American Public Health Movement," in *Medicine in America,* 126-138. John D. Davies skillfully chronicles the phrenology movement in *Phrenology, Fad and Science* (New Haven, 1955).

2. *Water Cure Journal,* 7 (1849), 18. (Hereafter cited as *WCJ.*) The Seventh Day Adventist publication, *The Health Reformer* claimed 11,000 subscribers in 1868. See Ronald L. Numbers "Health Reform on the Delaware," *New Jersey History,* 92 (Sept., 1974), 7.

3. For the convergence of health reform with other reform movements see Robert S. Flectcher, "Bread and Doctrine at Oberlin," *Ohio State Archeological and Historical Quarterly,* 49 (Jan., 1940), 58; Sidonia E. Taupin, " 'Christianity in the Kitchen,' or A Moral Guide for Gourmets," *American Quarterly,* 15 (1963), 85-89; Thomas H. LeDuc, "Grahamites and Garrisonites," *New York History,* 20 (April, 1939), 189-191; Michael Katz, *The Irony of Early School Reform* (Boston, 1968). For a thoughtful and highly provocative recent treatment see Ronald G. Walters, "The Erotic South: Civilization and Sexuality in American Abolitionism," *American Quarterly,* 25 (May, 1973), 177-201.

4. See Martha Verbrugge, "The Ladies Physiological Institute: Health Reform and Women in Ante-bellum Boston" (Paper delivered at Third Annual Berkshire conference on Women's History, Bryn Mawr, June, 1976). The one exception to this middle-class analysis may have been the Thomsonians, a health reform sect which has been tentatively linked to working-class elements. I would contend that the Thomsonians do not fall out of the mainstream of the movement I am discussing, because health reform could very well have played a similar role in "modernizing" native American workers in the ante-bellum period as I will argue it played for the middle class. As Paul Faler and Alan Dawley have recently shown, the internalization of "modern" values often transcended class divisions. See "Working Class Culture and Politics in the Industrial Revolution: Sources of Loyalism and Rebellion," *Journal of Social History,* 9 (June, 1976) 466-79. I am indebted to Irene Javors of City College for discussing her preliminary findings on the Thomsonians with me.

5. For the influence of the Enlightenment see Alice Felt Tyler, *Freedom's Ferment* (New York, 1944). For Christian perfectionism see James C. Whorton, " 'Christian Physiology:' William Alcott's Prescription for the Millenium," *Bull. Hist. Med.,* 49, (Winter, 1975), 466-81. For the decline of heroic therapeutics see Shryock, op cit. For anti-elitism see Richard Shryock, "Cults and Quackery in American Medical History," Middle States Association of History and Social Studies Teachers, *Trans,* 37 (1939), 19-30.

6. The most recent treatment of modernization in America does not refer to health reform at all. See Richard D. Brown, *Modernization, The Transformation of American Life, 1600-1865,* (New York, 1976).

7. The one exception is John Blake's excellent article on Mary Gove Nichols, "Mary Gove Nichols, Prophetess of Health," in *Proceedings of the American Philosophical Society,* 106 (June, 1962), 219-234.

8. Hebbel and Hoff, *op cit,* 701.

9. On changes, particularly in New England, which touched the lives of many in the reform leadership see the thoughtful introduction by Michael Katz to *The Irony of Early School Reform* (Boston, 1968). Also Stanley Engerman, Ed., *The Reinterpretation of American Economic History,* (New York, 1971), Stephen Thernstrom, *Poverty and Progress* (Cambridge, 1964); Stephen Thernstrom and Richard Sennett, eds., *Nineteenth Century Cities* (New Haven, 1969). Two recent articles on women and work before industrializaition are Joan Scott and Louise Tilly, "Women's Work and Family in 19th Century Europe," *Comparative Studies in History & Society,* 17 (Jan., 1975) 36-64; Alice Kessler-Harris, "Stratifying by Sex: Understanding the History of Working Women," *Labor Market Segmentation,* ed. by Richard Edwards, *et al.* (Lexington, Mass., 1975). For quote from Frances Dana Gage see *WCJ,* 17 (1854), 35.

10. Rev. H. Winslow, "Domestic Education in Females," I (1847), 259-61.

11. The concept of the "republican mother," which was given life during the ante-bellum period, gained momentum through several permutations until progressive era reformers and social workers recast it in the 20th-century notion of "educated motherhood." See Linda Kerber, "Daughters of Columbia: Educating Women for the Republic, 1787-1805," in Stanley Elkins and Eric McKitrick, *The Hofstadter Aegis,* (New York, 1974), and "The Republican Mother" (Paper read at the Southern Historical Association Meeting, November, 1975); Jill Conway, "Perspectives on the History of Women's Education in the United States," *Hist. of Ed. Quart.* 14 (Spring, 1974), 1-12. For the progressive period see Sheila Rothman, "Social History and Social Policy: The Case of Women, Children & the Family" (Paper read at the meeting of the Organization of American Historians, April, 1976, St. Louis). For an excellent discussion of the social and economic roots of American feminism, particularly the influence of education see Keith Melder, "The Beginning of the Women's Rights Movement in the United States, 1800-1840" (Ph.D. Thesis, Yale, 1964); Gerda Lerner, "The Lady and the Mill Girl: Changes in the Status of Women in the Age of Jackson," *American Studies,* 10 (Spring, 1969), 5-15.

12. *Letters to the People on Health and Happiness* (New York, 1856), 7. "Shall Our Girls Live or Die," *Laws of Life,* 10 (1867), 2; "To Sick Women," *WCJ,* 26 (1858), 96. See also Augustus K. Gardner, "The Physical Decline of American Women," *WCJ,* 29 (1860), 21-22, 50-51.

13. Striking evidence for the conviction of many women writers that their grandmothers enjoyed better health can be found in Catherine Beecher, *Housekeeper and Healthkeeper* (New York, 1873), 424-428. Another possible explanation for the increase in complaints is that women were no longer willing to tolerate their ill health. See also Carroll Smith-Rosenberg, "The Hysterical Woman: Sex Roles and Role Conflict in Nineteenth-Century America," *Social Research,* 39 (Winter, 1972), 652-678.

14. *WCJ,* 15 (1854), 74, 94.

15. Italics mine. *WCJ,* 20 (1855), 74.

16. *WCJ,* 15 (1853), 131. See also Harriet Austin, "Woman's Present and Future," *WCJ,* 16 (1853), 57.

17. "Woman's Dress," *WCJ,* 11 (1851), 30: "The New Costume," *WCJ,* 12 (1851) 30; Science and Long Skirts," *WCJ,* 20 (1855), 7.

18. *WCJ,* 16 (1853), 120; 11 (1851) 96, and *passim.* Most of the water-cure establishments encouraged their female patients to wear reformed dress. Almost every issue of any health reform journal had something about dress: *The Water Cure Journal* and *The Laws of Life* showed special interest in dress reform; the *Graham Journal* and the *American Vegetarian and Health Journal* less frequently. Dress reform was also a popular topic in women's rights journals like *The Una, The Lily,* and later *The Revolution.* Many of the articles in these journals pertaining to dress were written by health reformers. See especially *WCJ,* 12 (1851), 33 58; *WCJ,* 34 (1862), 1-2; *WCJ,* 15 (1853), 7, 10, 32, 34, 35, 131; *WCJ,* 13 (1852), 111; *The Laws of Life,* 10 (1867), 93-94, 129-130, 145-146; *The Revolution,* 3 (1869), 149-50; *Graham Journal,* 3 (1839), 301-2.

19. Boston, 1839, 265-266.

20. *WCJ,* 1 (1846), 29.

21. See "To Her Sick Sisters," *WCJ,* 26 (1858), 96. "A Bloomer to Her Sisters," *WCJ,* 15 (1853), 131. There are many examples. For a possible meaning to this sense of community see Carroll Smith-Rosenberg "The Female World of Love and Ritual: Relations Between Women in 19th Century America," *Signs,* I (A'1975), 1-29. For Nichols quote see *A*

Woman's Work in Water Cure, 14. See also Mary Gove Nichols, "To the Women Who Read the Water Cure Journal," *WCJ,* 14 (1852), 68: "We do not consider ourselves doctors in the common understanding of the word – though we shall not neglect to do the highest good in this department, but we consider ourselves educators – set apart and qualified by Providence for the work. We will educate men and women for Physicans and Teachers of health, and young women to be wise wives and mothers. We will make the most beneficial impression on the world that is possible to us."

22. See Martha Verbrugge, *op cit.* Hers is the first local study we have of the rank and file. One suspects others will yield similar conclusions.

23. Chapters on Food, Cooking and Domestic Economy in William A. Alcott, *The Young Housekeeper* (Boston, 1849); *Graham Journal,* "Keep Your Children Clean," I (1837), 176; Masturbation and Its Effect on Health," 2 (1838), 23. Mary Gove Nichols, *Lectures to Women,* passim. See also advertisement in the *Graham Journal,* II (1838), 288. For articles on fresh air and bathing: *WCJ,* (1847), 161-68, 177; *WCJ,* 4 (1847), 193; pregnancy, exercise and childbirth: *WCJ,* 3 (1847), 145, 151, 183-84; "Our New Cookbook," "How to Can a Fruit," *Laws of Life,* 10 (1867), 12: "Cleanliness and Healthfulness," *Laws of Life,* 10 (1867), 16; "Teething and Its Management," "Children's Dress," *WCJ,* 12 (1851), 101, 104. Martha Verbrugge has emphasized this practical dimension of the health reform program. She contends that the Ladies' Physiological Institute helped ordinary middle-class women adjust to the opportunities and the limitations imposed on them by modern life. Verbrugge is impressed less with the radical elements of the Boston group and more with the organization's goal of easing women into traditional role patterns potentially disturbed by changing social conditions. Her study is significant because it suggests that health reform appealed to several different types of women. She argues, for example, that only a small minority of the members of the Boston society were outspoken feminists. See Verbrugge, *op cit.*

24. Thomas Low Nichols, *"The Curse Removed; The Efficacy of Water-Cure in the Treatment of Uterine Disease and the Removal of the Pains and Perils of Pregnancy and Childbirth,"* (New York, 1850), 13; Trall, "Allopathic Midwifery," *WCJ,* 9 (1850), 121; Mary Gove Nichols, "Maternity and the Water Cure for Infants," *WCJ,* 11 (1851), 57-9; Eliza de la Vergue, M.D. "Infants, Their Improper Nursing and Meication," *WCJ,* 20 (1855).

25. See an interesting autobiographical sketch by Mrs. Mary A. Torbit, "Reasons for Becoming a Lecturer," *WCJ,* 14 (1851), 91. One of the health reformers' favorite arguments – that women had natural abilities to cure – led them to a desire to teach women medicine. Indeed, the entrance of women into the medical profession grew out of the cult of scientific domesticity popularized by the health reform movement. Reformers applauded the acceptance of women as medical students, chiding the regulars for their conservatism. In time these early female pioneers, who entered medicine convinced of their natural abilities, would be transformed into full-fledged professionals by their contact with an increasingly scientific and empirical discipline. They became exposed to a more modern system of values, their outlook permanently altered in the process. See Regina Markell Morantz, "Daughters of Aesculapius: The Entrance of Women into the Medical Profession in 19th Century America, Ideology and Social Setting" (Paper delivered at Minneapolis, Women Historians of the Midwest Conference, October, 1975).

26. Indeed, the attitude of the health reformers toward the relations between the sexes was innovative. They preached a version of companionate marriage. See Morantz, "Health Reform and Women: An Ideology of Self Help" (Paper presented at the symposium on "Medicine Without Doctors, Home Health Care in American History," Department of the History of Medicine, University of Wisconsin, Madison, April 14, 1975).

27. Henry C. Wright, *Marriage and Parentage* (Boston, 1855, Arno reprint, 1974), 5.

28. *Ibid.,* 91, 257. See also Orson Fowler, *Love and Parentage* (New York, 1847), 272-274,

passim. See Linda Gordon, "Voluntary Motherhood: The Beginnings of Feminist Birth Control Ideas in the United States," in L. Banner and M. Hartman, *Clio's Consciousness Raised: New Perspectives on the History of Women* (New York, 1974), 54-71. Not all advisors proscribed sexual intercourse without procreation. However all agreed that coitus should be approached with caution. Mechanical means of contraception were an anathema because such methods degraded women by encouraging overindulgence.

29. Wright, *Ibid.*

30. See Eliza B. Duffey, *The Relations of the Sexes* (New York, 1879), especially Chapter 13, "The Limitation of Offspring."

31. Although Carl Degler has rightly pointed out that at least some women did have orgasms in the 19th century, a fact which it would be silly to dispute, I would suggest that female orgasm was inherently more problematical than that of the male, and that the 19th century was generally ignorant of the more subtle nature of female sexual response. Marriage counselors in the 1920's and 1930's documented this widespread ignorance and tried to correct it. Alfred Kinsey's statistics show a gradual increase in the number of married women achieving orgasm in the years after 1900. Carroll Smith-Rosenberg has examined possible differences in male and female approaches to sexuality in the 19th century in greater detail in a recent paper, "A Gentle and A Richer Sex: Female Perspectives on Nineteenth Century Sexuality" (Third Berkshire Conference on Women's History, Bryn Mawr, June, 1976). See also Regina Markell Morantz, "The Scientist as Sex Crusader: Alfred Kinsey and American Culture," *American Quarterly* (Fall, 1977) See Duffey, Ch. 13. It should be pointed out that most health reformers were also eugenicists. See Henry C. Wright, *The Empire of the Mother Over the Character and Destiny of the Race* (Boston, 1863).

32. Moreover, social reformers of all types recognized that large families hampered upward mobility. The reputation of the Irish for their alleged indulgence of the sensual passions was widespread. They had nothing but "large," dirty" families to show for it:" Did wealth consist in children," asserted the *Common School Journal*, "it is well known, that the Irish would be a rich people; and if the old Roman law prevailed here, which granted special privilege to every man who had more than three, this people would be elevated into an aristocracy." Quoted in Katz, *The Irony of Early School Reform*, 123. Many of the early school reformers, including Horace Mann, had a lively interest in health reform. Largely because of this interest the Massachusetts legislature passed a law in 1850 requiring physiological instruction in the schools.

33. *Lectures to Women*, 20. *Water Cure for Ladies*, Preface, iii. See Charles Rosenberg, *The Cholera Years* (Chicago, 1962).

34. See Christopher Lasch on the problems of the modernization model in the first of three articles on the historiography of the family in *New York Review of Books*, (Nov. 13, 1975).

35. James T. Fawcett, "Modernization, Individual Modernity, and Fertility," in J.T. Fawcett, ed. *Studies in the Psychology of Population* (New York, 1973); Alex Inkeles, "The Modernization of Man," in *Modernization, the Dynamics of Growth* New York, 1966), 138-150, and "Making Men Modern: on the Causes and Consequences of Individual Change in Six Developing Countries," *Am. Jour. of Soc,* 75 (1969), 208-225; also Richard D. Brown, "Modernization and the Modern Personality in America, 1600-1865," *Jour. of Interdisc. Hist.* 2 (W' 1972), 201-227.

36. See for example, David J. Rothman, *The Discovery of the Asylum* (Boston, 1971)

37. "Excessive Application: A Cause of Insanity," *Monthly Miscellany and Journal of Health 1 (1846) 212.* See also Barbara Sicherman, "Paradox of Prudence; Mental Health in the gilded Age," *Journ. of Amer. Hist.* 62 (Mar., 1976), 890-912.

38. For other discussions of this personality type see Peter Cominos, "Late Victorian Respectability and the Social System," *Int. Rev. of Soc. Hist.* 8 (1963), 18-48, 216-50; Herbert Gutman, "Work, Culture, and Society in Industrializing America," *AHR*, 78 (June, 1973), 531-587; Michael Katz, *The Irony of Early School Reform;* Alan Dawley and Paul Faler, "Working Class Culture and Politics in the Industrial Revolution: Sources of Loyalty and Rebellion," *Journal of Social History* 9 (June, 1976), 466-79.

39. "Looking. . . at the social habits of the working people in some of our densely populated districts, it does indeed appear a hopeless effort to attack their vices, unless one could at the same time pull down their houses, and build them others adapted to a more perfect state of bodily and mental health," "Sanitary and Social Reform Coeval," by Mrs. Ellis in *Practical Educator and Journal of Health,* 1 (1847) 354-5. Charles Rosenberg has made this same point in connection with 19th-century prescriptions for male sexual purity. See "Sexuality, Class, Role," *American Quarterly* 25 (May, 1973), 131-153; also William Coleman, "Health and Hygiene in the Encyclopedie: A Medical Doctrine for the Bourgeoisie," *Jour. Hist. Med.* 29 (Oct., 1974), 339-412, applies a similar argument to the French bourgeoisie. See S. Weir Mitchell, "So great is my reverence for supreme wholesomeness, that I should almost be tempted to assert that perfect health is virtue." *Address on Opening of the Institute of Hygiene of the University of Pennsylvania.* (Phil., 1892), 4. A few health reformers merged the moral injunction to "guard the health of the race" with overt nativism. "Already," warned James C. Jackson,

> the decay of our women and the delicate constitutions of our young men are forcing the latter to seek revitalization by intermarriage with immigrant women from Europe. What with the decline of the Puritan and Cavilier stock on the one hand, and the great influx of foreign born on the other, it is not difficult to predict *our future.* In less than fifty years the New England type of manhood will have ceased to govern this Republic, and when once it ceases to govern it will cease to exist. . . . *Nothing but a bold and faithful advocacy of the laws of health can stop this ebbtide of human life.*

See *WCJ* 26 (1858), 4.

40. See James T. Fawcett, "Modernization, Individual Modernity, and Fertility." Also see Robert V. Wells, "Family History and Demographic Transition," *Jour. Soc. Hist.,* 9 (Fall, 1975), 1-20.

41. It should be pointed out that the domestic ideal had very different effects on working-class women. By encouraging them to aspire to an often impossible goal, the cult of domesticity helped keep married women out of the work force, or at least aspiring to be idle. This insured that working women would often be undependable allies in labor disputes. Believing that their primary commitment should be to the family, they accepted low pay and low status jobs, viewing their situation as only temporary. See Alice Kessler-Harris, "Stratifying by Sex." The domestic ideology also increased women's perceptions of class differences among themselves. Middle-class women were often advised to be cautious about the health of hired servants. Advice literature warned of the dangers of immigrant girls infecting the household. I am indebted to my colleague David Katzman for this information. For a stimulating discussion of the middle-class English woman's involvement in health reform see Patricia Branca, *Silent Sisterhood, Middle Class Women in the Victorian Home* (Pittsburgh, 1976), especially Parts II and III. Branca argues that middle-class Victorian women were the first large group to establish a modern outlook toward life and death.

42. William Alcott, *The Young Wife* (Boston, 1837), 87-89; *The Lily,* I (1849), 52; Nichols, *Lectures to Women,* 212, and "Woman the Physician," *WCJ,* 12 (1851), 75; Jackson, "The Women of the United States," *WCJ* 26 (1858), 3, and "Women's Rights," *WCJ,* 31 (1861), 61. For an excellent summary of hereditarian views in this period see Charles Rosenberg, "The Bitter Fruit: Heredity, Disease, and Social Thought in Nineteenth Century America," *Perspectives in American History,* 7 (1974), 189-238.

43. *WCJ*, I(1846), 29.

44. See Christopher Lasch, "The Woman Reformers' Rebuke," in *The World of Nations,* (New York, 1974).

Charles E. Rosenberg

AND HEAL THE SICK: HOSPITAL AND PATIENT IN 19TH CENTURY AMERICA

In the 1970s it has become fashionable to think of the hospital patient as inmate, subject to the psychic and physical discipline of some institution which shapes every aspect of his physical and ultimately emotional life. Though the most influential of such interpretations have been drawn from the world of psychiatry and the mental hospital, the analytical vision of a legitimating ideology united with an oppressive institutional order has been applied to prisons, to public schools, and to factories as well as to the mental hospital itself.[1] Institutions traditionally seen as expressions of reform and benevolence have increasingly come to be seen as modes of enforcing social control. Social historians, motivated by such politically-resonant views, have turned in increasing numbers to previously unfashionable institutional records as they seek to explain how Americans adjusted to a new kind of ordered, urban, and bureaucratized world.

Yet despite a parallel growth in interest in the social history of medicine during the past decade, we have had almost no historical attention paid to the 19th century general hospital (despite its prominence in contemporary dissections of medicine's social aspects).[2] There are obvious reasons. First, the hospital is a less ambiguous institution than an asylum or penitentiary. It is difficult to entirely deny the social necessity — and consequent legitimacy — of the hospital in the same categorical way that some sociologists and historians have questioned the social and moral logic of the mental institution or prison; typhus or cholera, fractures and kidney failure can hardly be dismissed as mere exercises in the labelling of deviance. Second, even if we see the early 19th century hospital as a total institution — if in some sense a necessary one — it still implies problems of historical documentation.[3] The vision of the hospital as total institution demands the analysis of a question ultimately emotional: how did the routine of a particular ward impinge on the individuals residing within it. Yet we have comparatively little evidence bearing directly on the patient's felt experience; like so many other objects of current historical interest, he was generally inarticulate. Case records, administrative records, statistical compilations, and the recollections of resident physicians do provide insight, but they are indirect and in some ways arbitrary. We must infer the nature of the patient's experience from chance remarks and patterns of institutional practice.

Moreover, the 19th century American hospital was neither uniform nor in any of its guises monolithic. It was a diverse and constantly evolving institution. In each generation, the hospital necessarily incorporated a number of variables:

the values and attitudes of society generally, changing levels of technical sophistication and the public awareness of such accomplishment, the demographic and ecological realities of the industrial city. The hospital embodies all these factors in a particular generation-specific configuration.

The following pages attempt to sketch the hospital's internal environment in the first three-quarters of the century — before the impact of these far-reaching changes which were to transform it into its mid-20th century shape. This early 19th century hospital was not at all the institution which our politically-sensitized expectations might have led us to assume. In its day-to-day operations, the hospital was no monolith contrived for the imposition of social control, but rather several different institutions, each of which was marked by a fragmented structure of authority.

At least two sub-cultures coexisted within the hospital: that of the patients and attendants who cared for them, on the one hand, and, on the other, that of the hospital's lay trustees and medical staff. And though physicians and trustees shared most of the values which characterized their class and time, the groups diverged sharply on many issues. The physician's allegiance to the institutionally-defined needs and priorities of medicine created priorities and perceptions inevitably different from those which informed the view of his lay superiors. The hospital in ante-bellum America can thus be more usefully seen as a battleground for the conflicting values of traditional stewardship and the priorities of an emerging profession than as the coherent expression of a carefully-articulated vision of society. In so diffuse a setting, the patient could still maintain a degree of psychological autonomy despite the pain and deprivation which might characterize his external life.

I

In the opening decades of the 19th century, the hospital patient's experience was shaped largely by social factors — those which determined the likelihood of his admission and those which shaped the hospital's internal organization. These were, of course, coupled with the biological impact of his illness; medicine was limited both in therapeutics and by its far from preeminent place in the hospital. Finally, the hospital was an urban institution, and even within this demographically atypical context treated only a minority of individuals suffering pain and disability. As late as 1870, only a small proportion of even urban medical care was provided in a hospital setting. A far greater number of the urban poor were treated as out-patients by dispensaries created, among other reasons, in the hope of keeping the working man and his family safe from the hospital's pauperizing influence.[4] Some dimension of the patient's experience must necessarily have been shaped by the stigmatizing expectation of failure and misery associated in his mind with hospital residence.

Even in the opening years of the century, America's prototypical hospitals assumed no uniform shape. The major distinction which has come to characterize 20th century hospitals, that between private or "voluntary" hospitals and the municipal hospital, had already come into existence. Conditions in the two kinds of hospitals differed markedly. Though the patient population in both was drawn largely from the city's workers and artisans, America's pioneer voluntary hospitals – the Pennsylvania, New York, and Massachusetts General – always contained substantial numbers of private patients.[5] Even more important to contemporary social sensibilities, free patients in the private hospitals were – at least by intent – drawn from among the worthy and industrious poor, individuals whose style of life, religious affiliation, or personal contacts in a small and still deferential society singled them out from among those dependent individuals whose appropriate place was the almshouse. Though it was difficult for contemporaries to accept the idea that an industrious laborer would not be able to provide for himself,[6] they conceded there were cases in which such prudent workers – and aged, widowed or unfortunately married women – might through illness find themselves destitute. As late as 1888, the New York Hospital's executive committee required that

All persons applying for free service must bring a note from some well-known citizen, or present other evidence that their inability to pay does not arise from improvidence or dissipation.

Or, alternately, when the Boston Children's Hospital was being organized in 1869, its founders contended that they would draw their patients from among the laboring class "who are doing their best to live respectably; whose dwellings, though humble, are neat and orderly; who have a laudable desire to rise out of their present condition." Indeed, one clearly expressed motivation for the establishment of both private hospitals and dispensaries in the late 18th and early 19th centuries was the need for an institution in which the worthy and hard-working, the widowed and incapacitated of good family, might be cared for without having to suffer the humiliation of almshouse incarceration.[7]

At least in terms of conventional social categories, the almshouse was a "receptacle" for the inadequate and to some extent the delinquent. However, in Boston, in New York, and in Philadelphia, the almshouse hospital had by 1820 already assumed the functions of a general municipal hospital in all but name.[8] Originally this was an unsought consequence of increases of scale within the almshouse. In the larger cities increasing numbers of the dependent sick and aged implied the development of separate wards for their care. Coupled with the institutionally-defined needs of the medical profession for teaching opportunities and the acquistion of clinical experience, the rapidly increasing numbers of paupers in these sick wards had created *de facto* hospitals in New York and Philadelphia by the end of the 18th century. In smaller communities, the few chronically-ill or aged patients in the local almshouse hardly justified a separate institutional arrangement; a local physician might call several times a week and the acutely-ill patients were simply sequestered in a few ward-like rooms.[9]

The almshouse was the hospital of last resort. Private hospitals throughout the century refused to accept either contagious or incurable cases as free patients — and in the case of chronic conditions would, in theory, discharge those who did not improve after a reasonable length of time. Venereal and alcoholic patients were admitted to voluntary hospitals on a pay basis only — though at suitably inflated rates and with demands for substantial payment in advance. If a patient developed a contagious disease while in a private institution, he or she might be transferred to the municipal hospital. The 20th century practice of transferring troublesome, chronic or even moribund cases from private to public hospitals has had a long, if not entirely admirable, pedigree.[10]

Nevertheless, the patient populations at both private and public hospitals had a good deal in common. Most significantly, they tended to suffer from semi-chronic and long-term ills and to remain in the hospital for many weeks or months. At the Philadelphia Almshouse, for example, for patients identified in an 1807 census, the average length of stay was a year in the general wards, three to five years in the incurable wards. At the Pennsylvania Hospital, a youthful resident could complain in 1808 that the in-patients were so routine, chronic and uninteresting, that his position would be intellectually barren without the variety provided by out-patient duties. A half-century later, MGH house physicians complained in similar terms of the chronic patients who cluttered their wards. Experienced hospital physicians contended in the fall of 1834 that the Philadelphia Almshouse was ill-suited to clinical teaching because "few acute cases are introduced into the Almshouse; they are generally old Chronic Cases, owing to the general disinclination to go to an almshouse. . . ."[11] Thus the patient's hospital experience was determined, first, by his location in society which defined the likelihood of his applying for admissions, second by the natural course of the illness from which he suffered. Most patients were simply not that sick; the critically-ill could not be kept alive by "extraordinary means" and most pre-bellum hospital patients were, in fact, not even bedridden. The Inspecting Committee at MGH could, for example, report after visiting every patient on October 27, 1826, that they found them all "comfortable not one very sick; Marcus Jones had walked out; and John Battiste gone home." Later in the century, in a similar vein, a PGH resident could in describing a typical day note that "most of the beds are now unoccupied, because many of the patients are convalescent and are out in the yard sitting, smoking, or reading."[12]

Our vision of the hospital as acute-care facility does not apply to their ante-bellum prototypes. Though it may have meant pain and long-term disability or discomfort, the patient's reality was determined — in addition to those social factors we have discussed — more by his physical sensations and his attitude toward these feelings, toward the sick role itself, than by the intrusions of medicine. We entertain a conventional picture of draconic bleeding and purging throughout the ante-bellum years, but it is much exaggerated. Hospital records indicate that bleeding was not routine for most of the period, but indicated only in certain well-demarcated conditions. And by the late 1830s and early 1840s, shifts in therapeutic views pointed toward an ever more lenient regimen, one emphasizing diet, rest, and the healing power of nature in place of the violent purges and emetics which had been more fashionable in the century's first quarter. By mid-century, beef tea had come to replace the previously omnipresent mercury.[13] Even surgery was limited largely to the setting of fractures, the treatment of superficial abscesses and ulcers — conditions not immediately life-threatening but implying lengthy hospitalization.[14] The relatively brief but highly intrusive works of the surgeon which have come to figure so prominently in the 20th century hospital were almost unknown. It was only natural that patients should have often been referred to as boarders and the fees of paying patients as board; it accurately reflected medicine's less than central role in defining the patient's hospital experience.

The line between sickness and dependency was revealingly ill-defined.[15] In the almshouse itself, the vagueness of these categories was exemplified in the loose way in which inmates were shifted from working wards to sick wards "if they are *much* indisposed" and then back depending both on their health and conditions of crowding in the different areas. Within the almshouse ward designations reflected ability to work as much as diagnosis. In 1835, for example, Philadelphia's Board of Guardians of the Poor suggested the following arrangement of women's wards in the Almshouse:

1. aged and helpless women in bad health
2. aged and helpless women who can sew and knit
3. aged and helpless women who are good sewers
4. spinners
5. scrubbers and washerwomen.

The logic of discharge as well as admission reflected non-medical criteria. At the Philadelphia General Hospital, for example, the chief resident complained as late as 1898 that his wards were crowded with patients who needed little or no treatment. "These people," he explained, "are sent to us because they have no one or no means to care for themselves and if we send them away when they are unfit to care for themselves we open the way for adverse criticism."[16]

A peculiar but parallel ambiguity surrounds venereal and alcoholic patients, conditions which were at once ailment and diagnosis of moral incapacity. In both public and private hospitals, such patients were treated differently from individuals suffering from other ills. (We have noted that venereal patients were admitted, at specially advanced rates in private hospitals and of necessity in municipal hospitals. The New York Hospital only accepted male venereal patients). At the New York Hospital, attending physicians were often unwilling to visit certain wards, particularly the black and venereal. At the Pennsylvania Hospital, blacks and patients suffering from a "certain disease" were housed in a small building separate from the main wing.[17] The physical isolation of venereal cases was seen by contemporaries as a precaution against contagion. (Both syphilis and gonorrhea were considered contagious in a period when most ills were not so regarded). However, the level of distaste and emotionality surrounding the enforced isolation of venereal cases indicates the moral as well as material contagion imputed to such sufferers.

Admissions procedures at the private hospitals incorporated both medical and social criteria. In the early years of the Massachusetts General Hospital, for example, patients had at first to make written application, then be visited by a physician, then be endorsed by the visiting committee of the Board of Trustees. Similar procedures were followed at both the Pennsylvania and New York Hospitals, in both of which institutions a written certificate from a board member or "contributor" could bring admission. (Cases of "sudden accident" could be admitted at any time, though even such trauma cases had retrospectively to be approved by formal action of the lay-boards' subcommittee). By the end of the century, only residual aspects of this deferential and particularistic system remained; the seemingly universalistic categories of medical diagnosis had replaced these older procedures.

Once admitted, the patient was treated as a moral as well as economic dependent. The internal routine of both municipal and private hospitals was as paternalistic and ordered as its managers could devise. Swearing, card-playing, drinking and "impertinence" were always grounds for dismissal. Managers and superintendents fought a similarly ceaseless battle against tobacco. Visitors were carefully regulated; as late as 1868, for example, the Pennsylvania Hospital limited visitors to the hour between twelve and one (except Sundays), while nurses and domestics were to have visitors only between two and six on Saturday.[18]

As noted before, convalescent and ambulatory patients were asked to work in the hospital. At New York's Bellevue Hospital, male patients helped row the boats which plied between the mainland and the hospitals and prisons on Blackwell's Island. At Bellevue as well, expectant mothers scrubbed floors within hours of their expected date of delivery.[19] At New York's municipal hospital on Blackwell's Island, venereal patients were expected to work a suitable length of time after their recovery so as to repay the city for the cost of their hospitalization. The Philadelphia Hospital maintained a punishment cell in which patients could be incarcerated for cause — usually impertinence, drinking, eloping, and fighting. At the New York Hospital, the inspecting committee early in the century occasionally found it necessary to punish intractable and profane patients by transferring them to the lunatic asylum and limiting them to a "low diet."[20] Discipline was complicated as we have seen by the fact that most patients were ambulatory, often egregiously so, in an institution which was as much boarding house and convalescent home as it was a means of treating the acutely ill.

But oppressive as is this picture of muscular stewardship, conditions in the 19th century hospital seem to have been a good deal less ordered than formal regulations might indicate. Enforcement was lax and throughout the first three-quarters of a century, physicians and trustees complained again and again of failures in discipline. Most of these were relatively minor. Patients spat where they were not supposed to, emptied bedpans with casual insouciance. Visitors represented a particularly vexing problem. In their numbers and behavior, visitors actively embodied a latent conflict in cultures as they pressed into the ward, bearing forbidden fruits and drink. As late as 1874, the Pennsylvania Hospital's Officer of Hygiene was dismayed to find patients sitting in their own clothes, receiving visitors at the wrong hours and in unacceptable numbers. One patient found room on his bed for four visitors and a dog.[21] Other infractions of discipline could be more serious. At the New York Hospital, the sailors paid for by the marine hospital fund created disturbances when placed among the other patients – and brawled and scaled walls for evenings of carousing when housed in their own building.[22] The longevity of the punishment cells in the Philadelphia Almshouse illustrate an endemic truculence among the patients – as do continuing complaints of the theft of food and supplies and the smuggling in of whiskey. There were even more direct modes of evading the hospital's stewardship. One was to elope, or, in the patronizingly whimsical terms of a Cincinnati General Hospital physician, "take French leave," "move the goods," or "give leg bond."[23] Patients might forcibly reject medicines proferred by attending physicians. An ultimately passive – but ultimate – mode of resistance was suicide, a problem which plagued the municipal hospitals throughout the century.

But the everyday realities of the ward were necessarily more significant than direct resistance in insulating the patient from the full impact of the social values which informed the attitudes of trustees and attending physicians. Both public and private hospitals seem to have been administered on a day-to-day basis by individuals who failed in some measure to share the moralistic assumptions of those individuals who wrote the formal rules. Moreover, the structure of authority in the hospital was such that no single group defined the environment confronting the patient. There were inevitable conflicts between medical boards and lay managers, between physicians and steward, between nurses and physicians. Order and "decent gratitude" might be expected of the dependent patient, but they could hardly be guaranteed in so fragmented an institution.

The hospital staff was organized and recruited in a fashion which implied such diffusion of authority. Most important, nurses and attendants were not, in the sense that we have come to understand the term, professional. In both public and private hospitals, they were drawn from among recovered patients – or from men and women with some nursing or housekeeping experience outside the hospital. Yet there was a certain *ad hoc* professionalism within the ante-bellum hospital and ward nurses often enjoyed long terms of employment. At the Pennsylvania Hospital, for example, Mary Falconer died in 1805 after having been "3 years a Patient, near two years Matron, and about 18 years a nurse in the house." At the Massachusetts General Hospital, wards had by the 1840s come to be called after those nurses identified so closely with their management; they were Becca Taylor's ward or Miss Styles', not the first medical or second surgical. In 1871, to cite another example, the medical superintendent at MGH presented to the trustees the case of Mary Sweetman who had worked in the hospital "for the past thirty-five years and is now broken down by age & infirmities & incapable of longer performing duty here or of doing much toward earning her living." She had — in the words of a Philadelphia physician describing the nurses at his own Episcopal Hospital — grown literally gray in service.[24] The relatively brief careers of *most* nurses and attendants only magnified the influence of that minority devoted for decades to the institution.[25] Such men and women were professionals in terms of length of tenure and accumulated skills; but their conception of their role did not imply a close identification with medical men and medical ideas. Servants, attendants, washerwomen and coachmen all encysted themselves within the hospital's wards. Most lived in and many were paid quarterly; an unquestioning patriarchalism was assumed, but as in many such relationships the would-be patriarchs were far away — either physically or emotionally. Physicians often complained of their inability to control and order servants, even their refusal to sweep floors or make beds when requested. In 1857, for example, the house physicians at the Massachusetts General Hospital complained vocally of the seeming disorganization which they encountered in the wards. "The servants clan together," as one put it, "and are not in subjection" to the steward. "There is no system or order & no one knows precisely his duty or keeps to it." When we learn from the parallel testimony of another resident that there were employed by the hospital "a brother & 3 sisters, a father 2 sons & a daughter, & several brothers & sisters," we can only assume that there was indeed a well-defined order in the hospital — but one for which the ambitious young physician felt neither empathy nor understanding.[26] Patients and employees were alike embedded in a specific hospital culture (in some degree a necessary characteristic of any institution with a majority of long-term inhabitants) which was largely lower-class in a society in which differing styles of life were a well-delineated indication of social-class identity.

The very paternalism of lay managers also helped create a degree of disunity. In both public and private hospitals (and especially and more lastingly in the private institutions) lay managers felt no temptation to subordinate their sense of personal responsibility to medical authority. Christianity and the imperatives of traditional stewardship, not the institutional needs of the medical profession, often determined particular hospital policies. This asymmetry of priorities was clear enough to contemporaries. When, for example, in 1846 the MGH attending physicians urged the erection of a medical college in the hospital's vicinity, the trustees voted flatly "that they cannot perceive any advantage to this institution to arise therefrom." As late as 1872, a trustees' committee at the same institution explained in attempting to clarify autopsy procedures:[27]

The trustees are to consider that their special duty is to make the Hospital useful to the greatest possible number of patients, as a curative establishment. This duty is paramount to the duty of making it subserve scientific purposes: and they must therefore remove from the popular mind all apprehensions which may deter persons from entering its wards.

Physicians throughout the century, and with increasing success, contended that a truer vision of social utility would grant investigation and teaching a higher value than the comfort of a particular patient population. Though lay managers accepted the need for the hospital to serve a role in medical education, they always assumed that this must remain secondary to that of succouring the needy. Through the first three-quarters of the century, conflict between lay and medical authority was endemic within both private and municipal hospitals. Were autopsies to be performed? And if so, under what conditions? How many medical students were to be admitted to the hospital's wards? And with what safeguards were patients to be utilized in clinical teaching? Like the fear of autopsy after death, the fear of being experimented upon during life was a widespread and much-apprehended aspect of the hospital's public image — a constant worry to lay boards and a necessary component in forming the patient's expectation of hospital treatment.

Lay managers assumed a personal responsibility for overseeing day-to-day affairs in the hospital. The standard mode of structuring this oversight centered on the role of an attending or visiting subcommittee chosen on a rotating basis from among the board members. Through the Civil War, all three pioneer voluntary hospitals — Pennsylvania, New York and Massachusetts General — benefited from weekly or biweekly visits by subcommittees of the trustees, called variously the attending or visiting committee, whose task it was to certify all admissions, determine whether they should be free or pay, and if pay at what rate. Until almost mid-century, the New York Hospital maintained a separate inspecting committee whose weekly task was to visit each patient, interview the medical staff, and ascertain that all the hospital's by-laws were scrupulously observed. At the Massachusetts General Hospital, the trustees voted explicitly that their rounds be made unaccompanied by medical staff so that patients and nurses might express potential grievances.[28] In particular cases, nurses and attendants could find in trustees a willing ear for complaints. The managers took their work seriously indeed; H.P. Bowditch could, for example, boast in 1851 that the attending managers had missed only twelve weekly meetings since the opening of the hospital in 1821. Visiting committee minute books preserved at both the New York and Massachusetts General Hospitals indicate the care with which this personal oversight was conducted; in the hospital's early years, for example, MGH visiting committee members would excuse themselves for not having visited particular patients — perhaps because they were bathing, or abroad on a pass, in one case because a female patient's complaint was of a "delicate nature." Lengthy terms of board membership allied with such personal involvement — both growing out of a generally unquestioned sense of responsibility for the execution of an appropriate stewardship — guaranteed trustees a strong voice in the hospital's day-to-day operations.[29]

The trustees' authority was exerted through a lay superintendent or steward who was responsible for the non-medical staff, purchasing, and discipline generally. It was assumed in the first half of the century that the superintendent would act as father of an extended family in the "house" he administered. These usages are not entirely metaphorical. The resident physicians ate at the steward's table, while the steward's wife normally served as matron in particular charge of the women's wards and such matters as laundering and cleaning. The qualities desired in a superintendent were neither hospital experience nor medical training — but rather the prudence, responsibility, and piety one might hope for in a business partner or vestryman.[30] The superintendent represented virtue and morality in an otherwise problematical environment — an ambassador from an ordered world to a culture ominously different.[31] It was inevitable that the steward should find himself beset by conflict as he sought to control the work of house-staff, on the one hand, and nurses, attendants, and workmen on the other.

Another factor diluting medical authority was the transitory quality of the hospital's resident staff. House physicians, young men who lived in the hospital and provided the great bulk of daily care, began their terms of residence with little clinical experience and small status in the medical community. On the other hand, the prestigious attending physicians and surgeons who frequently served long terms ordinarily appeared infrequently — to admit patients and oversee difficult cases — and in those few hours exerted comparatively small influence on the hospital's internal environment. Throughout most of the century, moreover, attending physicians and surgeons rotated responsibilities; three or four month periods of duty diluted still further the attending physicians' potential influence. Resident physicians came and went, attending physicians stayed but infrequently came; the Mary Falconers and Becca Taylors endured.

Still another aspect of the medical staff minimized their impact on the hospital's internal life; the recruitment of hospital physicians in the first three-quarters of the century guaranteed a maximum social distance between doctor and patient. Hospital internships were only for the ambitious and economically secure. At the Philadelphia Almshouse hospital a fee of $250 was required to secure the place. At the New York Hospital, house physicians through the first two-thirds of the century were drawn from among those young men who had been fee-paying pupils of the institutions' attending physicians (then served as "walkers" in the hospital for a year). Until the end of the century, house positions at both the Massachusetts General and Pennsylvania Hospitals were dependent upon election by their socially-prominent boards; men with no social standing or contacts in the community would have had a difficult time finding a place (or supporting themselves while they did so). Even for young men of good family and appropriate social connections, the lobbying for votes among board members could be an arduous and unpleasant task.[32]

The "young medical gentlemen" successful in their quest for a resident physicianship, tended to see their hospital charges in terms either of aversion or condescension. The attitude of house physicians veered erratically between the sentimental depiction of an occasional winsome lily, sullied by the soot of the venereal ward or genteel maiden-lady sunken in fortune – to a visceral revulsion at the habits of the brutes "kenneled" in the city's slums and who found their way into the hospital's wards. A resident physician, as one who served in the Philadelphia Hospital in the 1870s warned, would have to "be wary if he wants to have control of his wards, for the vicious and often criminal characters therein will stop short of nothing to circumvent him."[33] The stylized distance between doctor and patient is apparent in a number of ways. It can be seen in the formal and sentimentalized terms in which young physicians chose to recall or describe particular patients or incidents; it is apparent in their casually cynical comments on case records; it is apparent as well in the formal and stilted language of hospital regulations which implored staff members to be "patient and forebearing," "indulgent," to make every effort to treat hospital patients as though they were private patients. As late as 1889 a San Francisco hospital could warn its young clinicians that patients must be "treated with the dignity befitting sick people."[34] The house physicians' contacts with his ward patients might often be characterized by a casual brutality, but its casual aspect was as significant as the brutality itself. (Youthful Americans, moreover, who studied in European hospitals in this period, often recoiled from the far greater degree of inhumanity which characterized doctor-patient interactions in old-world hospitals).[35]

Ethnic and religious differences between physician and patient also widened the social distance between them. As early as 1807, for example, the patient population at the Philadelphia Almshouse was over 50% foreign born, more than half of them Irish. At the New York City Almshouse in 1796, of 622 inmates only 102 were American born. By the early 1840s – before the height of the famine immigration – the Irish rivalled the native-born in numbers even at the conservative and Quaker-dominated Pennsylvania Hospital. In 1851, a Brahmin trustee alarmed at the numbers of Irish laborers treated at the MGH, suggested that it might be advisable to build a "cheap building" or rent one in the vicinity of the hospital in which these ignorant immigrants might be treated. "They cannot appreciate," he explained, "& do not really want, some of those conveniences which would be deemed essential by most of our native citizens." In the same year, the Governors of the New York Hospital barred priests from routine visiting when, as diocesan protests emphasized, the great majority of its patients were Catholic.[36] And though it surfaced infrequently in administrative records, there must have been frequent misunderstanding and even hostility between Catholic nurses and attendants and Protestant administrators.[37]

There were indeed differences between the almshouse and the voluntary hospital in the first two-thirds of the century – differences perhaps obscured in this synoptic discussion. (Though the differences were not as marked as trustees of private institutions assumed and hoped they would be). Perhaps most significant, there were always pay patients in the voluntary hospitals. Bachelors, for example, travelers without domestic arrangements, small shopkeepers and artisans able to pay some small amount for board, and – in great numbers in the early years of the New York and Pennsylvania Hospitals — the chronic insane whose families found it easier to pay than to cope with them at home.[38] In all the private hospitals, income from private patients was carefully calculated in chronically-straitened budgets as they sought each year to arrive at a level of free-bed use consistent with their income.

Class lines did not end at the gate-keeper's office. A central aspect of the private hospital throughout the 19th and into the 20th century were the distinctions between pay and pauper patients which shaped every aspect of their hospital experience. In all private hospitals in the opening decades of the century and in some until its end, pay patients might bring their own servants (causing occasional problems with regard to hospital discipline).[39] They were not called upon to perform the cleaning and nursing demanded of free patients, nor were paying patients exposed to the eyes and hands of medical students as "teaching material." Private patients might supplement their diet with wines and other delicacies, while even medical treatment was to some extent shaped by their class identity. Reformer Elizabeth Blackwell, for example, could write enthusiastically about her sister's growing mastery of surgery — emphasizing that Emily would soon perform her first operation on a private patient.[40]

In addition to the existence of two classes of patients within the same walls, there were other characteristics which distinguished the municipal from the private hospitals. Perhaps most significantly, the municipal hospital was never to escape the almshouse stigma; it was and is a hospital of last resort. The voluntary hospitals seem also to have experienced a lower level of conflict between medical staff and lay managers. One explanation lies in the greater degree of identity between the elite members of such governing boards and the elite physicians who populated their attending staffs. Physicians at these prestigious private hospitals might have served as family physician to board members of their friends; in a few cases they might even be related; their children might attend the same schools and dancing classes. Lay members of municipal hospital governing boards were — from early in the century — men of a rather different sort. Though the mechanisms through which such positions were filled varied, they consistently reflected a much closer relationship to the political process. Such realities implied a greater degree of conflict between politically appointed trustees and the prominent medical men whose interests dictated a willingness to accept attending positions at municipal hospitals.[41]

II

Though the American hospital at the beginning of the 20th century had not assumed the dominant role in medical care that it would occupy by mid-century, major changes had already begun to manifest themselves in the last decades on the 19th century. Every aspect of such change not only altered the likelihood of a particular individual becoming a patient, but also the nature of his or her experience as a patient.

The factors reshaping the hospital were of two different sorts. One kind of factor was social and ecological. Most urban families could not withstand an extended siege of illness; a good proportion depended on more than one income even to maintain the tenuous level of economic stability they enjoyed when all family members were in good health. In the second half of the century, the numbers of such individuals and families increased inexorably.[42] A second source of change must be sought within the world of medicine, in those intellectual and institutional changes which made early 20th century medicine objectively different from medicine a century earlier — ultimately offering a different kind of social image and creating new popular expectations. A changing universe of ideas and technological realities also reshaped morbidity patterns and thus the prevalence of particular ills; the germ theory, for example, and related innovations in areas as diverse as immunology and civil engineering changed incidence and death rates in the acute infectious ills. Anaesthesia, antisepsis, and increasing anatomical and physiological knowledge made surgery a central aspect of hospital practice. (Technology in a more general sense — refrigerator cars, better ventilation, cheaper soap and plumbing — also played a role in changing morbidity patterns). In experiential terms, this meant that hospital patients were, by the first decade of the 20th century, more likely to be surgical patients, that their average stays were likely to be much shorter, that the hospital's intrusion into their identities was much more likely to be biological and physician-shaped — as exemplified literally in the surgeon's knife — than primarily social as shaped by the routine of the ward.

Such changes in morbidity and technical capacity were paralleled by a growing bureaucratization of the hospital staff. Lay boards played an increasingly distant role. No longer did managers from visiting committees, meet each week at the hospital, superintend individual admissions. Medical men and medical criteria had come to dominate both the admission process and the consequent treatment of those admitted. Nurses too identified more closely with the medical profession as they began to define themselves as professionals, their status based to a good extent on the prestige increasingly accorded the new medical knowledge. Ward nurses might still exert some of that day-to-day hegemony they had in earlier generations, but they drew that authority from a clearly subordinate position in a medically-oriented hierarchy of authority. Another significant influence on the internal organization of the hospital grew out of post-bellum attempts to control and rationalize the administration of charity — efforts which impinged on every benevolent endeavor, but within the hospital manifested themselves in an attempt to define appropriate chains of command, to end the casual patterns of patient-staff interaction which had characterized the pre-bellum hospital. Such informal ways seemed increasingly indefensible as would-be experts on benevolence sought to bring order and efficiency to the hospital. A newer sense of professionalism helped create an increasingly novel hospital environment — one in which the pre-bellum ward culture could hardly survive. Conflict between patients and nurses, between physicians and lay authorities, between physicians and nurses hardly ended with the 19th century — but the structure within which such conflict occurred did change.

At the beginning of the 19th century, as I have tried to suggest, the hospitalized poor were to an extent buffered by the social distance which separated them from physicians and trustees, by the physician's somewhat tangential relationship to the hospital, and by the consequently fragmented structure of authority within the institution. Poor patients were insulated as well from the institution's potentially intrusive impact by their identity with a lower class (and often ethnically or religiously diverse) sub-culture – but nevertheless a stratum from which nurses and attendants were ordinarily recruited. If and when they did find their way into a hospital, the dignity of pay patients was protected by their class identity; the possession of their own servants and consumption of their own wines symbolized the ability of paying patients to bring into the status of patient the deference accorded them in the world outside the hospital. The poor, on the other hand, had always found the hospital a place of misery, but a novel texture undoubtedly characterized that discomfort in the early 20th century hospital. If they were warmer and better-clothed, their food more nourishing, their likelihood of survival better, their identity was subject to increasing pressures from an ever-more bureaucratized institution – one, moreover, in which the quality of his or her experience was increasingly likely to be shaped by medical men and medical measures. The rich had always fared better than the poor – but now both rich and poor shared the hospital experience to a greater extent; not only were the moderately prosperous more likely to be hospitalized but the nature of their experience was in at least some ways increasingly similar to that of their less prosperous fellow patients.

University of Pennsylvania   Charles E. Rosenberg

FOOTNOTES

*This discussion is based on materials from a larger study in progress on medical care in America, 1790-1910. I should like to acknowledge the support of the Rockefeller Foundation Division of Humanities in the academic year 1976-77 and the National Institutes of Health, LMO2826-01.

1. We have, at the same time, become accustomed to a reductionist sociology of knowledge which dismisses the views of reformers and physicians as ideology, as more or less consciously self-serving efforts to legitimate the social control of behavior – and thus particular relationships of power and status. Though not consistent in tone or emphasis, the works of Michel Foucault, Thomas Szasz, and R.D. Laing have exerted a parallel *political* impact, undercutting the legitimacy of the putatively value-free formulations of 19th and 20th century psychiatry. Similar arguments have been employed widely in other areas of social policy and historical interpretation, as, for example, the debate over public schools and schooling generally and, more recently, in the women's movement. See, for example, Michel Foucault, *Madness and Civilization: A History of Insanity in the Age of Reason* (New York, 1965); Szasz, *The Myth of Mental Illness: Foundations of a Theory of Personal Conduct* (New York, 1961); *The Manufacture of Madness: A Comparative*

Study of the Inquisition and the Mental Health Movement (New York, 1970). The sociological discussion of labelling has become voluminous in the past decade. For a recent attempt to outline such approaches, see: Robert Perrucci, *Circle of Madness: On Being Insane and Institutionalized in America* (Englewood Cliffs, 1974). David J. Rothman's *The Discovery of the Asylum: Social Order and Disorder in the New Republic* (Boston, 1971) has been the most influential attempt to apply these concepts to ante-bellum America.

2. There have been several recent exceptions: Morris Vogel, "Boston's Hospitals, 1870-1830: A Social History" (unpublished dissertation, University of Chicago, 1974) and Vogel, "Patrons, Practitioners and Patients: The Voluntary Hospital in Mid-Victorian Boston," in Daniel W. Howe, ed., *Victorian American* (Philadelphia, 1976), 121-138 and William H. Williams, *America's First Hospital: The Pennsylvania Hospital, 1751-1841* (Wayne, Pa. 1976) have both been useful as has the earlier study of *New England Hospitals 1790-1833* (Ann Arbor, 1957), by Leonard Eaton. We have no synthesis of American hospital history comparable to those by Brian Abel-Smith, *The Hospitals 1800-1948. A Study in Social Administration in England and Wales* (Cambridge, 1964) and Gwendoline M. Ayers, *England's First State Hospitals and the Metropolitan Asylums Board. 1867-1930* (London, 1971).

3. Though the concept of "total institution" was employed in Bruno Bettelheim's classic studies of behavior in German concentration camps, it has been presented most systematically by Erving Goffman: *Asylums: Essays in the Social Situation of Mental Patients and other Inmates* (Garden City, 1961). Allied with the critical interpretations of medicine's objective diagnostic categories cited in note 1, the concept of the total institution has had a powerful social impact in the past decade.

4. For a unique study of hospital statistics in 1873, see: J.M. Toner, "Statistics of Regular Medical Associations and Hospitals of the United States," *Transactions of the American Medical Association,* 24 (1973), 287-333. On dispensaries and the motivations for their founding, see Charles E. Rosenberg, "Social Class and Medical Care in Nineteenth-Century America: This Rise and Fall of the Dispensary," *J. Hist. Medicine,* 29 (1974), 32-54.

5. This practice was sharply distinct from English prototypes which in this period were still exclusively eleemosynary; only the Royal Infirmary of Edinburgh seems to have constituted an exception in the late 18th century. Williams, *America's First Hospitals,* 15. Abel-Smith, *The Hospitals* emphasizes that the poorest among the English poor populated the workhouses when sick, not the voluntary hospitals. In America, the categories of pay and free were complicated by the admission of seamen as pay patients in both the Pennsylvania and New York Hospitals. Beginning in the late 1790s, merchant seamen were required to contribute twenty cents a month into a fund used to underwrite the costs of their hospitalization. The New York Hospital always cared for especially large numbers of such patients and both it and the Pennsylvania Hospital squabbled intermittently with the collectors of their ports over rates and speed of payment until the 1880s. At the Pennsylvania Hospital between its opening in 1752 and December of 1830, 28,105 patients were admitted, and of these 13,604 were pay patients. W.G. Malin, *Some Account of the Pennsylvania Hospital, Its Origin, Objects and Present State* (Philadelphia, 1831), 14. By mid-century, the balance had changed decisively toward the free side: for the three years ending in December of 1852, the average number of patients in the hospital was 154, of whom 115 were free and 39 pay patients. April 25, 1852, Minutes, Board of Managers, Pennsylvania Hospital Archives (hereinafter PHA).

6. "In our country," as prominent Massachusetts General Hospital physicians James Jackson and John Collins Warren put it in 1822, "there are few persons, few men at least, who would ever stand in need of public or private charity, after their entrance into active life, if they were uniformly virtuous and industrious." Jackson and Warren to Richard Sullivan and Theodore Lyman, October 30, 1822, Venereal Disease File, Massachusetts General Hospital Archives (hereinafter MGHA).

7. Entry for June 2, 1888, Minutes, Executive Committee, Board of Governors, New York Hospital Archives (hereinafter NYHA); Francis H. Brown, et al, *A Statement made by Four Physicians, In Reference to the Establishment of a Children's Hospital in the City of Boston* (Boston, 1869), 2. For other representative discussions of the need for hospitals appropriate to the legitimate needs of the worthy poor, see: MGH, *Address of the Board of Trustees of the Massachusetts General Hospital to the Public...* (Boston, 1814), 5-6; N.I. Bowditch, *A History of the Massachusetts General Hospital. To August, 5, 1851.* Second ed., with a Continuation to 1872 (Boston, 1872), 4n-5n; Williams, *America's First Hospital,* 14, 125-6, 148.

8. The almshouse continued to care for the dependent, the aged, and the insane as well as minor offenders, most prominently prostitutes and the alcoholic. Later in the 19 century, the almshouse function gradually differentiated itself into more specialized forms: infant asylums, insane asylums, homes for the aged and incurable, contagious disease hospitals and outdoor relief.

9. This was true even in cities as large as Boston or Charleston. One of the reasons for the founding of the Massachusetts General Hospital was the inadequate hospital facilities at the Boston Almshouse. This generalization is also based on a reading of the Charleston Almshouse managers' minutes, South Carolina Historical Society, Charleston.

10. Robert J. Carlisle, *An Account of Bellevue Hospital with a Catalogue of the Medical and Surgical Staff from 1736 to 1894* (New York, 1893), 42; Society of the Alumni of City (Charity) Hospital, *Report for 1904. Together with a History of the City Hospital and a Register of its Medical Officers from 1864 to 1904* (New York, 1904), 35.

11. The Almshouse census is included among the papers of the Philadelphia Board of Guardians of the Poor, Philadelphia City Archives (hereinafter PCA); Samuel C. Hopkins to Board of Managers, January 25, 1808, Medical Staff Papers, PHA; "Report of the Committee appointed to confer with the Trustees of the University and the Jefferson College," October 27, 1834, Minutes, Board of Guardians; Testimony of Drs. Courcillon and Hooker before Committee on Internal Affairs, January 22, 1858, House Officers-Administration, File, MGHA. I should like to thank Priscilla Clement for the analysis of the 1807 Philadelphia Almshouse census; it is drawn from a thesis on the pre-bellum almshouse currently in progress.

12. Entry for October 27, 1826, Minutes, Inspecting Committee, MGHA; John Roberts, "Notes of Life in a Hospital by a Resident Physician, January, 1877," Historical Collections, College of Physicians of Philadelphia.

13. At the New York Hospital, beef tea was not prescribed at all between 1820 and 1837, while 5630 prescriptions were recorded in 1858. New York Hospital, *Report of the Committee on Retrenchment. May 3, 1859. Printed by order of the Board* (New York, 1859), 11-12. For a general discussion of this shift in therapeutic practice, see: Charles E. Rosenberg, "The Therapeutic Revolution: Medicine, Meaning and Social Change in Nineteenth-Century America," *Perspectives in Biology and Medicine* (forthcoming, 1977).

14. ,This pattern was not altered by the availability of anaesthesia. In October of 1858, for example, a dozen years after the introduction of ether, a typical month at New York Hospital's First Surgical Division saw 109 patients treated – and only eight operations performed. Three of these were for compound fracture of the skull (presumably desperate and perfunctory procedures on moribund accident victims). The management, that is, of most "surgical conditions," was largely expectant and emphasized regimen. Thomas Markoe to Board of Governors, December 3, 1858, Papers, Board of Governors, NYHA.

15. Until the middle third of the century, specific diagnosis and – indeed – the very concept of most ills being differentiated in terms of a specific cause and course and characterized by specific lesions was atypical in the medical profession. Holistic definitions of sickness as a total state of the organism were consistent with social definitions of need and dependency; both were inclusive and anti-reductionist and emphasized the continuing interaction between organism and external environment. The contrast with most mid-20th-century views needs no underlining.

16. May 8, 1809, Minutes, Board of Physicians, Board of Guardians, "Report on Womens' Wards;" July 20, 1835, Minutes, Board of Guardians; D.E. Hughes to J. Musser, February 9, 1898, Chief Resident Physician, Letterbook. See also a parallel memorandum of the chief resident physician, dated July 21, 1902, and indicating the persistence of the problem. Chief Resident Physician's Memos, 1897-1904. All PCA.

17. In revealingly parallel incidents at the Massachusetts General and Pennsylvania hospitals, patients admitted as venereal cases had their rates of board lowered when attending physicians found that they had mistaken their diagnoses. December 3, 1832, Minutes, Board of Managers, PHA; March 23, 1827, Visiting Committee Minutes, MGHA. For the unwillingness of the New York Hospital to receive female venereal patients, see: New York Hospital, *Report of a Committee of the Governors on the Occasional Prevalence of Erysipelas in that Hospital. . .* (New York, 1836). Alcoholics, significantly, were treated with a punitive attitude similar to that shown venereal patients. The Managers of the Pennsylvania Hospital, for example, decided that any patient admitted as a result of the intemperate use of strong drink would be denied "free intercourse" and the privileges of the House, including the use of pen and ink or visitors without the express permission of one of the attending managers or physicians. January 29, 1821, Minutes, Board of Managers, PHA.

18. March 30, 1868, Minutes, Board of Managers, PHA.

19. Case of Margaret Henry, November 6, 1851, Casebook kept at Bellevue Hospital, R.L. Brodie, Waring Historical Library, Medical College of South Carolina, Charleston; Charles E. Rosenberg, "The Practice of Medicine in New York a Century Ago," *Bulletin Hist. Med.* 41 (1967), 239.

20. Entries for November 9 and November 20, 1813, Minutes, Inspecting Committee, NYHA; Charity Hospital Alumni, *Report for 1904,* 38-9. The "black book" in which the names of those punished at the Philadelphia Hospital and their infractions were maintained as late as the 1890s. Surviving volumes are preserved in PCA.

21. July 7, 13, 1874, Daily Report Ledger, Office of Hygiene, PHA. D.B. St. John Roosa, *The Old Hospital and other Papers,* Second rev. ed. (New York, 1889), 12.

22. "Report of Committee to Consult with Physicians and Surgeons on Opening the New House," Fall, 1841, Papers, Board of Governors, NYHA; Charles Starr to Isaac Carow, June 28, 1842, Papers, Board of Governors, NYHA.

23. These phrases were all drawn from Casebook, Female, 1837-40, Cincinnati General Hospital Archives. See also, W.G. Thompson, "Odd Remarks of Dispensary and Hospital Patients. 1883-1885," Rare Book Room, New York Academy of Medicine.

24. Mary Falconer's executrix asked for payment of her salary for the years between 1802 and 1805. August 26, 1805, Minutes, Board of Managers, PHA; N.I. Bowditch to Marcus Morton, Feburary 29, 1844, N.I. Bowditch Biographical File, MGHA; Benjamin S. Shaw to Board of Trustees, August 31, 1871, Personnel File, MGHA; Elliston Morris, "Episcopal Hospital in 1888 and 1912," *Episcopal Hospital Reports*, 2 (1912), 101-2. The New York Hospital provided in 1821 for an increase in salary of 50% for nurses after five years service, an increase of another third after ten years service, and after twenty years an annuity of $25.00 and, in case of need, "support in the hospital during life." In 1845 the New York Hospital employed three female nurses with over ten years service, and three female and two male nurses with more than five years service. T.R. Smith and W.A. Stewart, "Report of Committee of Revision on 13th Chapter: also resolution respecting nurses passed Feb. 6, 1821," Papers, Board of Governors, NYHA.

25. At night even the normally tenuous structure of authority disappeared. Nursing was a five A.M. to nine P.M. occupation and "watchers" were engaged to oversee only the critically ill after nine. Convalescent patients routinely cared for their more severely-ill ward mates at night. At the Pennsylvania Hospital, medicines were to be administered by the night watchman if required. May 29, 1848, Minutes, Board of Managers, PHA.

26. The description of the hospital's network of relatives is drawn from the testimony of house physician Hasket Derby, fragment dated 1857-58, "Statements of House Physicians &c," House Officers-administration of, File, MGHA. Other testimony at the same hearing refers to the ability of the servants to "clan together" and thwart the will of the youthful physicians. The sense that a well-conceived and intractable underground dominated ward life was not infrequently expressed by lay authorities. As early as 1808, for example, a committee of Philadelphia's Board of Guardians reported that they could no longer tolerate the theft, introduction of whiskey, "drunkeness, elopement and fornication, and the perfectly systematized and good understanding which exists between the persons concerned, . . . " Charles Lawrence, *History of the Philadelphia Almshouses and Hospitals . . .* (Philadelphia, 1905), 52.

27. February 22, 1846, cited in Bowditch, *History,* 197; Samuel Eliot and S.G. Howe, "Report of Committee on Autopsies, December 27, 1872," Autopsy File, MGHA.

28. Bowditch, *History,* 71.

29. The visiting committee reported on November 17, 1826: "Saw all the patients excepting David Foley who was absent and Mrs. Damon whose complaint being of a delicate nature, it was deemed expedient not to obtrude upon her." Minutes, MGHA; Bowditch, *History,* 383. Samuel Coates' forty-one year tenure on the Pennsylvania Hospital Board of Managers, 1785-1825, was an extreme example of such lengthy tenures – but not entirely atypical. In 1857, for example, George Newbold and Benjamin Swan retired from the New York Hospital's Board of Governors, Newbold after forty-eight years on the Board and having served as its president for twenty-four, Benjamin Swan after thirty years of membership. George Newbold to the Governors of the New York Hospital, October 5, 1857; Swan to Governors, January 5, 1857, Papers, Board of Governors, NYHA.

30. The nature of the steward's personal responsibilities is symbolized neatly by the MGH visiting committee when they recorded the start of a new steward's tenure: "Nathan Gurney Esq. & his wife took possession of the Hospital as Superintendent &

Matron, of this Institution and keys of the Building were delivered to them with the inventory of the furniture. The several officers & servants of the institution were introduced to Mr. & Mrs. Gurney as Superintendent & Matron & requested to conform to their orders as such." July 1, 1825 Minutes, MGHA. Nathan Gurney's biographical file in the MGHA includes a revealing series of letters of recommendation.

31. When, in the mid-1850s, the MGH trustees appointed a salaried "resident physician" to undertake the steward's traditional duties it marked a first step toward unification of authority lay and medical under the trustees; it was not entirely popular with the hospital's attending staff. A similar proposal two decades earlier at Philadelphia's Almshouse Hospital had also been opposed by the board of attending physicians. November 2, 1835, Minutes, Board of Guardians, Philadelphia City Archives.

32. October 19, 1835, Minutes, Board of Guardians. As late as 1910, the superintendent of the Pennsylvania Hospital warned applicants without suitable Philadelphia connections that it would be fruitless to apply. D. Test to G.H.R. Ross, February 25, 1910, Superintendent's letterbooks, PHA. In the second half of the century there was a movement toward the instituting of competitive examinations for hospital appointments; the Boston City Hospital, for example, followed such a system from its founding in 1864. Examinations did not, of course, guarantee equal access to young men of all classes and backgrounds.

33. The term "kenneled" is from an extraordinarily enlightening diary kept by a resident in Philadelphia's municipal hospital: Arthur A. Bliss, *Blockley Days. Memories and Impressions of a Resident Physician, 1883-1884* (Philadelphia, 1916), 35, cf. 63 and *passim* for many such quotes; Roberts, "Notes of a Hospital Resident," 17.

34. February 19, 1889, Minutes, Committee on Clinics, Cooper Medical College, Lane Medical Library, Stanford University.

35. "For brutality I do not think his equal can be found," a young Bostonian wrote of one of Paris' leading clinicians in 1832: "If his orders are not immediately obeyed, he makes nothing of striking his patient and abusing him harshly. A favorite practice of his is to make a handle of a man's nose, seizing him by it and pulling him down on to his knees ... " Howard Payson Arnold, *Memoir of Jonathan Mason Warren, M.D.* (Boston, 1886), 85. Hospital records do indicate occasional specific examples of brutality toward patients as well as formal prescriptions against disciplining patients without the concurrence of steward or managers; it is difficult to judge, however, as to the frequency of the physical abuse of patients.

36. Philadelphia Almshouse Census for 1807; Carlisle, *Account of Bellevue* 10; Charles Jackson to N.I. Bowditch, October 1, 1851, Administration, Care of Patients, General Statements File, MGHA. Bowditch himself was appalled at the number and condition of the Irish who had begun to fill his hospital. *History*, 366, 454-5; J. Roosevelt Bayley to Board of Governors, January 6, 1851; Henry J. O'Neill to Board of Governors, 1851, Papers, Board of Governors, NYHA.

37. See, for example, the comments in an Irish nurse's diary at the New York Hospital who, though repelled by rancid butter at dinner, felt it "useless to complain because if we do it may irritate the religious feelings of our superintendent and he will soon point out the way to the gate.... our butter is rotten and stinks worse than a Sconk but it must be borne with for like everything else if we complain our godly Superintendent will tell us you may consider yourself discharged for the Lord sent it and you must eat it." James Duffe, Diary, New York Historical Society, March 30, 1844. This diary by a male nurse in the New York Hospital's Marine House — in which seamen on government contract were treated — provides a unique insight into the ward routine of an ante-bellum hospital.

38. Care of the insane was an explicit and prominent motive in the founding of all three pioneer voluntary hospitals. The Massachusetts General Hospital's "insane hospital" was opened before the general hospital itself (1818 as opposed to 1821), while the New York Hospital's first separate building was established on the hospital grounds as early as 1808. The possibility of adjusting rates according to the means of insane paying patients, allowed trustees to maintain a sanguine attitude toward their financial problems. Society of the New York Hospital, *An Account of the New York Hospital* (New York, 1820), 12.

39. In at least one case, difficulty arose from the disparity in pay between the private servant and the institution's nurses. June 24, 1805, Minutes, Board of Managers, PHA: W.F. Otis, N.I. Bowditch, and Wm. F. Otis, "Report of Trustees Committee. . .," 1841-45, Lawsuits File, MGHA.

40. Elizabeth Blackwell to Sara Elder, October 16, 1857, Archives, Medical College of Pennsylvania.

41. The older histories of almshouse hospitals all contain appropriate documentation. See, for example, the histories by Carlisle, Lawrence, and that compiled by the Alumni Association of New York's Charity Hospital, all cited previously and: John W. Croskey, ed., *History of Blockley. A History of the Philadelphia General Hospital from its Inception* (Philadelphia, 1929). It should be emphasized, however, that the political atmosphere of the municipal hospitals so galling to young residents and visiting physicians alike, did not necessarily provide worse medical care. As one resident confessed, his decisions were on occasion far less humane than the political appointees with whom he worked. "It must be confessed that the yound medical man was too often disposed to be sarcastic, cynical, suspicious, and drive away every applicant who did not bear in his or her body the symptoms of being an interesting medical or surgical case." The admissions officers, on the other hand, would often ignore his verdict that the patient was "not sick enough" and admit the poor sufferer anyway. Bliss, *Blockley Days,* 14. Morris Vogel's, "Boston Hospital," also emphasizes the way in which the Boston City Hospital was more open to pressure from Boston's less-than-Brahmin elements than the comparatively rigid and unresponsive MGH.

42. This variable is extremely difficult to weigh — for there were particular areas of dense population in the pre-bellum city and this congestion did not guarantee high rates of hospital utilization. Though significant, the ecological variable does not correlate in any simple way with the changing propensity of individuals to seek medical care within a hospital setting. It nevertheless remained significant, even into the twentieth-century. As late as 1905, for example, male admissions outnumbered female 5,243 to 2,780 at the Cincinnati General Hospital, while single men outnumbered married men almost four to one (2,696 to 741), Cincinnati General Hospital, *Annual Report, 1905* (Cincinnati, 1906), p. 23.

Arthur E. Imhof

THE HOSPITAL IN THE 18TH CENTURY: FOR WHOM?

The Charite Hospital in Berlin, The Navy Hospital in Copenhagen, the Kongsberg Hospital in Norway

I. The Problem of Health and Disease.

Many a historian is at present occupied with the phenomenon of death. To a large extent, this boom is due to the progress of historical demography within the last two to three decades and particularly the preeminent role of mortality, which served as the focus of some pioneering researches.[1] By refining the questions asked and the methods' employed, particularly by reifying death and subjecting it to the scientific method, which encompasses more than the act of dying – and its consequent rituals, the bier, the casket and the open grave – recent research encourages the comprehension both of death as a statistical unit, as a biological fact, and of the changing attitude of the living in the face of death up to the present day. Yet our understanding of death seems far from complete.[2]

An important aspect of the study of death which is the question that concerns us here is death's corollary sickness.[3] This is not to imply that every disease leads to death. However, in view of the inadequate medical cures, the loss of health was judged the first step to death more commonly than today. In his admirable study: *Western Attitudes toward Death from the Middle-Ages to the Present*, Phippe Aries suggests four successive basic attitudes. He starts with the medieval conception of death as the self-evident, accepted, collective destiny of the human species and ends with the tendency in our industrial societies to repress and hide death, as if it were a nasty, irritating, private affair. It would be necessary to do similar research over a long period of time concerning the development of the Western attitude toward health and sickness, the recuperation from sickness, the desire of the individual to get well, and the sense of social obligation. Concretely expressed: How does one deal with sickness, epidemics, accidents, the loss of one's own physical and mental capacities, psychic instability, suicide attempts and temptation to commit suicide? Had both the health and the sickness of one's own body already become a problem to be pondered and if this was indeed the case, at what point in time did they become such a problem? Were there, in this case, standardized, collective behavior patterns and if so on the part of what groups; and to what intent and to what purpose were they standardized and controlled? Following Alfred Perrenoud, who recently dealt with the social inequality before death in the 17th century, and Roger Charter and Daniel Roche who dealt with the art of dying from the 15th to the 18th century[4] one would have to conduct historical analyses specifically with reference to the "social inequality in the face of sickness. . . health" and the "art of being sick. . . of recuperating."

The omnipresence of death from the Middle Ages until modern times produced a "familiarity with death," a "coexistence of the living and the dead," even a "promiscuity between the living and the dead." This prompted Ariès to speak about a "tamed death" with reference to that era.[5] It may be assumed that the pervasiveness of sickness in the earlier period – the high infant mortality, the mortality of mothers in childbirth, the mortality of people succumbing to epidemics in their prime – had led to a familiarity with all forms of ill health. The certainty of death and the frailty of life from which we nowadays have become estranged due to individual and collective repression, were at that time self-evident and commonplace. No one ever thought of escaping or glorifying them. If they were able to interpret death as a kind of acceptance of the law of nature,[6] this concept with respect to sickness was probably not in the foreground. Certainly we would not go as far as Jacques Dupâquier, who speaks in this context of a kind of biologically terrorized population.[7] This explanation is too present minded. Even if the historian no longer interprets sickness in terms of theology, one must constantly make an effort to face sickness through the eyes of one's contemporaries. François Lebrun's view of the 17th and 18th centuries experience suffering and sickness as a mystery is more acceptable.[8] Sicknesses were willed by God. They represented either individual, or in the case of epidemics, collective punishments for the sins committed, or else they represented a warning toward proper preparation for death. The sickness of the body was supposed to help the recuperation of the soul. Even when a physician was consulted, his job was more the salvation of his patient's soul than that of his body.[9] "Suffering is bliss, the only pleasure in God," is the opinion of Jacques Revel and Jean-Pierre Peter in their study of the history of the sick and the changing conceptions of the frailty of the body.[10]

But as long as sickness was considered an expression of supernatural forces faith and superstition were closely linked. There was only one step between the concept of divine intervention and the intervention of the devil or of demons of disease, one step between the appeal to the church and the clergy or to magic, quacks and sorcerers, one step between prayer, confession and repentance as therapy or escape to magical rituals, vulgar resort to drugs of all kinds and evocation of archaic cultural values.[11]

But even among the few laymen who were able to grasp somatic illnesses for what they were, namely disfunctions, we do not observe any specific interest in elaboration of the interlinkage of the biological functions until the middle of the 19th century. Well into the 19th century, for instance, tuberculosis of the lungs was as deadly as many varieties of cancer nowadays, yet neither the educated patient nor his family came to terms with the reason underlying the sickness or probed its scientific character. Patients who were treated by a physician or surgeon demanded no information from him, even if the subsequent course of the sickness had been evident from the diagnosis.[12] Frequently, several physicians were consulted, less because of medical reasons than to demonstrate the life-style which was commensurate with the status one occupied in society.[13] People died in accordance with a traditional ritual, and just as a person presided over his own death [14] so he presided over his own sickness.

Aside from the economic and social barriers between the trained doctor and large parts of the population (paramedics were not only socially closer to the people, but were also cheaper, hence more attractive)[15] there existed in the 18th century a mental schism between the doctor and the patient. As long as the disease had a magic-supernatural character and no scientific interest in sickness itself prevailed, there was no logical reason to be treated by a rationalistic physician or surgeon who gave exact and comprehensible instructions, quite apart from the fact that even with medical treatment the prospects of getting well were scanty. The typical sentiment was that: "If I lie on the bier, no one can help me. If not, I could get well in any case."[16] There was suffering, but it was largely undifferentiated, as in cases of high fever, unknown children's diseases, old age and infirmity.[17]

With this in mind, two possible avenues of study are suggested. One could start from the premise of *man's suffering* and try to differentiate the sickness and investigate the specific possibilities of cure, tracing both back to the 18th century. However, a retrospective diagnosis of this sort for the 18th century, in effect a retrospective epidemiology, risks running aground on epistemological issues stemming from the gap between the nosological system in 18th century medicine and the etiological system of the 20th century. Further, a descriptive, natural history of morbidity is liable to abstract the human content considerably and in consequence entirely disregard the patients and the doctors.[18] This was certainly the case of the plague. "Human beings are here only a part of a system of living things which was defined by the internal equilibrium, antagonism and biological adaptation."[19] For the pest-flea, the human being is only an object of interest if the rat, otherwise preferred, or some other rodent is absent.[20] This is not to undermine the importance of the study of carriers of disease, which is a vital element of retrospective ecology, but it would not touch upon the essential focus of the present essay, the patient.

The second possibility is to start on the premise of *the suffering man* and to attempt an "anthropocentric" investigation as a key element of a social history of disease, an historical anthropological approach only recently conceived at least in Germany. This approach is that of the sociologist Wolf Lepenies, who delineates the pressing topics to be dealt with in the framework of an interdisciplinary historic-anthropological cooperation and assigns to the historians the areas of reproduction and the threat to life, and the related subjects of sexuality, birth, family and childhood — in other words the topics of sickness and death which as we have pointed out, dominated the Middle Ages and into the early part of the modern era.[21] Jacques Revel and Jean-Pierre Peter go even a step further. Within the framework of their socio-historical investigation of morbidity, illnesses become significant factors that constantly demand the demographic, economic, institutional, political, administrative, religious analysis for their explanation.[22] Jean-Pierre Goubert speaks, in this connection, about an "integrated history of health".[23] It is to this approach that investigation has to turn. Starting from the premises of historical demography, three different systems of reference were developed which the components "morbidity", "mortality" and "socio-economic structure" are interconnected along with a selection of further components derived from a "total history."[24]

Having outlined the topic to this extent, we are now in the position to give a first answer to our question: "The hospital in the 18th century: For whom?" In terms specifically of stratification only members of marginal groups were involved, people for whom in case of loss of health there remained no other choice: military personnel of the lower ranks as well as their families; single apprentices and journey men; the service personnel in households that were not well off; the lowest strata within the purview of a charity organization; the aged and the infirm without family; and finally lower-class groups who, for reasons of work depended on permanent health and their physical well-being and could not avoid the hospital.

The hospitals of the 18th century were organized to meet the needs of these groups: military hospitals, hospitals for the care of the aged and the infirm, hospitals for the poor. In the 18th century it would have been meaningless to establish a hospital for the middle or upper class given the preconceived attitudes toward hospital and their organizations. They would have remained empty or, like the health baths, they would have been changed into establishments of acceptable social interaction. In a functioning hospital, the physician presides over the course of recuperation in an authoritarian manner. Tolerance of authoritarianism in the 18th century was reserved for the marginal groups who lacked any other choice.

In order to relate these reflections to the empirical material, three hospitals from the 18th century European scene were selected: The Charité-Hospital in Berlin 1731-1742, the Navy Hospital in Copenhagen 1788-1791 and the Hospital of Kongsberg (a mining town) in Norway 1769-1773.[25] The Charité Hospital was at the same time a military hospital, a hospital for poor sick people, and a hospital for the aged and the infirm with a capacity of 400 beds; it was simultaneously a clinical training center. Its management was technically under the jurisdiction of the alms administration. The Navy Hospital in Copenhagen, which goes back to the 1650's, was intended mainly for sailors wounded in wartime. It could house up to 1,000 persons. In times of peace, it was used partly as a hospital, partly as a shelter for the poor or workhouse for the impoverished relatives of the sailors. The institutions of both Berlin and Copenhagen were modern in the sense that they pursued curative aims; therapy was used where there was a prospect of cure. The task of the Hospital in Kongsberg, the miners' city in Southern Norway with a population of about 8,000, was mainly to give shelter and sustenance, not to treat patients. With its 12 beds, it was in no position to do that, in view of the numerous miners' casualties and diseases. We are dealing here with a type of hospital which goes back hundreds of years and in which the doctor's care did not actually exist.

II. The Thresholds of Disease

One of the problems of health and its complementary concept of disease lies in the fact that both are so difficult to define. According to the World Health Organization, the state of health is not characterized merely by the absence of sickness. Complete physical, mental and social well-being is essential.[26] This ideal postulate is seldom accomplished, since the plurality of all people has in some sense been "sick" at all times. "Health" and "sickness" have been defined repeatedly for daily use in less absolute terms.[27]

In the light of the practical work stemming from the material on 18th century hospitals, it seemed most appropriate to take over the model of the so-called "morbidity-onion" developed by the Norwegian physician Øivind Larsen and to develop it further for our specific interests (see Figure 1).[28] According to Larsen, every person moves constantly between two poles throughout his life-time: "absolute health" and "final death." While the extreme case of death, i.e., the innermost skin of the "morbidity-onion," is easy to grasp — given source material such as church books, vital statistics, and so forth — the border line between well-being and sickness is quite fluid, depending in the final analysis on the individual perception of each person, i.e., on his subjective consciousness of suffering.

Figure 1: "Morbidity-Onion" according to Øivind Larsen

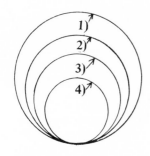

The Thresholds of Disease

1) The patient feels sick
2) The physician's help is required
3) The patient is brought to the hospital
4) The patient dies

The threshold of disease (stage 1) is reached at the first contact with the disease, i.e., the subjective recognition of the symptom or the feeling of being sick. Both may disappear by themselves or be cured through self-help, or they may be too insignificant to require help from the outside. To cross to the next stage of disease an act of will-power is needed, which necessitates overcoming psychological, social, or economic limitations. Concerning admission to a hospital — the

3rd stage of a sickness — the patient no longer decides, but a medical or health organization or — in the 18th century — a council concerned with treatment of the poor. For the patient this is psychologically aggravating, especially for the one who will reach the final stage — death in the hospital. For him, the general practitioner or the old family doctor, even the quack who formerly, together with the family clergyman, attended the dying person, are being replaced by the anonymous, scientifically oriented clinical physician.[29] In combination all the stages of disease depend on the condition of a civilization defined in time and space, in its social, medical and hygienic aspects as well as by the specific status of the patient (e.g., with reference to the expectation as to what role the sick person has to play, whether his sickness is light or severe, etc.).

To further the assessment of the 18th century generally as well as the three institutions selected for study, the "morbidity-onion" was modified to illustrate stratification (see Figure 2). This has been done in accordance with a rough socio-professional-economic classification of the population in six parts. Since the focus of this study is the interval that precedes death as stated at the beginning, the primary concern is with stage 5 — that stage of disease which led to hospital admission. Depending on the social stratum and those specific factors promoting (=+) or diminishing (=−) health, the "morbidity-onion" looks different. The subjective feeling of being sick appeared — in the presence of the same objective symptoms — at varying times, and the patients followed different procedures in the attempt to get well. This means that depending on the stratum one belonged to, morbidity, letality, and mortality, varied for the same disease.[30] From the literature concerning the 18th century we know that members of the upper class did not make the effort to visit the doctor's office, but that the contact between the doctor and the patient always developed in the direction of the patient.[31] Any treatment, even the most difficult operation, took place in the house of the patient. Accordingly, stage number 5 of disease appears seldom among members of the upper class, almost as seldom as premise number 3, where a patient tried to get amateur help and was treated by a quack or a bungler. Financial capacity invariably allowed the members of this class the best available medical and drug services. Minor illnesses were cured by the layman himself through reading medical literature (because of his library).[32]

A relatively large percentage of hospital patients can be predicted for those classes of the population for whom such institutions were established (Military Hospitals, Navy Hospitals, Hospitals for the aged and the infirm, Insane Asylums and the like), or those who turned to a track or social organization in case of sickness, because the organization held in reserve a certain number of hospital places or else took over the hospital expenses (the guild for their masters, orders for their friars, the upper classes for their servants, the army for soldiers, charity organizations for members of the lowest marginal classes).[33]

The lowest marginal strata were not altogether the worst off — i.e., those who frequently acknowledged poverty and therefore enjoyed the traditional help for the poor. Very badly off were those members of the lowest strata who were hiding their poverty and believed they could make ends meet without public support. To these people no one had an obligation. In the urban setting this

ure 2. Variable "morbidity-onions" in accordance with the socio-professional-
nomic class of the patient.

'esholds of Disease:

The patient feels sick   4) The patient seeks expert outside help
The patient tries self-help   5) The patient is admitted to hospital
The patient seeks non-expert outside help 6) The patient dies

Class of Patient	Health promoting (=+), resp. health
Upper Class	diminishing factors (=−)
Can afford medical and drug treatment available at that time (medication, attendants). Every treatment at home	+ wealth, hygiene, sustenance (qualitative and quantitative), medical education in alphabetical order, social proximity to expert curative personnel, good relations, geographic mobility possible. − relatively low immunity because of less frequent contact with infectious diseases
Professionally secure Groups (Army, Service personnel of upper classes, Members of Orders and Guilds). Own hospitals, a number of reserved beds, secure wages.	+ often in the "prime of life", natural resistance great, sustenance secure. Established capital investment. Larger number of doctors and surgeons, spatial proximity with reference to doctors. Special hospitals (e.g. Military hospitals) − specially exposed to damages, partly higher danger of venereal diseases. "Camp-sicknesses", eventual professional diseases.
Aged and Infirm People Special Foundations, Hospitals (without therapy)	+ often long experiences with miserable hygienic conditions. Special institutions for old and infirm people. Partly established in multi-generative families. − natural aging process, higher susceptibility to sickness, senility. Low earning power, eventual reduction of will-power to continue living.
Lower Marginal Stratum Acknowledging Poverty Disposition of means by way of charity (for physicians of the poor, medication, hospital expenses)	+ greater immunity because of greater contact with infectious diseases; higher mobility. Low psychological threshold for claiming charity. − Sustenance (quantitative and qualitative) very insecure, hygiene lacking. Dependence on support. Frequent contact with disease.
Lower Class	+ relatively good immunity, pressure to be well. − Sustenance (quantitative and qualitative) very insecure, hygiene lacking, frequent contact with disease. Greater proximity (social and geographic) to non-expert practices. Scanty self-observation.
Children "Stages of sicknesses" are largely determined by environment. Eventually special institutions.	+ "Discovery" of childhood through adults. Pediatric interest. − exposed to numerous "unknown children's diseases," "infant and child turnover" (new procreation) instead of infant and child care.

refers in the main to the small independent bread-winners (without membership in any guild) — plus their families — such as shoe repairmen, broom producers, book dealers and others, plus people in transient working conditions such as journeymen, handymen, many working men and finally numerous surviving orphans and widows even from well-to-do classes. Members of these groups sought admission to hospitals only in case of serious, often permanent loss of health. They went to a physician or surgeon if they could afford to.[34] They visited the doctor treating the poor or they were in touch with the board of directors governing the affairs of the poor, if it was possible for them to overcome the psychological threshold and if the restoration of their health was, for whatever reason, more important to them than the "shame" of acknowledging their poverty publicly.[35] It is to be noted that in this category the percentage of "healthy" people was as large as that of people in the upper class who could live "healthier lives" because of their wealth, or in the army where most members were in the "healthiest" years of their lives. Since in the lower strata disease is tantamount to lack of earning power, the pressure to be well was essentially greater. Thus the threshold of sickness in these groups was decisively higher than that of the other strata.

III. The Hospital Patients

Having identified the patient, the task is by no means complete. In fact it now becomes more difficult since for the most part we are dealing with the "inarticulate," the patient in history has remained silent.[36] Medical records concerning people treated by physicians as out patients or who remained in a hospital are rare for the 18th century.[37] We therefore have to do with other sources, and must try to reach our goal through skillful questioning and by juxtaposing findings from varied data.

Records of the patients who died in the Charité Hospital and who were listed in the registers starting with the year 1727 allow the serial approach. They contain, to begin with, information concerning sex, socio-professional as well as geographic origin, the date of burial and the age of the deceased.[38] Registration on admission provides not only the same data contained in the death-register, but also notation of the disease of the patient, who had admitted him, whether he was admitted to the ward for the sick or the ward for the old people, the duration of stay at the Charité Hospital and the reason for dismissal (dismissed as healthy, escaped, deceased). For the Navy-Hospital in Copenhagen, we relied on the computerized evaluations of a hospital protocol from the years 1788-1791 conducted by Øivind Larsen and published in 1970.[39] This protocol contains the names of each patient, geographic and military origin, the disease involved, and the nature of release from the hospital (whether judged as recovered or incurable or dead). As to Kongsberg, the most important sources are the statements of accounts as well as some correspondence. The names of those admitted are known, as well as their time of confinement. Known also is the cost of nursing and the working hours of the personnel. Aside from receipted pharmacy bills, it was not possible to locate specific medical archival material. The entire material, covering the 68 admitted hospital inmates during the period

1769-1773, has also been evaluated by Øivind Larsen in a quantitative series published in 1967.[40]

The available records allow us to offer a whole series of answers to our question: "The hospital in the 18th century: For whom"? They offer details on the following factors: the geographic, and the socio-professional-economic origin of the patients; age and sex; seasonal variations in the number of those admitted and dismissed; medical or social indications, such as the nature of the disease (which, in the case of death, was often identical with the cause of death) and prognosis (whether healed, incurable etc.); reasons for admission, duration of hospitalization; and the specific cause of disease and death, plus percentage of death cases in connection with the diseases.

Just as we have determined the stages of diseases and the specific strata variations determining hospital admission, it is possible to consider the projected results with reference to various ",morbidity-onions," before we present the empirical results. A series of factors shaped the selection of patients to be admitted to hospital. The nature of disease was a decisive element here, that is, whether the illness was short and vehement or protracted and difficult to cure. A severe epidemic of typhus might have passed so quickly and led to so many cases of sickness and death in a short time that the clumsy mechanism of admission to the hospital could not be brought to bear, except in military hospitals which were bent on preventing the onslaught of the spreading epidemic at any price. It was different in the case of protracted diseases, damages or accidents as well as in cases of a difficult pregnancy or of the deterioration connected with progressing age that does not kill the patient, at least not immediately, but impairs the habitual rhythm of life sufficiently to render him unfit to earn a living and make him dependent on support. The duration and course of an illness plus the professional, familial, economic and social consequences connected with it lent themselves to an evaluation of the assistance then available, some forms of which might be repugnant from a psycho-economic aspect, but responsive to the pressure for recovery (e.g., head of a family belonging to the lower strata).

In addition to the type of disease as well as the evaluation by specific strata criteria, factors of age and sex must be taken into consideration. Liability to disease may vary according to sickness, type of accident and infirmity. Diseases like smallpox, measles or whooping cough created a reservoir of patients only in the lower age groups. The so-called "camp epidemics" such as typhus led to widespread illness among the age cohorts of the conscripted personnel (above all among men between the ages of 15 and 35 years). Venereal diseases were naturally frequent among men and women in the procreative age range. Work accidents happened mainly among the gainfully employed and so on.

With these points of reference in mind, the following picture results:

1) Most patients were admitted to hospital because of protracted diseases, damages or accidents, and age and infirmity; plus relatively few women entered because of difficult pregnancy and, finally, still fewer people entered because of acute sickness. All this resulted in a stay of medium to long duration.

2) Most patients were young and middle-aged adults (between roughly 15

and 40). On the other hand, only few belonged to the youngest while the elderly fell in the middle range.

3) Most patients were either professionally secure or members of the lower order who were supported by charity. Very seldom did they originate from the remainder of the lower strata, and they practically never belonged to the upper stratum.

III.1 The Admission Office

As already mentioned, the Berlin Charité Hospital had two main functions: It served both as a curative and nursing institution for the city's (poor) population and as a military hospital. Accordingly, there were three groups responsible for admissions: the board of directors governing the affairs of the poor (of the 7,365 admissions in the years 1731, 1733-1742, a subtotal of 3,673, or 49.9%), and the physicians and surgeons employed within the Charité organization (2,696 admissions, or 36.6%). Remaining admissions stemmed from commanders of regiments and other high ranking officers (272 admissions, or 3.7%).[41]

The number of admissions in the Charité Hospital per year varied greatly, from 499 in the year 1741 to 776 in the year 1737. Furthermore, the proportion of new patients was rarely over 10% (1740: 10.7%). Because of the varying duration of confinement in the individual departments of the Charité Hospital, these figures reveal rather little about the rate of occupancy of the total of 400 beds (in the Charité Hospital each patient, in principle, had his own bed). The most frequent duration of confinement in the ward for the sick was between one and two months (23.8%), while in the ward for the old people the most common duration was between 2 and 5 years (= 16.2%). It is astounding that the number of civilians admitted fluctuated in absolute terms as well as in terms of percentage of admissions to the ward of the sick (admitted by the charity board, 58 patients in 1732, or 9.2%, but 564 in 1737, or 72.7%; admitted by the Charité physicians, 4 in 1738, or 0.6%, but 530 in 1731, or 70.3%).

There is no need to discuss the controversies over jurisdiction among the institutions allowed to admit patients to hospitals. The topic has already been studied[42] and we are only interested in the situation of the patients in any event. It is obvious that in an admission by a physician or surgeon the medical symptoms must have predominated whereas the charity organization was primarily guided by social and economic factors. More simply expressed: the candidate for admission in the Charité Hospital up to 1736 had to be *sick and needy*, while from 1737 and on, when the charity board assumed the authority over most of cases, he had to be *needy and sick*.

The numerous admissions through physicians and surgeons in 1731 and 1733-1736, compel attention to which physicians or surgeons were guided by the patient's viewpoint. The individual training and medical interest of the admitting doctor might have played a role at the selection, along with his specialty and professional ethics, while the sense of obligation could affect the prospects of recovery. Thus Dr. Johann Theodor Eller (1689-1760) called in 1724 to the Berlin medico-surgical College and active there as the first medical director of the Charité-Hospital, between 1725-1735 had received a well-rounded, indeed unusual training, at the best known Prussian and foreign centers of medicine and the natural sciences (Halle, Leiden, Amsterdam, Paris, London). Stimulated by the famous clinic of Hermann Boerhaave (1668-1738) in Leiden, Eller built the Charité-Hospital into the largest clinic in Germany. He personally prompted a considerable share of admissions up to the year 1734.[43]

After his departure, the two doctors Otto Theodor Sprögel (1699-1759) and Samuel Schaarschmidt (1709-1747) divided the care of the patients between them. Both were responsible for numerous new admissions to the ward of the sick of the Charité-Hospital at that time. Sprögel who had studied in Hamburg but, like Eller, had received further training abroad, was appointed royal physician at the Berlin Court. In 1737, he was released from his function as a Charité-Hospital physician because the charity board did not want to pay a second doctor's salary. Although Eller held the lead in knowledge and activity, the Charité-Hospital patient was probably in better hands with Sprögel. Eller initiated the scientific-literary approach at the Charité-Hospital,[44] while Sprögel's research contribution was limited to the description of the sicknesses of three patients in 1740. The latter was not a scientist but rather a thoroughly practical doctor. He opposed daring therapeutic experiments at the sickbed and depended solely on his experience and the traditional methods of cure. From our contemporary viewpoint, wherein medical research enjoys higher prestige than patient-oriented treatment, we know only too well that the doctor's interest as a scientist is not directed toward the patient per se but toward those patients suffering from a disease he (the doctor) is doing research on. The research physician is not in his own view, geared to the patient; rather, the patient is geared to the doctor's research.[45]

After the dismissal of Sprögel and until 1744 Schaarschmidt, a product of the University of Halle, was the sole medical director of the Charité-Hospital. He paid little direct attention to admissions at that time.

In terms of biographical data, there is little known about the surgical directors at the Charité-Hospital. In chronological order there were Gabriel Senff (? -1738): 1727-1737; Johann Daniel Neubauer (? -1739): 1737-1739, and Simon Pallas (1694/95-1770): 1740-1770. Senff and Pallas are supposed to have received part of their training in France. While Neubauer hardly ever exercised his right to admit patients, Senff made ample use of it at least until 1736 and even Pallas admitted a number of patients during the first and second year of his activity. As to the other doctors, the numerous admissions of Dr. Ehrenreich Wilhelm Kaatzky during 1734 and 1735 should be emphasized. Kaatzky, a member of the Royal Prussian Chief Medical College, was in charge of the poor but was not personally active in the Charité-Hospital.

III.2 The Classification of Patients According to Disease, Age, Sex as well as Socio-Professional Origin.

The historian must be aware of the difficulties involved in evaluating causes of diseases or detailed causes of death for past centuries where an entirely different approach to systematizing prevailed. Yet we need not be overly concerned with this problem.[46] Moreover, since the admission registers of the

Charité-Hospital and the Navy-Hospital in Copenhagen were not available in the original, we were forced to take over the classification of such medical doctors as Stürzbecher, Böhme and Larsen. Unfortunately, the same holds true for the division of patients according to socio-professional groups by the above mentioned authors.

There were four or five main reasons and groups of causes for an admission to the ward for the sick of the Charité-Hospital on medical grounds. With males, the rank order was 1) Injuries (506 from a total of 3.607 = 14.0%), 2) "infected" (464 = 12.9%), 3) Chest diseases (447 = 12.4%), and 4) Fever (380 = 10.5%). With females: 1) Pregnancy (494 from a total of 3.160 = 15.6%), 2) "Infected" (444 = 14.0%), 3) Injuries (342 = 10.8%), and 4) Fever (284 = 9.0%). No further malady reached the 5% limit for either males or females. In the discussion of the various categories of ill-health wounds were subsumed under "injuries" while "infected": comprised venereal diseases, above all, and "chest diseases" meant tuberculosis and malaria predominantly.

The frequency of the leading illnesses is of little surprise; the previous discussion suggested them already. If the cases of pregnancy led among female patient population, it should be remembered that obstetrics played an important role in the Charité Hospital almost from the beginning, and that this was organized in an exemplary fashion with a midwife on permanent call plus an obstetrician for severe cases. In accordance with the function of the Charité-Hospital, poor and single women primarily benefited from the service. Of a total of 550 pregnant women admitted, 57 were married, 9 widows, 23 single, 452 out of wedlock, and 9 unaccounted for.[47] The groups of causes, with the exception perhaps of intestinal and women's diseases, fit the category of protracted disease (skin diseases, ulcers, consumption, swellings, dropsy,), plus disease aggravated by injuries and accidents and deterioration with advancing age (rheumatic pains and arthritis).

The medical indications in the Navy Hospital in Copenhagen are different. However, in this case it should be noted from the start that the record of this hospital better reflects general morbidity than does the patient population of the ward for the sick in the Charité-Hospital. The Hospital in Copenhagen served a clearly defined segment of the population. Although the institution was called "Quaest-Huuset" (accident-house) the patients admitted for injuries only amounted to a total of 2.4% of the overall patient population (81 of a total of 3,327 admissions). The injured remained, however, in treatment for a rather long time, claiming 4.3% of the total sickdays. Yet while the training of physicians devoted to the care of military personnel emphasized surgery, one must ask if this was appropriate. For the personnel drafted into the Navy in times of war, the infectious diseases obviously constituted a greater danger than the weapons of the enemy. Yet the stress in surgery had a definite effect. Mortality rates among the injured, in spite of the risk of complicating infections, was rather low (7.4% in comparison to 15.2% with stomach and intestinal diseases).

With 50.9% of all admissions, the soldiers hospitalized because of stomach and intestinal diseases formed the largest group. They were also of great importance in terms of maintenance since they required over one-half of the total sickdays (51.7%). Without question, in a military hospital acute injuries were treated far less than illness stemming from epidemics, both small and large. Hence admissions of patients suffering from stomach and intestinal ailments tended to bunch up (especially in the summers of 1789 and 1790) — which was liable to lead to a disproportionate occupation of the number of beds and accordingly to bottle-necks in care and control. The admission of patients with respiratory ailments and fever were more evenly divided over the years. At 23.0% of the patient population, they formed the second main category. In maintenance, however, they occupied the place behind skin and venereal diseases (16.8% of all maintenance days compared to the 18.7% devoted to skin and venereal disease, which clearly demanded prolonged hospitalization. Within this latter group of diseases, scabies were dominant, with 54.6% of the total).

As to age and sex classification, every third person admitted to the ward for the sick of the Charité-Hospital was between 20 and 30 years old (33.0%), every fifth one between 30 and 40 years old (21.3%). More than half of all inmates were here in their "prime." This fact is scarcely surprising in view of the age-specific medical reasons for admission of these age groups: venereal diseases and pregnancies. As to gender, it is noteworthy that in the age groups 10-20 and 20-30 years, the share of women was distinctly higher than that of men (12.7% as compared to 8.6% and 37.3% as compared to 29.2% respectively). This re-flects the importance of the pregnant cases admitted. However, in the age groups between 30 and 70, the percentage of men predominates. This is especially so in the 40-50 and 50-60 age categories (15.1% compared to 10.0% and 12.5% com-pared to 8.0% respectively). The males outranked females in the categories of "injuries" and "accidents." Their percentage share is therefore notably higher than that of the women (for injuries, 14.0% for males as compared to 10.8% for females; for accidents, 3.3% as compared to 1.1%).

In terms of age cohorts in admissions to the ward for old and infirm people, older people have of course a preponderant share. Only one out of ten was, as a rule, under 40 years of age, and many of these reflected admission of orphans or young mental patients. Of all those admitted, 82.9% were over 50, and almost every third person was between 60 and 70 (30.8%). In the Navy Hospital in Copenhagen, on the other hand, only two patients admitted in the years 1788-1791 (of a known total of 2,999 in a specific age group) were over 55. As can be expected, the patient population derived from those able to serve in the Army, i.e., those between 15 and 35 years. Of all those admitted, 83.2% be-longed to this age group; patients between 20-29 amounted to 62.3% of the total.

In the Charité-Hospital the military personnel comprise by far the largest part in the ward for the sick and the ward for the old (40.6% resp. 35.1%). Clearly the Charité Hospital was a military institution above all, an Army Hospital for the sick and wounded, active as well as retired soldiers and their wives who often lived in poverty, or their widows and daughters. The Charité Hospital served also as a military institution of public relief for the aged. Hence the occupational category of next importance, the textile industry, lagged far behind the military. Textiles did enjoy a preferential position in 18th century Berlin (processing of wool, weaving, embroidering, knitting, fabrics and others). At 8.1%, textile workers formed the largest civilian group in the Charité, followed by the day-labourers (7.8%), and workers in processing daily (5.4%; brewers, bakers, inn-keepers) or luxury items (5.0%; glove, hat and sock makers, furriers, tailors etc.). None of the remaining socio-professional groups reached the 5% limit.

III.3 The Duration of Stay.

Additional data deal with the duration of stay of patients at the Hospital in Kongsberg as well as in both wards of the Charité Hospital. As one would expect, the duration of stay of patients in the ward for the old in the Charité Hospital must be figured in terms of years rather than months, while the patients in the ward for the sick were more frequently discharged to make room for new applicants. It is, however, surprising that the Hospital in Kongsberg, with all its non-therapeutic treatment, housed numerous patients who did not stay longer than one month (16.2%), two months (22.1%) or three months (16.2%). The figures are more comparable to data of the ward for the sick of the Charité than those of the ward for the old. Thus 20.4% stayed in the ward for the sick of the Charité Hospital up to a month, 23.8% up to two months and 13.5% up to three months. If there are protracted stays of several years' duration, they may be due to the circumstance that some patients who may have been hospitalized for a long time were finally transferred to the ward for the old, but not registered as new admissions.

The data concerning the duration of stay reveal little about the course of treatment or its success. It is not at all certain that patients, especially those of the ward for the sick, were dismissed as cured. They may have died of their disease or released as incurable. They may also have been transferred to the ward for the old. Runaways also were frequently noted. On the other hand, some patients may have simulated sickness in order to stay on longer because of assured food and shelter. Certain able-bodied inmates may have been kept on in order to partially pay back the hospital expenses they had incurred by temporarily assisting in the maintenance of the hospital. Thus the duration of stay actually recorded cannot usually be equated with the time actually necessary for treatment.

III.4 Mortality.

Considerable data exist concerning the mortality in the hospitals of the 18th century. For patients admitted to the ward of the sick of the Charité Hospital, in the case of women, every 4th admission (25.1%), in the case of men, every 3rd admission (31.2%) ended in death. For the younger age groups (aside from infants and small children), the prospects of cure were higher; for the more advanced age groups they were significantly lower. In the Charité Hospital, "consumption" and "dropsy" represent by far the most dangerous diseases: 73.8% and 70.1% of all cases, respectively, led to death. However, the treatment of "tumors" was fatal in every second case (at 54.7%). Since a high percentage of the patient population, particularly men, suffered from "chest diseases", this category was the most important in terms of absolute numbers (282 deaths of a total of 581 patients). On the other hand, the Department of child delivery (pregnancy) of the Charité Hospital can claim a good record. At 4.9%, "pregnancy" produced the lowest percentage of death (of the mother).

The percentage of deaths in the Navy Hospital in Copenhagen was generally lower, at 11.7%, which is not surprising in view of the age structure of the patients. There were a number of diseases with frequently fatal results here too, particularly in the respiratory and fever category (tuberculosis of the lungs 80.6%, peripneumonia 32.7%) as well as among the stomach and intestinal diseases (febris putrida 42.4%, dysentery 38.7%). In both institutions skin and venereal diseases (16.5% mortality) and likewise "injuries" (Navy Hospital at 7.4% resp. "accidents" in the Charité Hospital at 14.6%) normally yielded to treatment.

Finally, mortality can be linked to socio-professio-economic status. At the Charité Hospital the percentage of soldiers admitted, at 15.3%, was equal to the number of soldiers' wives (15.8%).[48] Active soldiers obviously received treatment even for minor ailments, while the illness on the part of their wives had to be more serious, thus the share of the dead varies between 9.9% (males) and 11.3% (females). Other occupational groups among whom the percentage of admissions is notably higher than that of the mortality are instructive also. This is the case in agriculture and forestry (4.6% as compared to 1.9%), also in the processing of wood and paper (3.1% as compared to 1.2%). Evidently we are dealing here with groups that were particularly exposed to job-related accidents. These accidents frequently caused transfer to a hospital, but were seldom fatal.

Finally, we turn to the question of the effectiveness of the Charité Hospital in terms of the health systems available in the 18th century. To this end, we have specifically compared all mortality cases in this hospital during the years 1731-1742 in terms of month and age at death, to an analogous classification of all cases of death in the town parish of Giessen (60 km north of Frankfurt on the Main) for the entire 18th century.[49] The correspondences are astounding. Just as in Giessen, the percentage value of all deceased in the Charité Hospital starts at a medium level at the beginning of the year (8.6% and 8.1% respectively), and slowly increases in the spring up to a maximum in May (9.9% and 10.5%). During the summer and fall it falls only to rise again later in the year. We seem to be facing the same structure of mortality variation in the Berlin Hospital as in a whole urban parish community. Admission to a hospital did thus not essentially alter the overall mortality pattern. Specific reference to age confirms this impression. Thus the hospital in the 18th century was not the place where the risk of death in case of a grave loss of health had appreciably diminished; rather, it served those age groups that were predisposed to admission largely as a place of withdrawal prior to death (especially adults between 20 and 40 years of age).

So if the hospital in the 18th century could not show any outstanding success in terms of therapy, it was nevertheless a forerunner of the hospital in the second half of the 20th century. For it was modern in the sense that it began to attract the dying in the intensive stage of illness, providing a structure for death removed from the normal community.

IV. Conclusion.

During the Middle Ages and the early modern era, the hospital served mainly as an ultimate refuge for those marginal groups of people who, for various reasons, were dependent on the care of others (due to poverty, physical or mental infirmities, lack of family, age). It offered shelter and care, but no special treatment by doctors and no medication. The idea that the seriously ill should be concentrated in a special institution for therapeutic care began to come into its own only in the 17th/18th century, at first as a result of the state initiative, in order to guarantee the health of a military contingent as much as possible, for military reasons (= Military Hospital); later because of the need to create a continuous patient population for the purpose of medical education and training (= Clinic).

In this study, the three types, medieval, military, and clinic, were analyzed, for they coexisted in the 18th century. Kongsberg turned out to be an old-type hospital without therapy; the Navy Hospital in Copenhagen was strictly the military type, with a patient population well defined in terms of age, sex and profession; the Clinic type, with a broad spectrum of diseases, was found in the Berlin Charité Hospital (which simultaneously maintained military hospital and general hospital functions).

Any hospital study for the century which centers on patients encounters the essential problem of data that the patients remain mute. It was, however, possible to find a series of answers to the question: "The hospital in the 18th century: for whom?" indirectly by means of theoretical conjectures. It was furthermore possible to answer this question empirically, testing a number of factors (on the basis of a differentiated registration at the point of admission as well as discharge of the patients).

The group able to value the hospitals of that time with new functions held secure jobs (mainly members of the Army: in the Charité Hospital 41.1%). But members of the lower marginal strata who openly acknowledged their poverty and who were eligible for the traditional charitable care of the poor at that time (such as day-labourers in the Charité Hospital: 7.8%, or third rank) also loomed large. In terms of age, those in their prime were heavily represented, since they were exposed to "camp-diseases," venereal diseases, work accidents and pregnancies with complications (share of the 20-40 years old in the Charité Hospital: 40.6%, in the Navy Hospital: 78.0%). As to disease, the ailments of long duration (e.g., venereal diseases in the Charité Hospital: 13.4%, skin and venereal diseases in the Navy Hospital: 13.8%), injuries and accidents including dangerous pregnancies (Charité Hospital 15.6%), and in the case of inmates of the ward for the old hospital, age and infirmity were preponderant. The highest mortality rates were found in the ward of the sick of the Charité Hospital, particularly among patients suffering from consumption and dropsy. In the Navy Hospital, lung tuberculosis had an 80.6% mortality rate. Overall, in the Charité Hospital every fourth admission of women, every third admission of men ended in death; in the Navy Hospital with its favorable age structure, only every ninth admission. The most common duration of hospitalization in the ward for the sick of the Charité Hospital was 1 to 2 months (23.8%), while the most frequent confined in the ward for the old varied from two to five years (16.2%).

The answers to such specific questions relate to two problems currently under intense scrutiny. Hospitalization is obviously linked to possible changes in the attitude towards death. It relates also to the mentality of significant groups confronted with an anonymous medical technology. Both issues found their forerunners in the new therapeutic hospital of the 18th century. Not only were the admitted patients selected on definite principles of disease, social strata and so on, but also selectivity itself was practiced despite the fact that the prospects of cure of those admitted was not essentially different than among those who did not go to the hospital. Indeed the mortality rates of those Charité Hospital patients who died in their prime (20-40 years old) are very high compared to a general urban population. And for these people death no longer occurred in a familiar surrounding or among relatives, but under routine clinical observation and in the anonymous death cell of the hospital.

Free University Berlin   Arthur E. Imhof

FOOTNOTES

For the cooperation in Berlin, the author wishes to thank Dorothee Koppes, Angelika Kater, and Thomas Kühn. They carried through the computer evaluation and the comprehension of data with reference to the cases of death in the Charité Hospital that occurred during the years 1731-1742. Thanks also to Dr. Paul Neumarkt, Duquesne University, for translating the manuscript.

1. Jean Meuvret, "Les crises de subsistance et la démographie de la France d'Ancien Régime," *Population* 1 (1946) 643-650; reprinted in *Etudes d'histoire économique* (Paris, 1971) 271-278. See also the work of Pierre Goubert on the peasants of the Beauvaisis, where death often was more central than birth [*Beauvais et le Beauvaisis de 1600 a 1730*, 2 vols. (Paris, 1960)]. The first International Colloquium for historical demography, April 18th-20th, 1963, in Liège, was devoted to the problems of mortality; [*Actes du Colloque International de Démographie Historique*, Paul Harsin and Etienne Hélin, eds. (Paris, 1965)]. At the last International Colloquium for historical demography (October, 1975, in Montreal), one of the three main sessions was again devoted to the crises concerning mortality. One of the principal organizers, Hubert Charbonneau, had shortly before published a new work entitled *Vie et mort de nos ancêtres: Etude démographique* (Montreal, 1975).

2. Selected studies on this topic can be cited: Philippe Ariès, *Western Attitudes toward Death from the Middle Ages to the Present* (Baltimore, 1974); The French version of *Western Attitudes* (Paris, 1975) contains 12 additional essays on this subject, published between 1966 and 1975); *Autour de la mort*, special number of the *Annales E.S.C.* (1976), 3-240; *Leichenpredigten als Quelle historischer Wissenschaften*, Rudolf Lenz, ed. (Cologne-Vienna, 1975); Emmanuel le Roy Ladurie, "Chaunu, Lebrun, Vovelle: La nouvelle histoire de la mort," in *Territoire de l'historien* (Paris, 1973), 393-403; Alfred Perrenoud, "L'inégalité sociale devant la mort à Genève au XVIIᵉ siècle," *Population* (November 1975)

221-243; Michel Vovelle, *Piété baroque et déchristianisation en Provence au XVIIIe siècle* (Paris, 1973); Michel Vovelle, *Mourir autrefois. Attitudes collectives devant la mort au XVIIe et XVIIIe siècles* (Paris, 1974); Michel Vovelle, "La redécouverte de la mort," *La Pensee* (1976), 3-18.

3. It is not surprising that the investigators of death and mortality as well as historic demographers have voiced their opinions on this topic: Philippe Ariès, "Le malade, la famille et le medecin," *Essais sur L'histoire de la mort* (Paris, 1975) 198-209; Jacques Dupâquier, "Démographie historique et médecine," *Introduction à la démographie historique* (Paris, 1974) 93 ss.; Jean-Pierre Goubert, *Malades et médecins en Bretagne 1770-1790* (Paris, 1974); François Lebrun, "Les hommes devant la maladie," *Les Hommes et la mort en Anjou aux 17e et 18e siècles* (Paris-The Hague, 1971) 391-415; Emmanuel le Roy Ladurie et al., eds. *Médecins, climat et épidémies à la fin du XVIIIe siècle*, (Paris-The Hague, 1972).

4. Perrenoud, "L'inégalité," 221-243; Roger Chartier in *Annales E.S.C.* (1976), 51-75; Daniel Roche in *Annales E.S.C.* (1976) 76-119.

5. Ariès, *Western Attitudes*, 1-25, the quotations on 14 and 25.

6. Ibid., 28, 44.

7. Jacques Dupâquier, *Introduction à la démographie historique* (Paris, 1974) 93.

8. Lebrun, "Les Hommes," 391 ss.

9. While the doctor had become the sole person concerned with cure, a clergyman was simultaneously called in. Thus, during the 18th century, a clergyman was present at severe cases of surgery in the Charité Hospital in Berlin "for the comfort of the patients". Cf. Ingrid Lobbes, "Die Entwicklung des Berliner Krankenhauswesens" medical dissertation, (Berlin 1955) 23. Concerning the role of pastoral medicine, Heinrich Pompey furnishes detailed information: *Die Bedeutung der Medizin für die kirchliche Seelsorge im Selbstverständnis der sogenannten Pastoralmedizin. Eine bibliographisch-historische Untersuchung bis zur Mitte des 19. Jahrhunderts* (Freiburg im Breisgau, 1968). See also Robert Heller, "'Priest-Doctors' as a rural health service in the age of enlightenment," *Medical History* (1976), 361, 383.

10. Jacques Revel and Jean-Pierre Peter, "Le corps; l'homme malade et son histoire," *Faire de l'histoire, nouveaux objets* by Jacques le Goff and Pierre Nora, eds. III (Paris 1974), 175.

11. On the position and the lasting prestige of non-medical personnel, the folklorist Marcelle Bouteiller has written in detail: *Medecine populaire d'hier et d'aujourd'hui (Paris, 1966)*. Cf. the critique by Robert Mandrou from an historical aspect, in *Revue Historique* (1967), 214-217. With reference to the problem of subcultural medical behavior, cf. Franz Grass, "Volksmedizin, Sakralkultur und Recht," *Volksmedizin, Probleme und Forschungsberichte* Elfriede Grabner, ed. (Darmstadt 1967), 399-412; Robert Jalby, *Sorcellerie, médecine populaire et pratiques médico-magiques en Languedoc* (Nyon 1974); Lutz Röhrich, "Krankheitsdämonen," *Volksmedizin*, Elfriede Grabner ed. (1967), 283-288; Helmut Paul Fielhauer, "Voksmedizin-Heilkulturwissenschaft. Grundätzliche Erwagungen-anhand von Beispielen aus Niederosterreich," *Mitteilungen de Anthropologischen Gesellschaft in Wien* 102 (1972), 114-136; Rudolf Schenda, "Volksmedizin – was ist das heute?" *Stadtmedizin-Landmedizin. Ein Versuch zur Erklarung subkulturalen medikalen Verhaltens* (Stadt-Land-Beziehungen. Verhandlungen des 19. Deutschen-Volkskunde-Kongresses vom 1. bis 7. Oktober, 1973) (Gottingen, 1975), 147-170. It should be noted that the last mentioned essay by Schenda was severely criticized. Having made popular medicine an indicator of medical subsistence or progressive deterioration within the area of education, prevention and cure (152), he has been rightfully reproached for the fact that his topic deals

not so much with popular medicine but represents a "critique of the system".

12. Ariès, *Essais sur l'histoire,* 199 ss. According to the observations of Ariès who is supported by literary sources in this respect, the change seems to have come about in the 2nd half of the 19th century. At that time, people were conscious of going to the doctor and of observing his advice strictly with reference to hygiene and medication. To judge on the basis of these sources, the interest in sickness and health began at that time. Cf. especially 204.

13. Concerning the specific behavior of classes with regard to health and diseases from the 16th to the 18th century cf. Otto Döhner, Jr., "Historisch-soziologische Aspekte des Krankheitsbegriffs und des Gesundheitsverhaltens im 16. und 18. Jahrhundert," *Leichenpredigten als Quelle historischer Wissenschaften,* Rudolf Lenz, ed., 442-469, especially 443, 459. It should, however, be noted that Döhner's source, the printed death-sermons, represented a class phenomenon per se, since they were essentially limited to the urban upper stratum in Protestant areas.

14. To preside over one's own death is, according to Philippe Ariès, one of the most essential features of dying within the family and a close social network context, before death was forced into the framework of the hospital, where it is possible to become frustrated about one's own death. Philippe Ariès, *Western Attitudes,* 1974, op. cit., special chapter 1-3, 1 ss., (11), 27 ss., 55 ss., as well as Philippe Ariès, *Essais sur l'histoire de la mort,* 209.

15. Concerning the doctor's fee in the 18th century, cf. Manfred Stürzbecher, *Beiträge zur Berliner Medizingeschichte. Quellen und Studien zur Geschichte des Gesundheitswesens vom 17. bis zum 19. Jahrhundert* (Berlin 1966), 97 ss., as well as Chart IV, 148-149 where the doctor's fee is compared to the servants' wages according to the medical regulation dated 1725. Concerning the social gap and the resultant lack of confidence between large parts of the population and the trained medical personnel cf. Alfons Fischer, *Geschichte des deutschen Gesundheitswesens,* vol. II (Berlin, 1933), 64. The attitude toward the doctor is further evaluated by Ernst Heinrich Rehermann, *Volkskundliche Aspekte in Leichenpredigten protestantischer Prediger Mittel-und Norddeutschlands im 16. und 17. Jahrhundert* in *Leichenpredigten* op. cit., 289 ss.

16. Statement of a patient directed at the assistant medical officer of the city of Nyköping in Sweden, end of January 1743. Cf. chapter 6, "Countermeasures against the Spread of Epidemics leading to infectious Diseases," in Arthur E. Imhof, *Aspekte der Bevölkerungsentwicklung in den nordischen Ländern 1720-1750* (Bern 1976), 681. During the period of bad harvest 1740-1743 which afflicted large parts of Europe, it was entirely possible that patients refused medication distributed free of charge, fearing that it could stimulate their appetite. Cf. op. cit., 680 ss. Concerning the refusal of medical consultation as well as hesitation to take medication in urban upper classes, cf., *Historisch-soziologische Aspekte 6. bis. 18. Jahrhundert,* 463.

17. As is well known, the medical terminology in the 18th century was oriented along nosological lines, i.e., the recognizable symptoms were described and the disease was named accordingly. Today's medicine proceeds in an etiological manner, i.e., the main focal point lies in the biological causes. In the 18th century it was possible to get sick from a high fever and die from it. For today's medical doctor high fever involves little more than a prevalent symptom behind which many different diseases could hide (according to today's terminology). "Fever" today points to a sickness, the same as "dropsy" or "jaundice" which were sicknesses in themselves during the 18th century. It is instructive to state that even in the mortality register of the first statistical central bureau of the world (in Stockholm/Sweden since 1749), set up by a medical professor at the University of Uppsala/Sweden, the terms "unknown children's diseases" and "old age and infirmity" appear as undifferentiated causes of death (in a total of 33 different cases). "Infirmity due to age" is to be found in

this register even until 1830, while the "unknown children's diseases disappear with the 2nd edition of the register 1774, to be replaced by specific diagnoses. Cf. Arthur E. Imhof and Øivind Larsen, *Sozialgeschichte und Medizin. Probleme der quantifizierenden Quellenbearbeitung in der Sozial-und Medizingeschichte* (Oslo, 1975, Stuttgart, 1976), 244-245.

18. Cf. here Frank Macfarlane Burnet, *Natural History of Infectious Disease* (London 1962), especially the chapters about the ecological aspects as well as chapter 12, concerning the spread of infections among different species – animal reservoirs. Cf. furthermore the exciting and often republished little book by Hans Zinsser, *Rats, Lice and History,* (8th printing, New York, 1971), especially chapter XI ("Much about Rats – a little about Mice").

19. Revel and Peter, *Le corps, 172.*

20. Jean-Nöel Biraben, *Les hommes et la peste en France et dans les pays européens et méditerranéens,* I; *La peste dans l'histoire* (Paris-The Hague, 1975), 12 ss., on epidemiology.

21. Wolf Lepenies, in his lecture "Historical Anthropology," June 4, 1976, at the Institute for Historical Sciences of the Berlin Technical University. Cf. also Wolf Lepenies, "History and Anthropology," *Geschichte und Gesellschaft,* 1, vol. 2/3 (1975), 338.

22. Revel and Peter, *Le corps, 173.*

23. Jean Pierre Goubert, "Methodologische Probleme zu einer Geschichte des Gesundheitswesens. Frankreich am Ende des 18. Jahrhunderts als Beispiel," in: *Historische Demographie als Sozialgeschichte,* ed. by Arthur E. Imhof (Darmstadt and Marburg, 1975), 627-638. Cf. in this connection, the "Bibliographie sommaire d'histoire de la médicine 18-19 siècles) in: *"dh,"* *Bulletin d'information* (April 12, 1974), 27-30.

24. Arthur E. Imhof,"Sosioøkonomisk struktur, morbiditet og mortalitet," *The Journal of the Norwegian Medical Association* (Nr. 5, 1976), 278-282; also in *Historische Demographie als Sozialgeschichte,* 257 ss., particularly the figures 9-11, 259-261.

25. The results of the investigation presented here are based partly on the investigation of archives carried out with the help of students in Berlin, partly on data already collected by others. Recent descriptions of all three institutions are available, excusing us from elaborate introductions. With reference to the history of the Charité Hospital as well as the health-care system in Berlin in the 18th century, cf. Paul Diepgen and Edith Heischkel, *Die Medizin an der Berliner Charité bis zur Gründung der Universität. Ein Beitrag zur Medizingeschichte des 18. Jahrhunderts* (Berlin, 1935); Ingrid Lobbes, *Die Entwicklung des Berliner Krankenhauswesens* (Medical Dissertation in manuscript, Berlin, 1955); Ludwig Formey, *Versuch einer medicinischen Topographie von Berlin* (Berlin, 1796); Manfred Stürzbecher, "Über die medizinische Versorgung der Berliner Bevölkerung im 18. Jahrhundert," *Beiträge zur Berliner Medizingeschichte* (Berlin, 1966), 67-155. Detailed bibliographical data on the topic can be found in: *Berlin-Bibliographie (bis 1960),* revised by Hans Zopf and Gerd Heinrich (Berlin, 1965), 648-665; *Berlin-Bibliographie 1961-1966,* revised by Ursula Scholz and Rainald Stromeyer (Berlin, 1973), 259-272. We are indebted for numerous statistical data to Karlheinz Böhme, *Untersuchungen über die Charité-Patienten von 1731 bis 1742. Eine Studie zur Funktion und Soziologie eines Krankenhauses im 18. Jahrhundert. (Sociological Function of a Hospital in the 18th Century). (Inaugural Dissertation, upon receiving the doctorate of Dental Medicine at the Medical Faculty of the Humboldt-University Berlin; in manuscript) (Berlin 1969).* Concerning the history of the hospital in Kongsberg, as well as the Navy Hospital in Copenhagen, *cf.* Oivind Larsen, "Sykehusets funksjon i bergstaden Kongsberg i årene 1796-1773," *Medicinhistorisk Årsbok* (1967), 10 pages with independent page numbers; as well as Øivind Larsen, "'Söe-Quaest-Huuset' – des Marinespital zu Kopenhagen und seine Funktion 1788-1791," *Medizinhistorisches Journal* (1970), 247-267. Both articles contain far-reaching bibliographical data.

26. Cf. the recent article of the Frankfurt medical sociologist Armin Menz, "Gesundheit und soziale Verantwortung," *Neue Zürcher Zeitung, Fernausgabe,* Nr. 133 (June 11, 1976) 29.

27. Well known, even if controversial, is, e.g., the clarification of the concept of disease by the American sociologist Talcott Parsons: *"Definition von Gesundheit und Krankheit im Lichte der Wertbegriffe und der sozialen Strucktur Amerikas,"* in *Der Kranke in der modernen Gesellschaft,* by Alexander Mitscherlich (Cologne, 1973). Concerning the change of the delineations between "Health" and "Sickness" from a historic-sociological aspect: Döhner, Jr., *Historisch-soziologische Aspekte,* 443 ss. Cf. for the rest of the handbooks and introductions, e.g., Karlheinz Engelhardt, Alfred Wirth and Lothar Kindermann, *Kranke im Krankenhaus* (Stuttgart, 1973), especially chapter 7: "Das Krankheitsverstandnis des Patienten und seine Erwartungshaltung," 120 ss.; or Asmus Finzen, *Patient und Gesellschaft,* (Stuttgart, 1969) *(Medizin in Geschichte und Kultur,* Vol. 10 especially part II: "Arzt und Patient in der modernen Gesellschaft," 74 ss.). 28 Øivind Larsen, "Die 'Morbiditäts-Zwiebel' in: Imhof and Larsen, *Sozialgeschichte und Medizin,* 180 ss.

29. This is especially valid for medical university clinics "in which the practical and scientific work concerning anthropological, psychological and social groups of topics is not modern and not questioned." Cf. "Ursachen fur die mangelhafte arztliche Kenntniss" in: Engelhardt, Wirt and Kindermann, *Kranke,* 46 ss.; the quotation is on 49.

30. Cf. Arthur E. Imhof and Øivind Larsen, "Social and Medical History – Methodological Problems in Interdisciplinary Quantitative Research," – *The Journal of Interdisciplinary History,* (Winter, 1977), especially figure 2: "Mortality in correlation with important factors of human surroundings, which influence mortality."

31. Stürzbecher, *Über die medizinische Versorgung,* 81.

32. A compilation of medical handbooks put together by leading experts for the sake of the well-read layman such as "Anleitung für das Landvolk in Absicht auf seine Gesundheit" (by Simon Andre Tissot. (Translation from the French, Augsburg and Innsbruck 1772) in: Imhof, *Aspekte,* 335 ss.

33. Cf. Alfons Fischer, *Geschichte des deutschen Gesundheitswesens,* vol. II (Berlin, 1933) 251 ss; Ludwig Formey, *Versuch einer medizinischen Topographie von Berlin* (Berlin, 1796), 101, 268; Stürzbecher, *"Über die medizinische Versorgung,"* 105 ss.; P.F.C. Willie, "Soziale Krankenfürsorge vor zwei Jahrhunderten," *Medizinische Klink* (1950), 372.

34. For calculation of the doctor's fee in Berlin during the 18th century based on empirical material and converted to a so-called "egg-index", cf. Stürzbecher, *Über die medizinische Versorgung,* 97 ss., 148 ss. Thus, e.g., a doctor's single visit to a patient cost the equivalent of 240 eggs. Blood-letting on the arm performed by a surgeon had the value of 20-30 eggs.

35. The Charité Hospital doctors often complained that the patients came to the hospital too late and that the mortality was consequently high. Cf. Formey, *Versuch einer medicinischen Topographie,* 273.

36. This insight relates to the efforts of medical historian Erwin H. Ackerknecht "to write from the vantage ground of the patient", cf. Esther Fischer-Homberger, "Erwin H. Ackerknecht, zum 70. Geburtstag des Zürcher Medizinhistorikers," *Neue Zürcher Zeitung, Fernausgabe* (June 2, 1976), 23-24. In a similar manner, Revel and Peter note: "It is indeed a silent body which the archives convey to the historian," *Le Corps,* 177.

37. Cf. Øivind Larsen, "Medisinsk journalmateriale fra 1700-talet som utgangspunkt for historiske undersøkelser," Sydsvenska medicin-historiska Sällskapet, *Årsskrift* (1968), 79-95.

38. All these data were transferred on a magnetic tape by teleprint 390 and were evaluated by means of Fortran IV programs in the computer. The results were then combined with the data-series which Karlheinz Böhme developed a few years ago for every patient on the basis of the personal register of people admitted to the Charité Hospital during the year 1731, 1733 to 1742 (since published in manuscript). Böhme, *Untersuchungen.*

39. Øivind Larsen, "'Söe-Quaest-Huuset' – Das Marinespital zu Kopenhagen und seine Funktion 1788-1791," *Medizinhistorisches Journal* (1970), 247-267.

40. Oivind Larsen, "Skykehusets funksjon i bergstaden Kongsberg i arene 1769-1772," *Medicinhistorisk Arsbok* (1967), independent page numbers.

41. All data concerning the patient population in the Charité Hospital that are based on the entries for reception in the hospital, are gleaned from: Böhme, *Untersuchungen.*

42. Cf. Diepgen and Heischkel, *Die Medizin,* 22.

43. Concerning Johann Theodor Eller, see Diepgen and Heischkel, *Die Medizin,* 5-14.

44. Next to his activities as a practical physician and professor, Eller was very active as a lecturer and wrote large numbers of scientific works on the various areas of the natural sciences and medicine. In the light of his observations and experiences, made on the basis of numerous diseases and their treatment in the Charité Hospital, he published already in 1730 his "useful and selected medical and surgical notations about interior and exterior diseases and about surgery in some of these cases which, up to that point, had taken place in the large hospital of the Charité founded by His Royal Majesty in Berlin; also a short introductory description of the foundation, growth and present condition of this house," (Berlin 1730).

45. Concerning the specifically professional dilemma of the "physician" and the "scientist," cf. more detailed information in Finzen, *Arzt,* 126 ss., 137 ss.; as well as Engelhardt, Wirth and Kindermann, *Kranke,* 48 ss.

46. Cf. e.g., Studies with informative titles such as: Jean-Pierre Peter, "Les mots et les objets de la maladie. Remarques sur les épidemics et la médicine dans la société française de la fin du XVIIIᵉ siecle," *Revue Historique,* (1971) 13-13. A detailed discussion of this problem is also in Arthur E. Imhof and Oivind Larsen, *Sozialgeschichte und Medizin,* (1975-1976), 140 ss.

47. Böhme, *Untersuchungen,* 88.

48. Death Register of the Charité Hospital since 1727; archives of the Evangelic Church in Germany, Church Office Berlin West. (The difference in the sums of charts 8 (2834) and 9 (2836) stems from the fact that in two cases the sex of the deceased was not registered and therefore no first names were mentioned. Unfortunately, every 5th case of death (21.1%) was registered without any special reference to occupation.

49. The data concerning Giessen are taken from: *Historische Demographie als Sozialgeschichte,* ed. by Arthur E. Imhof, Darmstadt and Marburg (1975) 152 ss. The detailed classification with specific reference to age was carried out on the basis of the investigation for the particular purpose of this study.

50. Cf. the vehement accusation of Ivan Illich, *Medical Nemesis* (London 1975). Cf. also Alexandre Dorozynski, *Médecine sans medicins* (Ottawa, 1975).

Peter L. Tylor

"DENIED THE POWER TO CHOOSE THE GOOD:"
SEXUALITY AND MENTAL DEFECT IN AMERICAN
MEDICAL PRACTICE, 1850-1920

During the 19th century while medicine was supplanting theology as the touchstone of authority in matters of sexuality, the beliefs of physicians became a dominant part of America's sexual ideology. That 19th century physicians and their contemporaries were deeply concerned with the management of human sexuality comes as no surprise to social and medical historians.[1] These concerns were premised on the widely accepted belief that sexuality had to be rationally channeled into socially acceptable outlets. Anxiety arising over the proper control of sex was expressed in such diverse areas as dress and dietary reform, marital advice books, the sale of patent medicines, the popular and professional literature, and the daily practice of medicine. The challenge for historians is to discover to what extent medical concepts of sexuality influenced individual behavior or public policy. This paper will attempt to meet this challenge by examining the relationship of sexuality and mental defect, including an analysis of the institutionalization of deviant men and women.

Recently Carl Degler has challenged the proposition that 19th century marital advice manuals are a reliable guide to sexual behavior — even the behavior of the urban middle class women to whom they were directed.[2] Degler's study is most useful in calling our attention to the divergent views of authors of advice manuals concerning female sexuality. In the first part of the article, Degler argues persuasively that we badly misread the sources if we believe that the 19th century authorities unanimously agreed that women had no legitimate sexual desires, and hence had no need for fulfillment. What Degler does not point out is the general agreement among these authors on two points. First, that women's sexual needs were milder than men's, and secondly that sexual satisfaction could only be allowed within the framework of marriage and moderation. Any sexual behavior that violated these norms became deviant. In the second part of the article, Degler's findings, based primarily on his discovery of the Mosher survey, lead him to conclude "historians are ill-advised to rely upon the marital-advice books as descriptions either of the sexual behavior of women or of general attitudes towards women's sexuality."[3]

For the purpose of analysis we should separate Degler's first statement that the advice books serve as poor descriptions of sexual behavior in the Victorian era, from his second assertion that the advice books tell us little about attitudes toward women's sexuality. Degler's first assertion, even if true, does not mandate acceptance of his second. Degler's first point gives historians advice that they have already taken. Nathan G. Hale, Jr. has previously observed that "'Civilized' morality was, above all, an ideal of conduct, not a description of reality. In many respects this moral system was a heroic attempt to coerce a recalcitrant and hostile reality."[4] Degler's second argument — that the advice books reveal little about sexual attitudes — is weaker. Although he may demonstrate that some women did not fully internalize the ideology of passionless chasteness, the manuals nonetheless provide much evidence about the attitudes of the men who originated and perpetuated the ideology. Why some men created a sexual ideology that may have distorted female sexual behavior is an important question, but one that I cannot discuss here. My efforts in this paper will draw upon different sources and deal with broader groups of women to show that the sexual beliefs of physicians defined and shaped public policy.

My primary argument is that 19th century sexual norms and gender roles encouraged physicians to treat deviant female sexual behavior as evidence of mental retardation which warranted strigent measures of social control. Concern for the social and sexual influence of the retarded was reflected in the creation of custodial facilities for women, the study of defective families, the eugenics movement, and differential admission and retention of women in American institutions for the mentally defective. The dominant sexual ideology, which stressed moderation and self-control, supported the doctor's assertions that sexual sins — masturbation, incest, consanguineous marriage, overindulgence — were at once causes and effects of hereditary disabilities. For most of the century, these concepts flourished in an intellectual milieu which accepted belief in the inheritance of acquired characteristics, without denying the power of the environment, (physicians posited the duality of mind and brain, distinguishing the brain's functions according to notions of faculty psychology, while acknowledging the important relationship of physical and mental health).[5]

This study relies on two types of sources. One is the literature concerned with mental retardation which is to be found in governmental and institutional reports, professional medical journals, and in more general periodicals. This was written mainly by the physicians who were employed as the chief medical officers and superintendents of the facilities for the retarded. The second source is a quantitative analysis of the records of American institutions for the mentally retarded.[6] The data presented were gathered from the surviving materials of every institution which had been in existence for at least twenty years during the period from 1850 to 1920. There were twelve such institutions in eleven states.

Before proceeding, it is important to clarify the 19th century concepts of the etiology, diagnosis, and classification of mental retardation. Classification schemes were imprecise, and they reflected social, and not medical judgments in most instances. The most accurately classified were the lowest grade, which constituted approximately 30% of the institutional population. These cases were classified as idiots, a term sometimes used to refer to all levels of retardation. Generally included in the lowest grade were individuals suffering overt physical lesions such as cretins, microcephalics, and mongoloids (Down's Syndrome). Imbeciles, the next highest grade, were considered to have more ability and could assist the less able, or perhaps be self-sufficient with the proper supervision. During the 1850s a new term, the feeble-minded, came into use. Specifically the feeble-minded were the highest grade, although the appellation was also used generically in reference to all grades of mental defect. These classifications did not correspond to any verifiable mental hierarchy. Until the development of the intelligence test, there was no agreed-upon method of determining either the existence or the degree of mental disabilities. A determination of retardation depended upon reference to subjective standards; physicians relied upon their personal judgment of an individual's mental and social capabilities. The relative nature of retardation was apparent to physicians, as one remarked:

> It is well to bear in mind that feeble-mindedness represents a comparative condition of the mental faculties, and that the demands of our age, the various requirements of the time are largely responsible (aside from heredity) for the vast numbers of incompetents that exist.[7]

Because the most commonly used definitions of retardation were based on social performance, there is no way to establish whether the majority of the institutional populations were actually retarded, or if they suffered from some other developmental disability not then diagnosed, or if they had violated societal norms and were institutionalized as a consequence.

The etiology of mental defect as understood in the 19th century was variegated, although it ultimately served to reinforce the physicians' norms of moderation and self-control. Superintendents of schools for the retarded, almost all of whom were physicians, never claimed to be able to cure idiocy. They were always careful to define it as condition, not a disease, that could be ameliorated but never entirely cured. They believed the retarded had suffered some physical lesion which prevented them from developing, first their perceptual senses, and then from acquiring the faculties of will, reason, judgment, or intelligence. The antecedents of this defective condition were believed to be either hereditary predisposition, or accidental causes such as childhood illness or neurological injury. Little could be done to prevent accident, but the hereditary predispositions, which were thought to be the result of inherited constitutional weakness, could be substantially eliminated by parental obedience to the natural laws of health.[8]

Dr. Samuel Gridley Howe in his pioneering *Report on the Condition of Idiots* (1848) found that 355 of the 359 parents he examined had "widely departed from the normal conditions of health and violated natural laws."[9] This verified the established belief that "the tendency to constitutional disease is transmitted from parent to child."[10] An inherited predisposition did not guarantee the development of any specific condition, but there was general agreement among physicians that

> repeated abuse and indulgence establish a condition at variance from that which is normal. The enfeebled or congested brain becomes habitual, the diseased condition of the body becomes chronic, and the law of hereditary transmission explains like begetting like.[11]

"Abuse and indulgence" referred to many possible transgressions; however, the superintendents reserved their strongest criticism for those who partook in intemperate sexual activity.

Unlawful and excessive use of the organs and functions of procreation, probably stands at the head of all enervating and demoralizing influences. That self-prostitution of innocent childhood, early learned and secretly practiced, which can not be here described in its ghastly contamination of body, mind and morals, developing too often into prurient libertinism and licentiousness of later years, when men blindly enter "temples of pleasure" to find themselves and their guilty paramours ushered through "the gates of hell" or tainted forever, in blood, bone, brain and soul: and yet again, the same evil, potential for misery in another guise, when concealing its hideousness under the sanction of marriage, and making of the "divine institution" a cover for unrestricted and senseless self-indulgence; youth and adult, married and unmarried, alike yielding to their unregenerate natures, in the abuse of bodies that should be the white, pure temples for purified souls; sinning against their moral convictions in the rush of passion, and in the hour of physical enervation and self-loathing. [12]

In a single sentence (!) Dr. Isaac N. Kerlin of Pennsylvania identified the three primary forms of sexual dissipation — masturbation, prostitution, overindulgence — which 19th century physicians condemned as violations of the precepts of moderation and self-control. The consequences of these violations could be dire. Idiocy was only one manifestation of hereditary weakness which was a warning that society, through its individual members, had to redeem itself.

Like other newly established ante-bellum institutions, the schools for the retarded were opened with an optimistic, almost evangelical faith that their operations would regenerate their charges and restore them to society. The first American schools were opened in Massachusetts on an experimental basis in 1848. This followed early French successes in special education which were pioneered by Edward Seguin in the previous decade.[13] Through the trans-Atlantic community of reformers Americans learned of Seguin's new methods, which he terms physiological instruction, and they were inspired to duplicate his achievements. The schools' founders and supporters believed

that in almost all cases, and with very few, if any exceptions, those usually called idiots, under the age of twelve or fifteen, may be so trained and instructed as to render them useful to themselves and fitted to learn some of the ordinary trades, or to engage in agriculture. [14]

To insure that the schools would not be "a mere asylum for custodial purposes,"[15] the students were admitted while they were still young and malleable, adults and individuals who were not improvable were excluded, and the pupils were retained only so long as they continued to benefit from instruction. They were discharged at the end of this time to make way for others. Therefore the mean age of admission and period of retention are the lowest for those admitted to the schools in the 1850s and 1860s (see Table 1), and the most common form of disposition is discharge (see Table 2). It should be noted that for almost the entire period from 1850 to 1920, the schools could neither initiate admission nor hinder removal; they could only reject unsuitable cases. The institutions' capacity provided for the needs of approximately one-tenth of the number of the retarded. There were always waiting lists and considerable pressure on admissions. Generally the schools initiated discharge or transfer, while removal refers to individuals separated from the institution without its prior consent.

After 1870 a new system of institutional life emerged. The sexual attitudes of physicians would ultimately shape the crucial elements of this system. As the first generation of students approached the critical school-leaving age, the superintendents had begun to acquire a more complete understanding of their pupils' true capabilities. After working with the retarded on a daily basis for twenty years the superintendents discovered that their students' rates of development were steadily declining over time. Earlier improvements which had seemed so encouraging, were due to the combined influence of the natural process of growth and entry into the therapeutic environment of the school. The effects of both factors diminished with time. Except for a few cases, there were no continued improvements after the age of puberty. Instead, the superintendents now warned of regression and of dangers to their patients and to society if the retarded were denied the proper care and supervision. By the late 1860s, institutional officials acknowledged that only a small percentage of their students could ever be completely self-supporting, and that alternate provisions for the retarded would have to be made. [16]

The institutions for the retarded gradually assumed a more custodial character, retaining some, but not all, residents for increasing periods of time. That the superintendents accepted this development is evident from the increasing proportion of those who died within the institutions (Table 2), together with the lengthening mean period of retention (Table 1). The dramatic increase in mortality for those admitted after the 1870s could be attributed to disease and poorer standards of health (for which there is little evidence), or it could be explained by a change in the institution's retention policy. This latter hypothesis is confirmed by the data in Table 1 which shows that the mean period of retention more than doubled for those admitted in the 1870s and 1880s as opposed to those admitted in the previous twenty years. In fact the mean period of retention for those admitted in the 1880s was the highest of any decade for the entire time span. This is partly explained by the relatively lower mean ages of admission for those admitted in the 1880s when compared to admission ages in succeeding decades. As the mean admission age rises, there will necessarily be shorter potential periods of retention, as older admissions have fewer potential years to be institutionalized than younger admissions.

The schools became custodial in another sense as well; their daily routines became more regimented, and institutional life became more inwardly focused. As the institutions began to productively employ their inmates' labor, the educational emphasis shifted from academic achievement to vocational training. One superintendent noted that "the school exercises, in the early days of the asylum its most prominent feature, still fulfill their proper function, but now in subordination to the more practical objects of the institution." [17] In the 1870s plans for a custodial department were published in the schools' *Annual Reports*. By the 1880s custodial facilities were being built, uniforms were instituted for staff and residents, and there had been some successful attempts to abolish the annual vacation in July or August, and to extend the mandatory school-leaving age of sixteen or eighteen. The custodial character was acquired in a piecemeal fashion by the various schools. Since each institution was a separate entity, no unified policies existed, but officials shared information and ideas through professional associations.[18]

These institutions embodied an ideology which insisted that both the retarded and society be protected from retardation and no group required as much protection as women of child-bearing years. Women's special needs grew directly from the sexual vulnerability projected on them by the "cult of true womanhood."[19] Sexual stereotypes dictated that women be admitted older and retained longer than men. Institutional officials had a ready explanation for the differential in the admission ages of men and women. Dr. James C. Carson of Syracuse, New York recognized that "feeble-minded boys are more difficult to care for at their homes than are feeble-minded girls. Especially is this true in urban communities."[20] Superintendent, Dr. Alfred W. Wilmarth emphasized the importance of gender role in relation to mental defect when he said,

> the boy is more destructive by instinct, and more restive and active in temperment, demonstrates early that is he mentally inadequate, and should be placed in our care. The girl is more closely kept, and more easily controlled when small. Only when she is physically matured, does she arouse attention as a potent factor in the increase of the unfit and a menace to public morals. [21]

Reflecting widely held beliefs about the nature of the sexes, Wilmarth's comments distinguished between the need to restrain men for reasons of public safety, while women required supervision to prevent socially undesirable sexual conduct.

How successful the institutions were in providing special protection is revealed in a close inspection of Table 1. Both the mean admission ages and periods of retention were higher for women than for men. Since these statistical means are strongly influenced by extreme cases, Table 3 and Table 4 present these data in a different format. These tables were created by first examining the ranges of both admission ages and periods of retention for the entire sample, and then classifying these ranges into quartiles. In both tables men constitute 57%, and women are 43%, of the totals. If sex is the only variable considered, an examination of Table 3 and Table 4 can test the null hypothesis that sex had no effect on admission age or retention. In both tables the null hypothesis is substantially upheld in the first three quartiles, but not in the fourth. Women are over-represented among those cases admitted over the age of eighteen (the actual range is eighteen to seventy-two), and women are over-represented among those cases retained for more than sixteen years (the range is sixteen to seventy-eight). With reference to the fourth quartile of both tables, the null hypothesis, that sex had no affect on admission age or period of retention, must be rejected.

At this point one might ask if sex is really the critical variable, or if it is masking the effect of some other factor. One alternative explanation, women's greater longevity, was not a significant contributor to their longer periods of retention. Remembering that women have a mean admission age two years greater than men, the age of death for women is 31.5 years, while for men it is 28.1 years. Class or economic status, as determined by an analysis of the father's occupation, appeared to play little role in admission age or retention. There are other variables which do have a substantial effect on mean age of admission and periods of retention; these variables are degrees of disability, nativity, and parental longevity. It should be noted that not every institution supplied information concerning all of these variables, but the sample size is large enough to be considered significant. An examination of admission age and retention periods for all of these variables demonstrates that a gender-reflective differential is maintained. For almost every category within these variables, women have greater mean admission ages and retention periods than men.

Nativity or birthplace has an obvious affect on admission age. The native-born have a greater opportunity to be admitted while very young, thus affecting the mean, than the foreign-born. But while the native-born do have a lower mean admission age (Table 5) than the foreign-born, within both categories women have a higher mean admission age than men. Nativity has a lesser affect on retention, but the gender differential is maintained. Degree of disability, as it was contemporaneously diagnosed, had a strong influence on admission age and retention. The more profoundly retarded had the lowest mean admission age and period of retention (Table 6). A severely retarded individual would be diagnosed at a younger age, and be a greater burden, than someone with a lesser affliction. The lower mean period of retention for the profoundly retarded is attributable to a higher mortality at younger ages than other degrees of disability. As would be expected, gender differences in mean admission ages and retentions are least pronounced among the severely retarded, and then increase as the degree of disability lessens.

Parental longevity was identified by multiple regression analysis as the most significant variable in predicting admission age and period of retention. Only two institutions, those at Glenwood, Iowa and Faribault, Minnesota, supplied information stating whether or not the mother and father were alive at the time of admission. Unfortunately the records from Glenwood are not complete enough to be very useful in this study. However, by comparing Faribault's institutional population with those of other states, I have determined that it is a representative sample in respect to age, gender, and retention distributions. As Table 7 reveals, families with both parents living enrolled their children at the youngest age, and kept them in the schools for the shortest time. The period of retention and age of admission for individuals removed from the institution are the lowest for any form of disposition (Table 8). Removal is a more prevalent form of disposition with both parents living than with any other family structure. Two other variables encouraged early admission. The proportion of native-born, and of the most severely retarded, is highest from two-parent households. The higher mean admission ages and periods of retention for individuals from one- or no-parent households indicates an attempt to delay admission, to provide care at home, until the death of a parent made institutionalization necessary. It should be possible to cross-reference these cases with census data to determine how quickly admission followed the parent's death. For these cases the most frequent disposition is death, while the least common is removal. These individuals have few alternatives but to remain within the institution until death or transfer elsewhere. The gender differentials in mean ages of admission and periods of retention are roughly proportional to the increasing mean age of admission; young children have somewhat smaller differentials, while adults have the largest. These differentials reflect increased sexual concern directed at women after the onset of puberty.

The study of defective families confirmed for many late 19th century physicians the terrible consequences of unrestrained sexual behavior. The first of these studies, *The Jukes,* was published in 1875 by Robert L. Dugdale.[22] Dugdale's findings dramatized for many readers the long suspected linkage between heredity and deviant behavior. Dugdale traced the history of five generations of an upstate New York family whom he called the Jukes. He found that criminality, pauperism, and licentiousness were each confined to a single branch of the Jukes. Using a type of human cost accounting, Dugdale calculated the Jukes had cost the state $1,308,000. Although Dugdale was circumspect in attributing the responsibility for social blight solely to heredity, his readers focused upon the point that if the original Juke parents had been prevented from having children, the state would have saved over a million dollars. Dugdale certainly did little to lessen interest in timely prophylactic measures by remarking that the Jukes "are not an exceptional class of people; their like may be found in every county in the state."[23]

The Jukes became the model for the numerous studies of defective families which followed. Later authors dwelled increasingly upon incidents of immorality, rape, licentiousness, incest, prostitution, and child abuse. They concentrated upon mothers who were congenitally unwilling or unable to perform their functions as teachers of morality, custodians of spiritual values, and guardians of virtue – all tasks that the concept of women's role in the family demanded. The researches of Oscar C. McCulloch into the tribe of Ishmael, a degenerate Indiana family, appeared in the 1880s. Concern with the relationship of heredity and social problems intensified after 1900, when such varied groups as the Hill Folks, The Nans, the Dacks, and possibly the most renowned of all, the Kallikaks, were investigated.[24] Many of these studies were conducted by eugenic field workers trained by Dr. Charles B. Davenport at his Eugenics Research Station.[25] The investigators sought to document the assumption that retardation, crime and vice were hereditary traits subject to transmission from generation to generation according to laws of Mendelian biology. All of the defective family studies had long pedigree charts of genealogies, complete with ubiquitous abbreviation to record the individual failures and shortcoming of family members. These studies, employing the crudest sort of Mendelian determinism, were readily accepted by physicians because they reinforced their belief that

> the most serious social consequences of permitting the mentally defective to participate fully in all phases of community life grow out of their inability to establish and maintain happy and well-ordered homes. High infant mortality, neglect of children, unsanitary living conditions and low moral standards characterize the homes of the feeble-minded.[26]

In short, defective families were a perverse negation of proper family life.

Institutional officials were also well aware of the disturbing effect of mental defect on normal households. These concerns about the well-ordered family were intimately associated with popular beliefs about female gender roles and sexuality. Dr. Walter E. Fernald of Massachusetts plaintively referred to

> countless loving mothers have been worried into nervous breakdowns or insanity, or

an untimely grave by the ceaseless anxiety and sorrow caused by the presence of the blighted child in the home. Many fathers have been driven to drink, sons to the "gang" and daughters to the street to get away from the unnatural and intolerable home conditions caused by the defective one. [27]

The superintendents realized that the public accepted the importance of their work because "it reaches the homes, the primary units of society upon the perfection of which the highest type of civilization depends. Whatever affects the homes whether for good or evil affects the country, the state, and the nation." [28] Relieving the home or the community of the care of the retarded and protecting both from degenerate influences was an important function of the institution, one which fully justified the institutionalization of adults for long periods of time.

The rationale for the retention of adult retarded women is best illustrated by the founding of the New York State Custodial Asylum for Feeble-minded Women in Newark, New York. In 1878, Josephine Shaw Lowell, the first woman member of the New York State Board of Charities, and the spokeswoman of its committee on the Condition of the Poorhouses, suggested the creation of a separate custodial asylum for retarded women of child-bearing age. [29] Her recommendation was prompted by her investigation of county poorhouses where she encountered weak-minded women who repeatedly bore illegitimate children, fathered by male inmates or other unscrupulous men only too willing to take advantage of their condition. In the same year it was suggested that $18,000 be appropriated to open an experimental home, which would be operated for the next seven years under the control of the older institution at Syracuse. Newark was hailed by other state institutional officials as a model to be imitated. Massachusetts and New Jersey were the only states to establish a separate custodial facility; almost all of the other states did create custodial departments and colonies associated with their central institutions. [30]

Newark's Board of Trustees emphasized that the purpose of the asylum was to take women "who grade in mind from being erratic to idiotic, one-fifth of whom being mothers from no wedlock," and who because of mental defect were "ungoverned and easily yielding to lust, denied the power to choose the good," and to "see them sheltered and shielded from the vices of vicious men." [31] While there was general agreement concerning the necessity of segregating retarded women, there were occasional complaints "that a few of the cases sent here were committed because they are wanton in their habits rather than lacking in intelligence. . . . Their proper home is in a reformatory rather than in an asylum for the feeble-minded." [32] It obviously was difficult to determine if the cause of immoral, licentious behavior was mental defect or simple perversity, especially since promiscuous actions were one indicator of retardation. According to physicians, one way of identifying high-grade imbecile girls was that "they run after the male sex without shame and make opportunities for sexual intercourse readily, cunningly, and frequently. . . ." [33]

Complicating the problem of classification was the concept of moral imbecility. [34] It was believed that the moral imbecile suffered an irreparable defect of the moral faculties comparable to the affliction of the intellectual faculties sustained by the retarded. However, only the moral sense, not the intelligence was affected. The moral imbecile was identified entirely through actions, behavior and attitudes. Many criminals, tramps and prostitutes were actually moral imbeciles. The difficulties presented to institutions for retarded by questionable cases of moral imbecility were best expressed by the Board of Trustees of the Massachusetts school:

> It is difficult to draw the line between the girl who has gone astray, or may be led astray, by reason of mental defect, and one who is merely a person of uncontrollable sexual desire. But be the line a broad or a narrow one, is this school to become a convenient "home" for girls of confessedly the latter description. In other words, is inordinate sexual passion on the part of a young woman to be regarded by the trustees as sufficient evidence of feeble-mindedness to hold her as an inmate of this institution. [35]

The Board was not disputing if "inordinate sexual passion" in a woman was a legitimate indicator of mental defect. Rather, it was raising the issue if sexual activity by itself was sufficient evidence of retardation. These cases where "the mental defect is relatively slight, and the immoral and criminal tendencies are strongly developed," [36] were classified as defective delinquents, and were provided with special facilities which combined the security of a prison with the educational features of the school.

After 1908 when the Binet-Simon intelligence test was introduced to the United States, physicians and psychologists believed it was a simple matter to classify mental defect. According to their standards, anyone who scored more than three mental years below their chronological age was retarded. The widespread use of the tests did reveal a new higher grade of mental defect, then classified as the "moron." [37] Aside from this development, the tests generally confirmed what institutional officials thought they already knew: that a significant percentage of criminals, paupers and prostitutes were retarded. A well publicized example of these findings were in the Massachusetts *Report of the Commission for the Investigation of the White Slave Traffic, So-Called* of 1914. The commission found in its examination of 300 prostitutes that 154 were mentally defective enough to warrant institutionalization for their average mental age was 9.5 years; of those who were rated as normal, "no more than six of the entire number seemed to have really good minds." [38]

I have tried to show in this paper that there was a strong relationship between the sexual beliefs of 19th century physicians and the assumed necessity of institutionalizing retarded women. Although Carl Degler has questioned the usefulness of marital advice books as sources of attitudes about women's sexuality, my research indicates that the sexual ideology expressed in these books was readily accepted and employed by physicians in rendering judgments about deviant sexual behavior and mental defect. Physicians' attitudes about proper sexual conduct were derived from both their professional experiences and from the wider society in which they lived. During the 19th century there was little conflict between these two spheres. Many doctors wholeheartedly subscribed to the sexual ideology presented in the advice literature; in fact, some of the most popular volumes were written by physicians.

Victorian physicians believed that men had stronger sexual desires, that they were the initiators of sexual activity, and that men were less discriminating than women in their choice of sexual partners. These beliefs were implicit in Dr. Fernald's remarks that

> a feeble-minded girl is exposed as no other girl in the world is exposed. She has not the sense enough to protect herself from the perils to which women are subjected. Often bright and attractive, if at large they either marry and bring forth in geometrical ratio a new generation of defectives and dependents or become irresponsible sources of corruption and debauchery in the communities where they live.[39]

For these reasons physicians believed that female mental defectives would be the easy prey of unthinking boys or unscrupulous men, while they thought most unlikely that any normal minded woman would seek the attentions of a retarded man. Although it was desirable that both sexes be custodially segregated, it was more important to safeguard women than men. This policy was justified by the perceived need to protect society from the consequences of "inordinate sexual passion," and to protect the retarded woman from her greater sexual vulnerability. So long as these beliefs were dominant, institutional populations would reflect gender differentials.[40] Women who had been "denied the power to choose the good" would not be given the opportunity to make any selection at all. In this instance, the sexual ideology of the 19th century was powerful enough to transfer anxiety out of the bedroom and into the asylum.

Illinois Institute of Technology   Peter L. Tylor

TABLE 1.
ADMISSION AGE AND RETENTION

Decade	Sex	Admission Age			Retention		
		$\bar{X}$	SD	N	$\bar{X}$	SD	N
1851-59	Men	11.1	3.8	28	5.7	9.2	28
	Women	10.0	2.8	14	5.8	7.2	13
	Both	10.8	3.5	42	5.7	8.7	41
1860-69	Men	10.8	2.6	19	5.0	7.4	16
	Women	10.0	3.7	23	4.8	3.5	30
	Both	10.4	3.2	42	4.9	4.4	46
1870-79	Men	11.7	4.0	48	7.2	8.7	41
	Women	11.8	3.7	21	12.6	18.2	19
	Both	11.7	3.8	69	9.0	12.6	60
1880-89	Men	12.0	6.1	123	14.1	13.4	119
	Women	13.4	6.0	82	14.7	12.9	80
	Both	12.6	6.0	205	14.3	13.2	199
1890-99	Men	15.4	10.6	299	12.7	15.0	293
	Women	15.3	9.7	245	14.1	15.2	242
	Both	15.4	10.2	544	13.3	15.0	535
1900-09	Men	14.4	8.0	542	11.4	14.2	576
	Women	16.3	10.4	407	12.8	14.7	407
	Both	15.2	9.1	949	12.0	14.4	983

Decade	Sex	Admission Age			Retention		
1910-19	Men	14.4	8.8	783	9.9	12.5	851
	Women	17.6	9.8	605	12.0	14.0	655
	Both	15.8	9.4	1388	10.8	13.2	1506
1851-	Men	14.2	8.6	1842	10.9	13.4	1924
1919	Women	16.3	9.7	1397	12.6	14.3	1436
	Both	15.1	9.2	3239	11.6	13.9	3360

TABLE 2.

PERCENTAGES OF DISPOSITIONS FOR EACH ADMISSION DECADE

	1851-59	1860-69	1870-79	1880-89	1890-99	1900-09	1910-19
Removal	0.0	0.0	10.0	13.5	19.5	17.7	11.1
Discharge	86.0	78.9	55.0	31.5	14.2	20.3	25.5
Death	14.0	7.9	20.0	45.0	51.6	44.6	35.1
Transfer	0.0	13.2	15.0	10.0	14.5	17.2	18.3

TABLE 3.

ADMISSION AGES BY QUARTILES

	1-9 Years		10-13 Years		14-17 Years		Over 18		Total	
	N	% Col.	N	% Col.	N	% Col.	N	% Col.	N	% Col.
Men	521	62.3	520	60.6	427	59.6	374	45.1	1842	56.9
Women	315	37.7	338	39.4	289	40.4	455	54.9	1397	43.1

TABLE 4.

RETENTION PERIODS BY QUARTILES

	0-23 Mos.		2-6 Years		7-15 Years		Over 16		Total	
	N	% Col.	N	% Col.	N	% Col.	N	% Col.	N	% Col.
Men	416	60.6	562	58.8	534	59.1	412	50.6	1924	57.3
Women	270	39.4	394	41.2	369	40.9	403	49.4	1436	42.7

TABLE 5.

ADMISSION AGE AND RETENTION BY NATIVITY

Nativity	Sex	Admission Age				Retention		
		X̄	SD	N	X̄		SD	N
Native-born	Men	13.2	8.6	1309	9.3		12.2	700
	Women	14.9	9.0	549	10.6		13.2	475
	Both	13.9	8.6	1435	9.9		12.6	1175
Foreign-born	Men	17.4	10.5	60	9.2		13.4	51
	Women	20.9	11.5	66	12.0		13.9	61
	Both	19.2	11.0	126	10.7		13.7	112
Total	Both	14.4	9.0	1435	9.9		12.8	1287

TABLE 6.

ADMISSION AGE AND RETENTION BY CLASSIFICATION OF DEFECT

Nativity	Sex	Admission Age			Retention		
		$\overline{X}$	SD	N	$\overline{X}$	SD	N
Profound	Men	14.4	9.7	118	10.8	12.2	98
(Idiots)	Women	15.5	10.0	118	11.7	12.3	102
	Both	15.0	9.9	236	11.2	12.2	200
Moderate	Men	14.5	8.9	168	13.2	13.0	136
(Idiot-	Women	16.7	10.4	129	11.4	12.6	95
Imbecile)	Both	15.5	9.6	297	12.5	12.8	231
Mild	Men	14.7	6.5	68	14.5	15.0	62
(Imbecile:	Women	20.1	9.8	45	17.8	13.8	43
Moron)	Both	16.9	8.3	113	15.8	14.6	105
Total	Both	16.0	10.2	963	11.3	12.3	872

TABLE 7.

ADMISSION AGE AND RETENTION BY PARENTAL LONGEVITY

Family	Sex	Admission Age			Retention		
	X	$\overline{X}$	SD	N	$\overline{X}$	SD	N
Both	Men	12.7	6.5	188	6.4	7.1	161
Parents	Women	14.2	7.9	143	6.0	7.1	119
	Both	13.3	7.1	331	6.3	7.2	280
Mother	Men	12.9	8.6	62	10.6	13.1	47
Only	Women	17.2	10.9	48	11.0	10.0	39
	Both	14.8	9.9	110	10.8	11.8	86
Father	Men	17.6	11.3	61	12.0	10.4	48
Only	Women	15.3	8.3	53	13.3	9.6	39
	Both	16.6	10.0	114	12.6	10.0	87
No	Men	22.7	15.3	58	12.6	11.9	46
Parents	Women	24.4	14.0	60	14.3	10.6	48
	Both	23.6	14.7	118	13.5	11.2	94
Total	Both	15.9	10.4	673	9.2	9.8	547

TABLE 8.

ADMISSION AGE AND RETENTION BY DISPOSITION

Disposition	Sex	Admission Age			Retention		
		$\overline{X}$	SD	N	$\overline{X}$	SD	N
Removal	Men	12.4	5.1	290	4.7	6.0	307
	Women	13.9	6.4	152	5.5	7.3	161
	Both	13.0	5.6	442	5.0	6.5	468
Discharge	Men	13.4	6.5	519	10.6	14.7	563
	Women	15.1	7.6	374	11.5	13.7	404
	Both	14.1	7.0	892	11.0	14.3	967
Death	Men	15.6	10.5	679	12.9	14.3	771
	Women	18.0	12.0	505	13.7	15.1	587
	Both	16.6	11.1	1184	13.1	14.6	1358
Transfer	Men	15.2	10.2	250	12.8	12.0	282
	Women	17.9	9.7	246	15.2	13.7	276
	Both	16.5	10.0	496	14.0	13.0	558
Total	Both	15.3	9.3	3015	11.5	13.7	3351

FOOTNOTES

The author wishes to acknowledge the generous support of the Elwyn Institute of Elwyn, Pennsylvania which made much of this work possible.

1. See: Ronald G. Walters, ed., *Primers for Prudery: Sexual Advice to Victorian America* (Englewood Cliffs, 1974); Ann Douglas Wood, "'The Fashionable Diseases': Women's Complaints and Their Treatment in 19th Century America," *Journal of Interdisciplinary History* 4, no. 1 (Summer, 1973), 25-52; Regina Morantz, "The Lady and Her Physician," in Mary S. Hartman and Lois Banner, eds. *Clio's Consciousness Raised: New Perspectives on the History of Women* (New York, 1974), 38-53; Ben Barker-Benfield, "The Spermatic Economy: A 19th Century View of Sexuality," in Michael Gordon, ed., *The American Family in Social-Historical Perspective* (New York, 1973), 336-372; Nathan G. Hale, Jr. *Freud and the Americans: The Beginnings of Psychoanalysis in the United States,* 1876-1917 (New York, 1971); John S. Haller, Jr., and Robin M. Haller, *The Physician and Sexuality in Victorian America,* (Urbana, 1974); Carroll Smith-Rosenberg and Charles Rosenberg, "The Female Animal: Medical and Biological Views of Women and Her Role in 19th Century America," *Journal of American History,* Vol. 60, no. 2 (September, 1973), 332-357; Charles Rosenberg, "Sexuality, Class and Role in 19th Century America," *American Quarterly,* Vol. 25 (May, 1973), 131-154; Carroll Smith-Rosenberg, "The Hysterical Women: Sex Roles and Role Conflict in 19th Century America," *Social Research,* Vol. 39 (1972), 652-78.

2. Carl N. Degler, "What Ought to Be and What Was: Women's Sexuality in the 19th Century," *American Historical Review,* Vol. 79, no. 5 (December, 1974), 1467-1490.

3. Degler, "What Ought," 1489. The Mosher Survey included responses of women to questions concerning their sexual activities.

4. Hale, *Freud and the Americans,* 25.

5. See: Norman Dain, *Concepts of Insanity in the United States, 1789-1865* (New Brunswick, 1964); Gerald N. Grob, *The State and the Mentally Ill: A History of Worcester State Hospital in Massachusetts, 1830-1920* (Chapel Hill, 1966).

6. All records were used while preserving the strictest medical confidentiality. I used the records of the following states, the dates are the time span of the records, the figures in parentheses are the number of cases: Massachusetts, 1851-1919 (590); Syracuse, N.Y., 1851-1912 (292); Ohio, 1912-1919 (192); Iowa, 1876-1905 (173); Indiana, 1879-1919 (323); Minnesota, 1879-1919 (503); Kansas, 1881-1919 (156); Maryland, 1889-1919 (129); Michigan, 1895-1919 (351); Rome, N.Y., 1894-1919 (472); Nebraska, 1887-1919 (165); and Wisconsin, 1897-1919 (284). I microfilmed the records and selected every tenth case for analysis. The sample size was 3630 from a population of over 36,000. Most individual records begin upon entry, and conclude with disposition from the institution. In all cases the individual's name, county of residence, and sex are indicated, and only two facilities failed to give either age at admission or birth year. In every record, save those cases still pending, the year of separation from the institution is given, and in most instances some explanation of disposition, such as death, discharge, transfer or removal, is supplied. From these data I compiled such basic indices as mean ages of admission, periods of retention, and ages at disposition. Some institutions supplied such useful additional data as birthplace or nativity, the degree of disability, parent's occupation, and if the parents were living at the time of admission. There is very little other information about the residents either before they enter or after they leave the institutions. For these data one would have to cross reference the census, which I have not yet done. One important caveat about these data: they are quite heterogeneous, and they have large standard deviations. In most instances some degree of association or correlation can be inferred, but certainly not any proofs of causality. Like other forms of historical material, these quantitative data will not stand alone; other sources from different perspectives are required to make their significance clear.

7. A. E. Osborne, "Presidental Address," *Proceedings of the Association of Medical Officers of American Institutions for Idiotic and Feeble-minded Persons* (Faribault, Minnesota, 1894), 395, hereafter cited as P.A.M.O.

8. See the excellent article by Charles E. Rosenberg, "The Bitter Fruit: Heredity, Disease and Social Thought in 19th Century America," *Perspectives in American History*, Vol. 8 (1974), 189-235.

9. Massachusetts Commission on the Condition of Idiots in the Commonwealth, *Report of the Commissioners Appointed to Inquire into the Conditions of Idiots in the Commonwealth* (Senate Document No. 51, Boston, 1848), 57.

10. *Fifth Annual Report of the Board of Directors of the Pennsylvania Training School For Feeble-minded Children* (Philadelphia, 1858), 24.

11. *Seventeenth Annual Report of the Trustees and the Superintendent of the Ohio Asylum for the Education of Idiotic and Imbecile Youth* (Columbus, 1864), 19.

12. *Fourteenth Annual Report of the Pennsylvania Training School for Feeble-minded Children* (Philadelphia, 1867), 19.

13. Seguin's major work was *Traitment moral, hygiene et education des idiots et des autres enfants arrieres* (Paris, 1846). He modified this work and published it as *Idiocy and its Treatment by the Physiological Method* (New York, 1866). Also see, Ivor Kraft, "Edward Seguin and the 19th Century Moral Treatment of Idiots," *Bulletin of the History of Medicine*, Vol. 45 (September-October 1961), 393-419.

14. *Third Annual Report of the Trustees of the New York Asylum for Idiots* (Assembly Document No. 54, Albany, 1854), 5.

15. *Third New York* (1854), 19.

16. For representative statements, see: *Fourteenth Pennsylvania* (1867), 19; *Sixteenth Annual Report of the Pennsylvania Training School for Feeble-minded Children* (Philadelphia, 1869); *Fourteenth Annual Report of the Trustees of the New York Asylum for Idiots* (Senate Document No. 54, Albany, 1865); *Twenty-seventh Annual Report of the Trustees of the Massachusetts School for Idiotic and Feeble-minded Youth* (Boston, 1874), 22; *Eleventh Annual Report of the Board of State Charities* (Boston, 1874), lxxvii.

17. *Eleventh Annual Report of the Trustees of the New York Asylum for Idiots* (Senate Document No. 59, Albany, 1862), 13.

18. The primary professional group was the Association of Medical Officers of American Institutions for Idiotic and Feeble-minded Persons, which was organized in 1876. The National Conference of Corrections and Charities also provided a forum for the superintendents.

19. See: Walters, *Primers,* 6; Hale, *Freud and the Americans,* 24-47; Carroll Smith-Rosenberg, "Beauty, the Beast and the Militant Women: A Case Study in Sex Roles and Social Stress in Jacksonian America, *American Quarterly,* Vol. 22 (1971), 562-584; David M. Kennedy, *Birth Control in America: The Career of Margaret Sanger* (New Haven, 1970), 36-71; Peter G. Filene, *Him Her Self: Sex Roles in Modern America* (New York, 1974), 92-103; Barbara Welter, "The Cult of True Womanhood," *American Quarterly,* Vol. 18 (Summer, 1966), 151-174.

20. *Fifty-second Annual Report of the Managers of the Syracuse State Institution for Feeble-Minded Children* (Assembly Document No. 6, Albany, 1902), 30; for an earlier statement, See Isaac N. Kerlin, "Enumeration, Classification and Causation of Idiocy," *Transactions of the Medical Society of Pennsylvania,* Vol. 17 (1880), 9.

21. *Tenth Biennal Report of the Wisconsin Home for the Feeble-Minded* (Madison, 1916), 274.

22. The work was first published in 1875 as an appendix to the *Thirty-first Annual Report of the New York Prison Association* (New York, 1875), and was entitled, "A Record and Study of the Relations of Crime, Pauperism and Disease."

23. Robert L. Dugdale, *The Jukes: A Study in Crime Pauperism, Disease and Heredity,* 4th ed. (New York, 1910), 66.

24. See: Florence H. Danielson and Charles B. Davenport, "The Hill Folk: Report of a Rural Community of Hereditary Defectives," Eugenics Record Office, *Memoir No. 1* (Cold Springs Harbor, 1912); Arthur H. Esterbrook and Charles B. Davenport, "The Nan Family: A Study in Cacogenics," Eugenics Record Office, *Memoir No. 2* (Cold Springs Harbor, 1912); Anna Finlayson, "The Dacks Family: A Study in the Hereditary Lack of Emotional Control," Eugenics Record Office, *Bulletin No. 15* (Cold Springs Harbor, 1916); Henry H. Goddard, *The Kallikak Family: A Study in the Heredity of Feeble-mindedness* (New York, 1912).

25. On Davenport and biology, see Charles E. Rosenberg, "Charles Benedict Davenport and the Beginning of Human Genetics." *Bulletin of the History of Medicine,* Vol. 35 (1961), 266-276. The best general work on eugenics is Mark H. Haller, *Eugenics: Hereditarian Attitudes in American Thought* (New Brunswick, 1963); and see Kenneth M. Ludmerer, *Genetics and American Society: A Historical Appraisal* (Baltimore, 1972); and Donald K. Pickens, *Eugenics and the Progressives* (Nashville, 1968).

26. Thomas W. Salmon, L. Pierce Clark, C. L. Dana, *Outlines of a State Policy for Dealing with Mental Deficiency* (New York, 1915), 4.

27. Walter E. Fernald, "Care of the Feeble-minded, *Proceedings of the National Conference of Charities and Corrections,* XXXI (1904), reprint, 3, hereafter cited as *N.C.C.C.* The same theme is repeated by virtually every institutional official, a good representative statement is in the *Second Biennial Report, of the Nebraska Institution for Feeble-minded Youth* (Lincoln, 1888), 187.

28. Arthur C. Rogers, "Presidential Address," *P.A.M.O.* (Philadelphia, 1891), 29.

29. For an interesting biographical sketch, see the memorial number of *Charities and the Commons,* Vol. 15 (December 2, 1905), 309-335.

30. For representative statements, see: *Thirtieth Annual Report of the Trustees of the Massachusetts School for Idiotic and Feeble-minded Youth* (Document No. 28, Boston, 1877), 14; the *Twenty-seventh Annual Report of the Board of Directors of the Pennsylvania Training School for Feeble-minded Children* (West Chester, 1879); the *Eighth Biennial Report of the Illinois Asylum for Feeble-minded Children* (Springfield, 1880), 8, 16; the *Twenty-second Annual Report of the Directors and Superintendent of the Connecticut School for Imbeciles* (Hartford, 1880), 6; and the *Twenty-fifth Annual Report of the Trustees and Superintendent of the Ohio Asylum for the Education of Idiotic and Imbecile Youth* (Columbus, 1881).

31. *Second Annual Report of the Trustees of the New York State Custodial Asylum for Feeble-minded Women* (Albany, 1887), 7.

32. *Thirty-second Annual Report of the Trustees of the New York Asylum for Idiots* (Assembly Document No. 23, Albany, 1883).

33. William N. Bullard, "The Placing Out of High Grade Imbecile Girls," *Boston Medical and Surgical Journal,* Vol. 155, no. 24 (June 17, 1910), 776-79, reprint, 2. For differing opinions on the sexual desires of the retarded, see Martin W. Barr, *Mental Defectives: The History Treatment and Training* (Philadelphia, 1910), 126, who argues that defectives had exaggerated sexual desires; and Henry H. Goddard, *Feeble-mindedness: Its Causes and Consequences* (New York, 1914), 497, who asserts the retarded merely lack sexual self-control.

34. Moral imbecility was mentioned as early as 1848 in the *Report on the Condition of Idiots,* 19-20, but it was most strongly developed by Isaac N. Kerlin, in his *Annual Reports* at Pennsylvania (1886, 1887, 1888), and papers presented to both the A.M.O., Isaac N. Kerlin, "Moral Imbecility," *P.A.M.O.* (1887), 32-37, and the N.C.C.C., "The Moral Imbecile," *N.C.C.C.,* XVII (1890), 244-250. Also see: Charles E. Rosenberg, *The Trial of the Assassin Guiteau: Psychiatry and Law in the Gilded Age* (Chicago, 1968), p. 68; Eric T. Carlson and Norman Dain, "The Meaning of Moral Insanity," *Bulletin of the History of Medicine,* Vol. 36 (1962), 130-140; and Arthur E. Fink, *Causes of Crime: Biological Theories in the United States, 1800-1915* (Philadelphia, 1938), pp. 48-75.

35. *Fifty-sixth Annual Report of the Trustees of the Massachusetts School for the Feeble-minded* (Boston, 1904), 17.

36. *Sixty-third Annual Report of the Massachusetts School for the Feeble-minded* (Document No. 28, Boston, 1910), 18.

37. See the "Report of the Committee on Classification of the Feeble-minded," *Journal of Psycho-Asthenics XIV* (September-December, 1910), 61-67. There is a huge literature on intelligence testing and social problems. J.E. Wallace-Wallin, *The Problems of Subnormality* (Yonkers-on-Hudson, 1917), 123-188 reviews forty-three of the most prominent investigations, but as Binet testing was popularized, there were literally thousands of these examinations. See: Fink, *Causes of Crime,* 217-234 for a guide to the bibliography; also see Peter L. Tyor, "Segregation or Surgery: The Mentally Retarded in America" (unpub. Ph.D. diss., Northwestern University, 1972), 188-223, for a more detailed discussion of retardation, crime, psychology and genetics.

38. *Report of the Commission for the Investigation of the White Slave Traffic, So-Called* (Boston, 1914), 30.

39. Walter E. Fernald, "The History of the Treatment of the Feeble-minded," *N.C.C.C.*, XX (1893), reprint, 10.

40. In 1974-75 the sexual ratios of residential institutions for the retarded were 60% male and 40% female. Contrast this with the 55:45 ratio of the 19th century. In conversation with institutional officials, they all expressed the belief that today's sexual ratios closely represent the occurrence of mental defect in the population, while those of the past tended toward over-representation of women for social rather than purely medical reasons.

Matthew Ramsey

MEDICAL POWER AND POPULAR MEDICINE: ILLEGAL HEALERS IN NINETEENTH-CENTURY FRANCE

In the rise of the medical profession, the social history of medicine has found one of its standard themes. In every "modern" society physicians have won some form of monopoly for their version of medicine, and the victors, as usually happens, have figured most prominently in historical writing. Yet what we would now call "parallel" medical practice constituted a major part of the medical systems of Western Europe and the United States until recent times. Since it served the needs of much of the population, it is well worth studying in its own right, and the relations between popular and official healers form an important chapter in the history of professionalization. Modern medicine did not arise in a vacuum; it established itself by denying legitimacy to competing practitioners and medical cultures.[1]

This article will deal with one case: the history of unauthorized healers in the French department of the Bas-Rhin during the first decades of the 19th century. This administrative division, in the northern part of the old province of Alsace, owed many of its medical traditions to German institutions, which were marked by an early and strong concern with public health and the control of charlatanism and popular medicine.[2] In the Napoleonic period, the Bas-Rhin developed one of the most extensive systems of medical administration in France and produced the fullest police records on medicine of any department. These documents suggest the range of popular healers perceived by physicians and the local authorities, as well as the views of illegal practice taken by local doctors who may never have published on the subject or even corresponded with a learned society.[3]

My larger concern, though, will be with the workings of the nexus of professional and administrative authority which is sometimes known as *le pouvoir médical,* or medical power. Physicians in the French Enlightenment, who described themselves as *médecins éclairés,* insisted that the profession, in cooperation with the state, should oversee medical practice and public health. Both proponents and critics of professional monopoly agree that the apparatus of licensing laws and regulations adopted in the 19th century was translated into a form of social control. Physicians and hospitals pre-empted the delivery of health care, discarding traditional methods of treating and preventing disease as superstitious, and branding popular healers as deviants. Taking the argument one step further, Ivan Illich and Michel Foucault have suggested, in their different idioms, the extensive "normalizing" effects of modern medicine, which touch not only on popular medical practices, but on an increasing range of other human behavior as well.[4]

The new history of medical power parallels the history of professionalization. If the latter has tended to exalt the process through which a certified élite strengthened its grasp on medical practice, the more recent writings have stressed the repressive and coercive aspects of monopoly. I would like to examine here the early stages of medical power in one domain: the control of illegal practice at the local level. Although the campaign against popular healers was in fact a major preoccupation of the French medical élite in the 18th and 19th centuries, it is easy to confuse the repressive program with the effective suppression of deviance, especially when its history is written exclusively from literary sources. Medical power was never entirely a myth; but what were its limits?

I. Medical police

In the year XI of the French Revolutionary calendar (1803), as the last elements of the Napoleonic Code were being ratified, the Consulate adopted two laws on medicine and pharmacy. The statute known, according to the French custom of identifying legislation by the date of enactment, as the law of 19 Ventôse year XI (10 March 1803), was to govern the medical professions until 1892, despite several attempts at revision in the course of the century. The new provisions united medicine and surgery for the first time, but set up a special category of healers with less demanding training than the physicians received, not unlike the old country surgeons of the Ancien Régime; these were the *officiers de santé*, of whom Charles Bovary in Flaubert's novel is a familiar literary example. The law also standardized a system of licensing practitioners, with a view to ending the "medical anarchy" that was believed to have followed the abolition of the old medical faculties during the Revolution, without reverting to the confusing pattern of endorsements, patents, and local authorizations which had characterized the Ancien Régime. In each department a medical "jury" was to examine candidates and draw up a list of authorized personnel. Any healer not on the rolls was *ipso facto* an illegal practitioner and subject to prosecution.[5]

The juries shared the oversight of professional practice with the regular administrative network made up of the prefects, subprefects, and their aides, and in some areas with local health councils as well; collectively, these institutions constituted a new medical bureaucracy. One of its functions was to call the attention of the prosecutors and the courts to illegal healing. The phrase "medical police," which in the 18th century usually referred to what we would now think of as public health, sometimes took on this additional sense. (In French, writers often reserved the term "police médicale" for public health and spoke of the regulation of the profession as "la police de la médecine.") The policing of medicine called in theory for constant observation, for a *quadrillage* of the territory that would pinpoint the activities of authorized and unauthorized healers alike. The principle of total surveillance, which Foucault has called "panopticism," an allusion to Bentham's "panopticon" prison, found an almost rhapsodic expression in one early 19th-century French handbook of jurisprudence:

> You can judge that no part of the Empire escapes observation, that no crime, no offense, no infraction can remain unprosecuted, and that the eye of the genius who

knows how to shed light on everything takes in the whole of this vast machine, without, however, overlooking the least detail. [6]

Applied to medicine such a program would ideally have produced a complete census of illegal practitioners and even of their patients, enabling the police to identify and repress every instance of illicit practice.

The Bas-Rhin came as close as any French department to realizing a strict surveillance of medical practice. The School (later Faculty) of Medicine of Strasbourg, one of the major centers of official medicine, had a part in this program. The departmental bureaucracy played an even greater role, especially in the last years of the Empire, thanks in large part to the efforts of an aggressive prefect, Adrien Lezay-Marnésia, who was transferred to the post of Strasbourg from Coblenz in 1810. This scion of the Ancien Régime nobility, who had studied at the University of Göttingen and remained a fervent disciple of the *Aufklärung*, complained that "every good regulation exists in this world, and yet everything proceeds as if there were none." He undertook a complete reorganization of the departmental bureaucracy and a program of enlightened reform from above which, in the words of the historian of Napoleonic Alsace, was to lead to a "veritable intendancy."[7]

In the field of public health (as indeed in everything else), Lezay-Marnésia soon showed signs of what French functionaries would call *du zèle,* and perhaps even *du zèle excessif.* Partly as a result of his experience in Germany, he was keenly aware of the requirements of a good medical police. His creations included a network of cantonal physicians (*médecins cantonaux*) — salaried civil servants, named by competitive examination, whose role recalled that of the 18th-century German *Physikus* or *Landarzt.* They were charged with caring for poor patients, vaccinating the population (a high priority for the administration), regulating wet nurses and prostitutes, and preparing expert reports in forensic medicine. Medical practice also came under their supervision, and in principle their trimestrial reports to the prefect were to indicate the state of "empirical medicine" in their jurisdictions.[8]

The reports of the cantonal physicians form the basis of the following discussion of the range of illegal healers in the Bas-Rhin and the responses of official practitioners to quackery and popular medicine. Some additional information comes from the isolated reports of individual physicians, and some from legal proceedings initiated by local authorities. It was the cantonal physicians, however, who had the most regular contact with rural medical conditions and local healers. A few were zealous supporters of the Enlightenment campaign against popular medicine, while others cooperated only reluctantly. But they were all points of contact between official and popular medicine, and symbols of medical power in the countryside.

II. The Illegal healers

In its broad outlines, illegal practice in the Bas-Rhin recalled the traditional medical network of Ancien Régime France: unlicensed midwives, itinerant charlatans who set up theaters in public squares, local occult healers and quacks who "scanned" urine to diagnose disease, and the far less visible folk healers, including *devins-guérisseurs* who, as their dual title indicates, combined healing with divination.[9] Many popular healers had achieved some sort of official recognition or at least toleration in the Ancien Régime, among them surgical specialists (such as bonesetters and hernia operators), ecclesiastics and other charitable healers, and peddlers of orvietan and other licensed remedies. After the reforms of the Napoleonic era, these practitioners were in theory either coopted into official medicine (as by studying surgery at a regular medical school) or outlawed.

The police and most physicians distinguished between itinerants — who posed the clearest threat not only to the privileges of the medical corporations, but also to public order — and resident healers, whose less aggressive practice was nevertheless more insidious because more difficult to detect. (The police were on the whole more concerned with vagrancy — *vagabondage* — than with the regulation of medical practice.) Eighteenth-century commentators also made a rough distinction between *charlatans*, or quack doctors, and *maiges*, or popular healers who were part of the local village culture and practiced folk medicine. I would add a third broad category: occasional healers, mostly economic marginals, who practiced empirical medicine for the sake of a little cash income.

The following discussion will consider the itinerant and sedentary healers who appeared in the reports of the physicians and administrators in the Bas-Rhin through the first half of the 19th century. A separate section will treat censuses of unauthorized healers and their implications for the social interpretation of popular healing, since this development in information gathering is in itself an important problem in the history of medical power.

Itinerant quacks

Like members of other ambulatory trades, most quacks were forced to travel because they could not earn enough from their specialty in any one place. Many itinerants were not actually full-time charlatans. Some *colporteurs* peddled medicines among other wares, notably the "Tyrolians" who sold the herbal infusion known as "Swiss tea," together with more dangerous drugs.[10] The less successful quacks were barely distinguishable from the other migrants who wandered through the department when times were hard. The agricultural statistics for 1814 in the canton of Brumath, for example, lumped them together in a note which observed that "beggars, especially vagrant Jews, Bohemians, and quack doctors" infested the countryside.[11]

But the department also had its share of classic mountebanks. In order to attract a clientele, they made themselves deliberately conspicuous, announcing their arrival with printed flyers, dressing in elaborate costumes, and using carnival barkers' techniques to draw large crowds at fairs and other public places. It has sometimes been suggested that the old-fashioned itinerant charlatan disappeared at the end of the 18th century, when the growth of advertising in provincial journals allowed a mail-order trade in patent remedies to flourish for the first time. But the quacks survived, like other *colporteurs*, through the 19th century.[12] The Bas-Rhin saw at least one troupe of classic mountebanks during the Napoleonic period. In 1803, not long before the new legislation on medical practice, the subprefect at Wissembourg issued a decree against the Traber brothers, natives of Mutzig in the Bas-Rhin, who had adopted Altenstadt as their base of operations. They travelled "around the communes, accompanied by a harlequin, selling drugs and unapproved remedies in the public squares, and gather[ed] the people with clowning in order to sell them more readily."[13] A "Traber," possibly one of the brothers, reappeared in the police records five years later, when he was arrested and convicted of illegal medical practice in the annexed Rhenish department of the Roer (Rur). This healer identified only as a native of the Bas-Rhin, called himself a physician.[14] In 1810, finally, a certain "Tauber" from the Bas-Rhin appeared in the Napoleonic department of Mont-Tonnerre in the Rhenish Palatinate. He called himself a dentist and oculist – two traditional empirical specialties – and travelled on horseback from village to village, claiming, among other things, to possess a marvelous specific to cure chronic illnesses in twenty-four hours, and to make goiters disappear. A buffoon followed him to distribute his flagons.[15] If these cases involved the same man, he operated for a decade in several German-speaking departments on both sides of the Rhine.

An itinerant charlatan of the classic type appeared as late as 1844 at Schiltigheim in the Bas-Rhin, where he was denounced by the cantonal physician. Disguised as a Chinaman, he peddled medicine "to the credulous inhabitants of the countryside, to the sound of trumpet and drum," saying that he was a millionaire and that he came not to earn money but exclusively "to help suffering humanity." In the four villages around the town he sold "more than 400 flagons at 1 franc and 1 franc 50 apiece of a green water that he declared a universal panacea. . . ." Several of the cantonal physician's patients bought the alleged remedy and "became ill as a result."[16]

Two itinerants succeeded in winning so regular a following in the department that they effectively served a part of the population as physicians, as their nicknames of "Doctor Johann" and "Doctor Hans" suggest. In February of 1811, the cantonal physician of Sarre-Union denounced to the prefect a "quack and famous ignoramus who is called Dr. Johann."

> I have been told that he is from around Bischwiller, arrondissement of Strasbourg, travels around the region, works terrible havoc, and swindles money from the credulous and superstitious inhabitants of the countryside. The people, who are gladly drawn to miracles and extraordinary things, chase after him in a mob in order to consult him. He gives prescriptions transcribed from an old German medical book, which he has others write down . . . ."[17]

He required the assistance of others to record the prescriptions because, according to the mayor of Bergzabern, where Dr. Johann had his main practice, he could neither read nor write.[18] The quack's background is obscure. The prosecutor at Wissembourg reported that his real name was Johann Propheter (significantly he gave the forename as "Jean"), and that he came from Switzerland originally and was already "getting on in years."[19] Other accounts said that he was from Bergzabern (Wissembourg), or even from the environs of Strasbourg, although the subprefect of Wissembourg added that he had "long since lost his rights as a citizen and his domicile."[20] The cantonal physician at Wissembourg at one point called him a baker; this is the only reference to a previous occupation.[21] Propheter had travelled widely in the department, practicing medicine in the cantons of Sarre-Union and Wissembourg, as well as in the arrondissement of Strasbourg, and had previously been arrested several times at Deux-Ponts (Zweibrücken), just over the border in the department of Mont-Tonnerre. So well established was Dr. Johann's reputation that the local apothecaries filled the prescription he wrote for his patients.[22] His practice in the Bas-Rhin continued at least two years; he appeared again in a census of illegal practitioners in 1813.[23]

The career of Dr. Hans was both longer and more varied. Jean (Hans) Volk or Volck probably came from Freiburg in the Grand Duchy of Baden; originally a shoemaker, he sometimes went by the second sobriquet of "Schumacher Hans."[24] The first mention of Dr. Hans comes in a report of January, 1811, by Hoffmann, a physician at Wissembourg, on an epidemic in the communes of Ober- and Niederbetschdorf. Volk was a "foreigner . . . who after being driven from his own country, came to seek refuge in ours, where he wanders with no fixed abode and works hard at making dupes . . . ."[25] Volk's activities ranged so widely that he appeared in the reports of several different cantonal physicians in 1813. In the canton of Brumath, Dr. Hans had been "very much in vogue a year ago in and around Gambsheim," where he "kept hidden during the day and travelled at night to see his patients, who were sometimes very far away."[26] Buchholtz, cantonal physician at Wissembourg, also denounced Volk, noting that he had already cited him in his regular report to the prefect in January, 1811.[27] And at Woerth, the cantonal physician complained that the "vagabond who calls himself Doctor Hanz . . . works great havoc in my canton . . . ." In this report he was linked with a local cartwright as one who was "adept in magical arts and sorcery."[28] Volk became a notorious recidivist, probably the best known illegal practitioner in the Bas-Rhin. He was subsequently convicted of illegal medical practice in 1818 and denounced still another time by the cantonal physician at Soultz-sous-Forêts two years later.[29]

Sedentary Healers

The itinerants, with a few exceptions such as Dr. Hans, rarely succeeded in establishing a regular following in the regions where they worked; many, indeed, were careful not to visit the same place twice with the same bag of tricks. Some might establish themselves in or near a large town for as long as several months, like Albertine Dränkler, who settled at Bischheim-am-Saum near Strasbourg in 1801, boasting that she could cure more than twenty disorders using surgery or medication.[30] But the resident healers belonged to the community in which they found a clientele, and if they were to practice any length of time they needed a permanent pool of patients. Even with a loyal following it was difficult to maintain a full-time practice outside of a city such as Strasbourg, although some local healers in France enjoyed at least a passing vogue which enabled them to draw patients from towns and villages as much as a hundred kilometers away. In most cases medicine could only be a sideline.

The majority of sedentary healers practiced routine empirical medicine or simply sold a few secret remedies. But a justice of the peace at Strasbourg dealt with one case in 1799 involving a pair of occult healers: Jean-Frédéric Küchel (or Kiechel), a former notary, and Barbe Richert, wife of a hemp grower. Barbe Richert was a "somnambulist"; on emerging from a hypnotic trance she recommended remedies to her patients, who purchased them from local pharmacies. Küchel was a magnetizer (mesmerist); he induced the trances and noted the responses of his partner, who did not know how to write. Küchel's mesmerist practice was not limited to hypnotism; he reappeared in 1808 as the discoverer of a "new infallible means to cure most of the external disorders of the body promptly and radically, whatever may have produced them, without the help of medication, by a light laying-on of the hand, or by a simple touch."[31]

The Bas-Rhin seems to have had no well-known religious healers in the early 19th century, comparable to the "saint of Savières," near Troyes, who enjoyed a few years of notoriety in the 18th century.[32] The clergy continued to exercise their traditional healing function, and some were indistinguishable from the quack doctors, at least in the eyes of the medical profession. In 1818 the cantonal physician at Niederbronn denounced "two scourges of humanity": a Protestant minister at Barenthal (Sarre-Union) and the curé of Lichtenberg (Petite-Pierre), both of whom administered remedies after inspecting the patient's urine and saw to it that they were "paid well."[33] One inspired healer was seen as a deviant by the local communities as well as by the authorities. The son of a blacksmith in the Haut-Rhin, he settled at Sélestat in the Bas-Rhin in 1841, calling himself "brother Martin." According to the prefect, he had already lived in various parts of the arrondissement as a hermit and most recently at "a pilgrimage near Dambach, where the inhabitants expelled him for laxity of conduct . . . ." He even went to Strasbourg, according to the report of the cantonal physician, "where he must be treating several persons."[34] Marginals of this sort posed a ticklish problem for the authorities and for the new discipline of forensic psychiatry: were they madmen or impostors?[35] Clearly they were beyond the pale of both official medicine and folk culture.

As for folk medicine itself, it rarely passed into the records of medical police; when no injury was done and no money changed hands, a case was unlikely to wind up in the courts. One zealous cantonal physician, Lion at Soultz-sous -Forêts, did complain about the "unfortunate accidents that have befallen Jewish children, as a result of the ineptitude of the person who performs the operation of circumcision on them."[36] There was no mention, though, of the *schormer*, or mystical healer, who was consulted by Jewish and Gentile patients alike in Alsace.[37] Folklore practices usually became visible to the authorities only when they constituted a threat to public order. One such incident occurred in 1820, when a girl at Lembach developed symptoms which the local population attributed to demonic possession. The cantonal physician offered the opinion that she was suffering from delirium and convulsions; he attributed her condition to worms. But the girl's father, deciding that the "assistance of medicine" was useless, ascribed the disease to a "supernatural cause." It therefore became "a question of exorcising his child, who said that the devil was waiting for her at the door, and who blasphemed when other persons prayed." Although charlatans played no role in this religious cure, the authorities expressed alarm at the presence around the patient's bed, day and night, of "some thirty weak and credulous persons," in a market town of about 1,800 inhabitants. The prefect intervened and transferred the girl to the local asylum, where the resident physician found his own positivist explanation for her behavior: "symptoms which indicate strong pains in the head and perhaps a case of hydrocephaly."[38] Superstition, then, could become a police problem. Accusations of witchcraft and charges of swindling by local magicians could also provoke disturbances, and records of some of them turn up in the judicial archives. But of the world of witches and *devins-guérisseurs,* pilgrimages and healing saints, the medical bureaucracy of the early 19th century took little direct notice.

III. Censuses of illegal practitioners

From the records of the medical police emerges a fragmentary picture of a network of parallel healers, survivals of the traditional medical system of the Ancien Régime and rivals of the official personnel. The quacks and especially the itinerants have a major place — greater, indeed, than their role in parallel medicine would warrant. It is likely that the special reports from physicians or officials considered so far, which were intended to promote the prosecution of major offenders, introduce a distortion into the description of unauthorized healing. Only more systematic surveys of popular medicine could give a sense of the full range of parallel practitioners, particularly the less conspicuous sedentary healers. At least two such lists survive from the Bas-Rhin of the early 19th century. The first is a report to the tribunal at Strasbourg from the medical jury on those persons who "as a matter of common knowledge" practiced medicine at Strasbourg without authorization in 1805. The second dossier is actually a compilation of reports prepared by the cantonal physicians in 1813.

The medical jury's list for Strasbourg identified nine individuals, including two whose names are familiar: Küchel, the hypnotist, who according to the report practiced medicine and distributed an "elixir"; and the Richert woman, "known by the name of La Dormeuse, or Barbe la Dormeuse." The others included an abbé; a weaver who treated external conditions and consumption; a *graissier* (grocer dealing in grease) who treated cancers; a shoemaker who practiced medicine "without being on any list"; and a self-styled *officier de santé* who had signed a spurious certificate. Among those whose occupations were identified are two "clerks," the abbé and the former notary (Küchel); two artisans; a peasant; and a small tradesman. One was the wife of a hemp grower.[39] Medicine appears here chiefly as a secondary activity, sometimes linked to the principal occupation: the shoemaker made us of his manual dexterity, and the *graissier* no doubt applied lard to the cancers.

The 1813 list was compiled at the instigation of Lezay-Marnésia, who recognized the principle that in medical police, as in any administrative domain, information is in a sense power; repression could not be directed against invisible targets. In a circular of 29 May 1813, he complained that empiricism was still "ravaging" the countryside, in spite of his decree of 1810 and subsequent instructions on medical police, and asked the cantonal physicians for a detailed report on all persons who practiced medicine without authorization.[40] The physicians' responses touch first of all on a familiar range of traditional healers, among them itinerant *colporteurs* and quacks (including Dr. Hans and Dr. Johann),[41] barbers,[42] and an executioner at Memelshoffen (canton of Soultz-sous-Forets) who dabbled in surgery. In the Ancien Régime it was commonly believed that the *bourreau,* whose duties included torturing suspects, was familiar with human anatomy and could mend the same parts that he knew how to break. This one was called Henri (Heinrich) Heid and went by the name of Master Henner.[43]

Midwives and unauthorized *matrones* have a large place in the reports. Two of them, apparently authorized *sages-femmes,* were accused of practicing medicine; the others were charged with practicing midwifery without a license.[44] In general the physicians complained of the dubious competence of the local midwives, and according to some reports nearly all *accoucheuses* practiced medicine as well, bleeding patients, administering remedies, and dosing small children with opiates.[45] A small number of women healers (about a fifth of the women on the list) practiced only branches of medicine and surgery other than midwifery.[46] Women had enjoyed an important place in the traditional medical network, but the jurisprudence of the Ancien Régime held that they could not practice as physicians, a principle sustained by the courts in the 19th century.[47] In all, almost half of the practitioners on the 1813 lists were women.

For the remaining empirics, the reports usually indicated some primary occupation other than healing. The few exceptions may have been full-time quacks;[48] the reports also cited three surgeons whose names were not on the official rolls, including the grandson of a surgeon and a man referred to as a student of surgery.[49] One part-time healer was identified only as the mayor of the commune of Dürrenbach (canton of Woerth, Wissembourg).[50] Occasional healers also included three "clerks" – two clergymen[51] and a certain Mathieu Treibel, clerk to a schoolmaster in the canton of Soultz-sous-Forêts (Wissembourg), who, according to the cantonal physician, had practiced medicine "without the least knowledge of the subject" since the age of eight. He was commonly known as "Provisor," the German word for a pharmacist's aide, perhaps a reminiscence of an earlier calling, perhaps simply a tribute to his skill in dispensing.[52] These educated healers recall a time when any literate person in the countryside was likely to practice a little charitable medicine, drawing on printed handbooks like *Les Remèdes de Mme Fouquet.*

A larger number of popular healers covered in the 1813 survey were artisans or tradespeople, although in some cases they became so successful in their medical practice that they abandoned the earlier occupation altogether. The sobriquets by which they were frequently known usually referred to this calling – "Pfeifenschneider" or "Weber Jackel."[53] The regular métier did not necessarily dictate the decision to practice medicine or the choice of therapeutic methods. The 1813 cases do not even suggest a transfer of empirical skills; the part-time healers had recourse to the sale of remedies or to occasional practice simply as a source of extra income which required no additional training and almost no initial investment.[54] In folk medicine, the occupation might have been linked more closely with the healing vocation; certain trades – carpentry, for example – were believed to confer the "gift" of healing, sometimes through hereditary transmission from father to son.[55] In contrast to the occasional practitioners, the folk healers who possessed the "gift" often avoided taking payment in money and sometimes refused remuneration altogether, out of fear of jeopardizing the efficacy of the healing rite. Partly for this reason the folk healers remained less visible than the mercenaries and went almost untouched by the 1813 survey. It is significant that among the occupations mentioned we find one "gardener" but no farmer or peasant.[56] Indeed most of the healers were based in towns or resided there permanently. In the canton of Brumath, for example, three of the empirics cited by the cantonal physician practiced in the town of Brumath itself;[57] and in the arrondissement of Sélestat, none of the reported healers had a rural practice.[58] The most visible empirics, then, were urban, though they sometimes sought a wider market in the countryside.

In view of the types of healers on which the survey was likely to touch, it is not surprising that their healing methods rarely varied from what might be called normal empiricism — the sale of remedies, traditional internal medicine, and surgery, singly or in combination. The reports occasionally refer to mystical healing, amulettes, exorcism, and magical practices. A certain Blassing in the Lutheran village of Dürstel even used "so-called witchcraft" and aroused "implacable hatreds in the communes" (probably by accusing local inhabitants of casting spells on his patients).[59] But such cases are unusual.

The following table summarizes the findings of the 1813 survey:

UNAUTHORIZED HEALERS IN THE BAS-RHIN, 1813[60]

Sex		Occupation		Type of practice	
M	39	"Midwife"	26	Medicine and general empiricism	29
F	32	Barber	8	Surgery	24
		Artisan	9	Midwifery	24
		Other	10	Sale of remedies	7
		No second occupation, or not known	1	Magic/sorcery	5
Total	71		71		– –

The records of medical police suggest that a social interpretation of popular healing and its relation to medical power in the 19th century must consider medicine as an economic activity. The more conspicuous healers were in effect successful small-time entrepreneurs. The charlatan's tricks may seem like an elaborate confidence game, which of course in a way they were; but these were the marketing techniques used by tradesmen in the Ancien Régime who operated outside the restrictions (and protection) of the guilds. The charlatan had to find ways to extract money from a clientele which had little cash and did not part with it easily. An old peasant proverb had it that a wound in the body would heal with time, but that a "wound" in one's money (*plaie d'argent*) would never mend. The 19th-century quacks continued the entrepreneurial tradition. Successful practitioners may have helped the towns by linking the peasants to the market economy; certainly local apothecaries often profited from their practice, since they bought some of their supplies on the spot. But they became dangerous economic rivals for some physicians.

The 1813 survey reveals another sizable category — occasional healers who, while less likely than the quacks to turn up in the regular reports, probably outnumbered them in the parallel medical network. The nicknames by which they were known often indicated their primary occupation (just as the best known itinerants were called "Doctor"). For them medicine was a supplementary source of income; some were victims of economic dislocation and found themselves with no secure niche in either the traditional or the modern economies. Their healing practice, which clearly did not fit into the world of official medicine, showed no unambiguous affinities with folk culture either. While they may not have been as distressed as the wandering beggars described in the 1814 statistics for the canton of Brumath, they remained economic marginals. If the successful charlatans exploited the possibilities of an urbanizing society, many of the part-time healers were its victims. The notion that these people might once have had a secure niche in "traditional" society is, of course, largely a myth; but this myth had its place in the ideology of official medicine, which suggested that the popular healers were men and women out of place, set apart from the populace they duped and from the administration and profession whose functions they subverted.

As for the largely invisible activities of the folk healers, they fell into the domain of what contemporary observers called *l'économie domestique,* the daily management of the household in a traditional society. The folk healer did not solicit custom; to borrow another expression from the 19th-century commentators, he was not *entreprenant.* His healing function may have owed more to considerations of prestige and tradition than to economic need; the same was true, for that matter, of charitable healing by local notabilities. Not that physicians condoned popular superstitions or even empirical healing by philanthropic persons; but as long as the healers stayed within the bounds of the *oeconomia,* they were unlikely to enter the purview of the medical bureaucracy.

IV. The Physicians look at popular medicine

Taken together, the comments by the physicians on the unauthorized healers suggest a highly conventional rhetoric on quackery and popular medicine which the official personnel used to affirm its own legitimacy and elicit support from the administration. The stereotyped image is a dark one, reiminiscent sometimes of the classical *topos* of the world turned upside-down, in which the quacks were seemingly on top and the professionals on the bottom. Most cantonal physicians insisted that charlatanism was rife in their own jurisdictions. Lion, cantonal physician at Soultz-sous-Forêts, might have spoken for each of his colleagues when he complained that "there is perhaps no other canton in the department, where charlatanism is practiced with more audacity than in mine." [61] Lacking statistical evidence, physicians throughout this period usually saw illegal medical practice as on the increase, like the practitioner who in 1844 denounced "the swindling which continues to spread in these parts." [62] Quacks, moreover, completed successfully with official healers for a clientele. Even the one cantonal physician who reported no resident empirics in 1813, Buchholtz at Wissembourg, regretted that the inhabitants of the countryside were "always more inclined to pay for the pompous promises of a charlatan than to recognize the useful care that a man without pretentions can give them."[63] Often the physician went unconsulted, as the cantonal physician at Niederbronn noted in a report of 1818 on an "extraordinary mortality" in the commune of Rothbach. "As a result of unforgiveable negligence, as well as blind confidence in charlatans, most of the inhabitants of the commune do not ask for the physician's aid except as a last resort; others simply refer all care to Providence."[64]

The neglected official healers who suffered financially blamed the charlatans; some were even so poor that they could not pay the fee for the licensing examination and thus remained technically unauthorized.[65] The cantonal physicians enjoyed greater security; their state salaries of from 600 to 1200 francs sufficed to put them in a better position than the lower ranks of the *officiers de santé*.[66] But even for them the charlatan was a direct and sometimes dangerous rival, and the local population was often inimical to their efforts in a post which, in the words of one incumbent, was "especially onerous and thankless."[67] The cantonal physician of Sarre-Union begged the prefect to take steps "to stop this evil [charlatanism], which does more harm than an epidemic disease," adding that he would also "avoid the unpleasantness for the cantonal physician of being in disfavor with the lower classes by prosecuting this sort of quacks, who are ordinarily particularly skillful in winning the blind confidence of the people . . . ."[68] One reluctant functionary actually feared retaliation from the charlatans he denounced:

> I would not want to make a personal question out of what I have been obliged to report and say above, knowing the spitefulness and vengefulness of most men. For . . . my profession obliges me to be constantly on the road, often even at night, and I am a husband and a father; the preservation of my life is therefore of great importance to me.[69]

But the strongest argument that the physicians could advance against the quacks was that they were dangerous to the population as a whole. Something of the 18th century's fear of depopulation lingered on in this protostatistical era; the peasantry in particular, the "most precious class" in the view of the enlightened physicians, had to be protected as a national resource. That the quacks were a *fléau destructeur,* a devastating scourge, was a rhetorical commonplace, but many commentators who used the phrase believed it quite literally. With only the crudest notions of how to assess correlations and strong confidence in the superiority of their own methods, they saw the quacks' patients die and reasoned *post hoc ergo propter hoc.* When Dr. Johann established himself openly as the rival of Neurohr, cantonal physician at Bergzabern (Wissembourg), where the physician was treating patients afflicted with an epidemic disease which he diagnosed as dysentery, the mayor blamed him for the death of 40 patients."[70] Dr. Hans was similarly attacked by Hoffmann, a physician treating an epidemic of "typhus" in the canton of Wissembourg. At Oberbetschdorf, he noted, "among the nine patients I saw . . . , five seemed to me to be in great danger, especially two who had been treated, according to admissions made to me, by a foreigner named Jean Volk."[71] In the same way, one of the responses in the 1813 survey blamed a curé practicing medicine for the deaths of three out of the four victims of an epidemic at Rothbach. This sort of argument could be inflated almost at will. The curé and a Protestant pastor shared responsibility in one cantonal physician's view for three-quarters of the 159 deaths he attributed to an epidemic disease in the cantons of Bouxwiller and Petite-Pierre.[72] The cantonal physician at Marckolsheim underscored the connection between quack medicine and demographic decline in an attack on a healer at Schoenau, noting sarcastically that "a proof of the skill of this famous doctor is that in that commune the number of deaths last year surpassed the number of births."[73]

The physicians' sense of impotence in their relations with the quacks contrasts with their apparent sense of confidence in dealing with the literal *fléau destructeur,* epidemic disease. In the case of the Protestant pastor, for example, two victims of the empiric were said to have been rescued by timely attention from medical doctors.[74] To be sure the physicians' rhetoric owed something to political interest; they could not very well report to the administration that they were helpless to fight disease but all-powerful against charlatanism. Still, although many physicians may have adhered in principle to a doctrine of expectant medicine and in practice made little use of drastic treatment, they had a strong sense that their intervention was essential; the motif "if only a physician had been called in time" was a commonplace long before the age of scientific medicine. Physicians saved; quacks killed.

The quack, though, was more than a murderer; he was also — and in the eyes of the physicians this was an almost equal offense — an *escroc,* a swindler. Not only was his practice unauthorized, but in the Ancien Régime his *charlataneries* had run counter to the spirit of guild regulations on fair dealing; now he was guilty of a breach of what we would call professional ethics, which were intended to safeguard the rights of the practitioners as much as those of the patients. The great villain in the rhetoric of medical enlightenment was not the superstitious peasant but the schemer who knowingly exploited his "vulgar errors." The cantonal physician at Brumath reserved his severest censure for a woman healer who in his view did the most harm because she was "an old hypocrite."[75] His counterpart at Geispolsheim (arrondissement of Strasbourg) developed this theme in a section of his 1813 report in which he added to his list of illegal practitioners "a few general considerations" on what "universally constitutes empiricism in the countryside":

> Bigotry and ignorance are indisputably an enormous source from which arise the swarm of prejudices that infect the countryside and resist even the most persuasive statements by enlightened men. Nevertheless, it is not the stubbornness of the people that must be blamed the most; let us rather point the finger at the audacity of the impostors who know how to take adroit advantage of its credulity and dupe its good faith. In what class of men, then, do we find most of these artists of deception, of these swindlers, I venture to say?

> Leaving aside abuses in matters of empiricism which prevail exclusively in the domestic economy and which consist in the fact that many heads of families are possessors of a few universal remedies, good against all ills, and whose secret is transmitted only from father to son (we often see similar remedies advised, obtained and administered by a man or woman neighbor, result in fatal consequences); there are besides a certain number of dreamers, magnetizers, makers of sympathetic magic and others, for whom I cannot give the names or places of residence, places where they are best able to conceal their activities and escape the pursuit of the police. Strasbourg, they generally say, is the center. [76]

Although the comment treats domestic medicine as hazardous, the author singles out for blame the entrepreneurial activities of the city quacks, "artists of deception" and "swindlers." Medical charlatanism may be added to the long list of vices attributed to urban corruption. The wily empiric knew how to extract the peasant's small cash savings – better, indeed, than the physician did. His irruption in the countryside constituted a breach of the economic peace.

Without reducing all of the physicians' attacks on the quacks to a question of material interest, it can be argued that the charlatans affronted the official practitioners' sense of economic justice. Their profession had traditionally made a heavy investment in education and charges for membership in the medical corporations in the Ancient Régime; even under the new medical order costs were high, and they believed that the profession deserved an enforced monopoly of patients' fees. The history of illegal medical practice in the early 19th century suggests that medicine was given over (as some had wished to recognize explicitly during the Revolution) to "free enterprise" (*libre commerce*), just as much as other economic activities. The physicians, while hesitant to advocate reviving the old corporations in their earlier form, remained resolutely anticapitalist in their professional domain.

If the quacks appeared as economic deviants, so in their own way did the occasional healers who neglected or abandoned a regular trade. The physicians' comments are impregnated with a class morality which the French sometimes call *la morale du bonhomme Richard,* after Franklin's Poor Richard: indolence and vice explained a behavior which might well have resulted from economic necessity. Lion, cantonal physician at Soultz-sous-Forêts, remarked of "Weber Jackel": "laziness, mother of all the vices, has banished him from society; it is only through swindling that he supports himself." Material pressures may have forced Jacques Vern to abandon his "profession and trade"; he was possibly a victim of the economic crisis of 1810-11 in Alsace, which affected the textile industry. He may even have sought an "honest" supplementary occupation to help him sustain an adequate income when times were hard, since the general list of empirics for the arrondissement identified him as a shoemaker as well as a weaver. But in the physician's eyes he was unwilling to work. An even worse offender was the healer who had no recognized trade other than quackery, such as Justin Breit, known as "Justul." "Instead of working and earning his living honestly, he hurries from one village to another in order to carry out as many swindles as possible, using his poisoned remedies." [77] The descriptions of the offending popular healers recall a conventional image of the social deviant: crafty and indolent, the empiric was the very type of the bad citizens.

Indeed physicians could often accuse popular rivals of multiple forms of deviance. In one case, for example, the informant charged that a healer mutilated conscripts to make them unfit for military service – a crime which particularly attracted the attention of the administration to popular healers. [78] In another case, a barber practicing medicine at Huttenheim was said to be "under the influence of wine from the morning on." [79] Two stereotypes of the fringe healer, however, are absent from the police reports of the Bas-Rhin, although they were common in the medical literature of the time. Quacks sometimes appeared to contemporary observers as lunatics, especially when they claimed to be religiously inspired; but only the case of "brother Martin" approaches the conventional image of the madman. The misogyny which sometimes led a physician to say that medicine was practiced in his district by the most ignorant peasants "and even by women" is muted here; the commentaries include no general denunciation of *femmelettes* who meddled in the healing art.

Missing, too, are the stereotypes of the folk healer and *devin.* The silence of this archive of medical police on folk medicine is not characteristic of the medical literature of the late 18th and early 19th century. Popular healers appeared in the reports of the *médecins des épidémies* sent into the provinces by the Intendants in the Ancien Régime, and at the end of the 18th century in the correspondence of the Société Royale de Médecine, an Enlightenment model for the project of medical police.[80] In the early modern treatises on "vulgar errors" in medicine and in the first studies of medical folklore at the beginning of the 19th century, the discussions of *maiges* and their methods were often extensive.[81] Physicians began to recognize a system of thought and therapeutics radically different from official medicine. This new focus on popular behavior was in keeping with the transition, which Foucault has recently described in *Surveiller et punir,* from an emphasis on public retribution for public offenses (of which the shaming and expulsion of quacks was an example in the Ancien Régime) to the systematic surveillance and "normalization" of deviant behavior. Yet, while many official healers may have shared in this consensus, it is likely that the more securely established physicians took a stronger interest in medical folklore than did their more vulnerable colleagues, some of whom, among the *officiers de santé,* may have been closer in outlook to their peasant patients than to the professional élite. The lower stratum of official healers feared most of all the rivals who intruded on their precarious practice.

V. Medical power and popular medicine

The administration echoed the physicians' hostility to popular practitioners; in theory it was this nexus of governmental and professional organization that created *le pouvoir médical.* The Bas-Rhin had a consistent record of opposition to charlatanism. Even before the legislation of the year XI, the administration prosecuted quacks, invoking the statutes of the Ancien Régime, as in the case of the Traber brothers. In October, 1810, Lezay-Marnésia issued a decree on illegal medical practice, and subsequent instructions reminded his subprefects of the policy they were to enforce. The prefect put pressure on the courts as well; when Jean Volk was first arrested in 1811, Lezay-Marnésia sent a note to the Wissembourg tribunal exhorting it "to let the credulous inhabitants of the countryside enjoy the guarantee which the law promises them against these dangerous empirics, who are nothing more than assassins and swindlers."[82]

A successor issued a directive to the mayors in 1817 reiterating the call for a strict medical police in the countryside. They were to denounce any individual distributing drugs or practicing medicine, but their surveillance "must above all be applied to quacks in the proper sense, who by means of so-called sympathetic remedies, which they administer with mysterious procedures, take possession of the credulity of the country people and contribute to maintaining prejudices which it is important to destroy."[83] Here in brief was enlightened medicine's program of attack against its popular rivals. But the constant reiteration of directives, reminiscent of the pattern of repetitive decrees in the legislation of the Ancien Régime, bespeaks a record of frustration.

It is not very surprising that this program failed. Napoleonic France was far from having the resources to carry out a systematic program of social control in any domain — even military recruitment, which mattered far more to the state. Many popular healers simply remained invisible to the medical police, as in the canton of Wissembourg, where Buchholtz, the cantonal physician, reported in 1813 no resident empirics but only "a few from outside who carry out their fatal practices on the credulity of the inhabitants" (Doctors Hans and Johann).[84] His colleague from Geispolsheim made the general comments on rural empiricism already cited because, he said, he was "unable to report individual cases."[85]

Even when empirics had been identified, enforcement at the local level was uneven. When Dr. Hans, for example, appeared in the canton of Wissembourg in 1820, the division of the national police which had jurisdiction over the Bas-Rhin found it necessary to urge both the subprefect and the royal prosecutor to act.[86] Some frustrated cantonal physicians hinted darkly that a quack might have "protectors" in their region,[87] and in fact some mayors did support local healers. One mayor in the arrondissement of Saverne refused to divulge the name of an *accoucheuse* for the 1813 survey.[88] In keeping with the Ancien Régime tradition of local authorizations, many mayors gave quacks documents allowing them to practice in their towns and then travel on to other communities. The subprefect of Speyer in the department of Mont-Tonnerre wrote that the "Tauber" quack had, "besides illegally delivered visas . . . a superb certificate from the mayor of Landau which paid tribute to his talents and to the evidence he had given of them in the town entrusted to his administration."[89] "These kinds of quacks," the prefect of the Roer observed, "are ordinarily in possession of passports, so that the mayors and officers of the judicial police are unable to arrest them" (presumably for vagrancy.)[90] Dr. Hans was particularly successful in securing the cooperation of local mayors; their testimonials served in his 1811 trial, and the cantonal physicians complained about the mayors' support for him in 1813 and again in 1820.[91] The physicians were of course at the greatest disadvantage when the mayor himself was a quack healer, as in the commune of Dürrenbach.[92]

Even when a quack was prosecuted, convictions for illegal medical practice could be difficult to obtain. Before 1803, the courts hesitated to apply pre-Revolutionary statutes on medical practice; the year before the new legislation the subprefect at Wissembourg heaped scorn on the magistrates who could find "no legal disposition which authorized to inflict penalties on the children of [Paracelsus]."[93] Even under the regime of the laws of the year XI, the machinery of repression turned slowly and sometimes not at all, provoking a regular series of administrative exhortations to act. The physicians criticized what they saw as the laxity of the administration and the courts combined and denounced the apparent impunity with which their rivals practiced "medical vandalism."[94]

The official healers' indignation reached its acme in the cases of "Doctors" Hans and Johann, which followed divergent paths to very similar, and for the physicians equally frustrating, conclusions. At least at the outset the local authorities were inclined to show more leniency towards Volk (Dr. Hans) than towards Propheter (Dr. Johann), although the administration in Paris favored a uniformly rigorist interpretation of the law of 1803. When Aronsohn, cantonal physician at Sarre-Union, first reported Dr. Johann, the prefect was uncertain whether this man was the same as Dr. Hans, whom he had already arraigned in the Wissembourg court, and he asked the imperial prosecutor for a clarification. The healer denounced by Aronsohn, the prosecutor replied, was not "our Doctor Hans, but a true quack and dangerous empiric. Jean Volk, from whom I obtained this information, got to know him as a result of having been called to help people who had been crippled or ruined by this quack."[95] Here Dr. Hans was promoted, as it were, to the unofficial status of *officier de santé.*

Volk did in the end stand trial, but he emerged almost unscathed. For his defense he fell back on the empiric's typical self-justification: if the physician could cite his training and official authorization to legitimate his practice, the popular healer could invoke successful outcomes, a record of public service, and local approval. Volk insisted that the inhabitants of the village where he practiced had sought him out three times during an epidemic, adding that he had cured "fifteen to sixteen people from that place who [were present at the hearing] to confirm the truth of this fact, whereas the physician with their knowledge were unable to save anyone." The records of the session indicate that the defendant did benefit from the presence of more than twenty persons who said that they had been cured by him gratis, and that he made maximum use of more than twelve certificates from local mayors. Indeed in the Ancien Régime, Volk might have come close to establishing a prescriptive right to practice. Under the new dispensation his conviction was a foregone conclusion, and every favorable testimony was damaging evidence against him, since it confirmed the fact of illegal practice. Yet as a matter of law the court was willing to admit a distinction between two categories of healers: "vagabonds, charlatans, and swindlers"; and "persons who practice medicine without a diploma, but who cure their fellow men of certain diseases, using a sort of domestic medicine, and who add neither quackery nor swindling to this service which they render to suffering humanity." It imposed a comparatively light though not insignificant penalty (50-franc fine, 15 days in prison, and expenses) and ordered that he be transported across the Rhine after serving his sentence.[96] The court's decision recalls the jurisprudence of the Ancien Régime, which was usually ready to tolerate a disinterested and relatively harmless healer; expelling the offender, which had been a common device in the local police jurisdictions of the 18th century, made sense in Napoleonic France only in the case of a foreigner visiting a border region.

It is unlikely that the medical profession shared the administration's willingness to tolerate Volk in 1811, and certainly the 1813 reports do not depict him as the innocent exemplar of domestic healing. "He is more dangerous than murderous weapons in the hands of a madman," wrote the cantonal physician at Soultz-sous-Forêts.

Through the mysterious air that he gives to his dealings, through the words that he utters, through the lies and effrontery that he uses with the credulous inhabitants of the countryside, and through various other kinds of charlatanism, he has been able to win for himself authority and limitless confidence . . . . His principle is to have himself paid triple or quadruple the price of drugs. [97]

The final note was almost predictably an attack on the charlatan's commercial activity. Dr. Hans clearly appears here as a swindler. He was also by 1813 a *convicted* illegal healer. What distressed the physicians most was the recidivism of popular practitioners, who were apparently not discouraged from practicing even by successful prosecution. One cantonal physician complained that Volk had "already been arrested and even convicted for practicing medicine, an art of which he is totally ignorant," and yet had managed to escape a punishment which was "waiting" for him and which he "deserved."[98] Even after serving a prison sentence, a colleague noted, Volk still practiced "the infamous trade of quack more than ever."[99]

In contrast to Jean Volk, Propheter appeared to the authorities at the outset as an itinerant swindler — the prefect proposed punishing him equally "as an empiric and a vagabond" — and they blamed him for several deaths.[100] But the quack proved an elusive target. When he first appeared in the canton of Sarre-Union in 1811, he usually escaped detection by local mayors by practicing only at night and leaving again the next day.[101] Since he enjoyed popular support, the police found that they could only accelerate his travels without eliminating his practice. After he was threatened with arrest and fled towards Bitche in the Moselle, "the people" ran after him, begging him to return soon. Arrested in the canton of Wissembourg he returned in triumph a week later "on a cart, led by a crowd of children, who shouted in the streets . . . ." The local population, according to the mayor of Bergzabern, publicly mocked the authorities for making the arrest, as well as the cantonal physician who had first denounced Propheter. The penalties the courts imposed in this case were too slight to serve as an effective deterrent. Dr. Johann was fined less than Dr. Hans — only 12 francs, a sum which he could have shrugged off as a minor professional expense.[102] The physicians were outraged. "This man should have felt, when first setting foot in the department of the Bas-Rhin, that law and order reign there . . . . Surgeons, barbers, and midwives meddle in the practice of internal medicine. What will happen if vagabonds practice medicine publicly?"[103]

The litany of complaints continued into the Restoration. Schneider, cantonal physician at Lauterbourg and Setz, wrote in 1816: "Charlatanism continues at its former rate, and the number of male or female practitioners so lightly tolerated increases daily. Soon there will not be a village that does not have a similar "doctor" or physician.[104] And Lion, the zealous critic of empiricism in the 1813 reports, still cantonal physician at Soultz in 1820, saw no improvement: "the laws of medical police are threatened in a shocking way"; a disease that was not particularly dangerous in itself had "wrought havoc, because of the quacks . . . ."[105] In 1821, the Ministry of the Interior itself took the royal prosecutor at Wasselonne to task for having "in no way deigned to carry out the measures prescribed by law," and asked that local officials show more severity towards charlatanism — "without which it is to be feared that in the end charlatans will invade the surrounding area, and especially the canton of Wasselonne, where they exist in greater number than anywhere else." [106] The failure of enforcement had become a convention in the rhetoric on illegal medical practice.

Looking to the future of medical police, the physicians expressed only a guarded optimism. At best they expected a decline in classic charlatanism; the less visible forms of popular healing would be more difficult to attack. The strongest statement of this view came from Buchholtz, the one cantonal physician who (no doubt too sanguinely) reported no resident empirics in his jurisdiction in 1813:

> The extirpation of charlatanism is probably a difficult thing to attain in every country under an orderly government, as we learn from the example of other countries, and especially those of Germany, where for a long time the governments have dealt with it without having obtained a perfect result from their efforts up to now. Public quackery can be destroyed; the public displays of quacks can be forbidden; the very tendency of the age makes repressive laws on this matter almost superfluous, since these sorts of crude speculations can no longer find dupes; but empiricism that is domestic and, so to speak, legal, if I may express myself thus, is more difficult to strike a blow against, although it is the most dangerous of all where public health is concerned. [107]

The form of "hidden empiricism" which Buchholtz feared most of all was actually practice by unqualified *officiers de santé*; since they were often the closest rivals of the physicians in the countryside, it is not surprising that the subject became a kind of King Charles's head. But the inconspicuous popular healers proved a still more stubborn enemy.

In the early 19th century, the repression of medical folklore did not become a consistent objective of medical police; even the census of small-time healers never developed into a coherent program. The movement for reform produced only the jeremiads of official medicine, without the systematic surveillance that might have permitted effective repression. The means and motivation were lacking. Occasional practitioners were too difficult to distinguish from the rest of the population and constituted a slighter threat to public order than did the quacks. Although the prefects ritually denounced popular superstition in their departmental *Statistics*, [108] folk healing did not constitute a regular target of the police and administration. Or rather, it was not simply a question of medical police in the usual sense where the "credulous and ignorant" people and their superstitions were concerned; there was no need to identify individual delinquents where deviance was, so to speak, the norm, where an entire culture was deviant. To suppress popular medicine nothing less was needed than a reform of the peasant mind; and the institution of socialization best suited to this task, however much the physicians may have wanted to have a hand in it, was the school. [109]

Seen in the context of a local jurisdiction, the repression of popular medicine appears in the early part of the 19th century as an unrealized project. To be sure, medical power was not entirely a myth. A well-designed bureaucratic mechanism existed to combat illegal medical practice; individual healers did stand trial, and some of them went to jail. Yet the recidivism rate must in itself have suggested the inadequacy of what might have been called, to borrow an expression from the physicians, "heroic measures." If the Bas-Rhin, with its well-developed system of medical police, could not regulate medical practice effectively, then it is unlikely that any local administration could have done so in the first decades after 1803. It would be a mistake to equate a repressive program with the reality of social control.

On the local level, the representatives of official medicine found themselves obliged to compete for a space in medical practice occupied by a host of part-time medical entrepreneurs, as well as by the more conspicuous survivors of the traditional medical network of the Ancien Régime. In the medical literature of the 19th century, the contest between the physicians and their rivals sometimes appears as the heroic phase of professionalization, pitting medical enlightenment against popular superstition. But the protagonists in the local struggle were rarely the physician-scientist, on the one hand, and the witch-healer, rooted in folk culture, on the other. More often, highly insecure "professionals" confronted still more vulnerable marginals — vagrants, unsuccessful artisans, widows, people without a safe niche in a changing economy and society.

Some of the subsequent success of official medicine can be ascribed to the therapeutic advances of the late 19th and 20th centuries. Education and urbanization could be cited among the many forces which have broken down peasant resistance to official medicine; the regular medical network has become more accessible for most Frenchmen, and social security has provided a powerful financial incentive to consult licensed practitioners.[110] Repression of illegal practice played a small role in this transformation. It is of course true that social control can be realized through other means than direct police action, and the factors just cited contributed indirectly to what has been called medical power. But this study suggests that in the early 19th century there was a critical disparity between the aspirations of a group which proposed to exercise hegemony over one professional domain and the reality of frustration and social inertia. To read the later developments which privileged professional medicine into the earlier period would be anachronistic. Like medicine itself, medical power had its limits.

Harvard University   Matthew Ramsey

FOOTNOTES

*Research for this article was supported by a fellowship from the Social Science Research Council and a Sheldon Travelling Fellowship from Harvard University.

1. Popular medicine is not of course a new subject. The folklore movement of the late 19th and early 20th centuries began a tradition of empirical investigation into popular healing that continues to the present day, and there is also an extensive literature on quacks. Some of the French material is surveyed in Marcelle Bouteiller, *Médecine populaire d'hier et d'aujourd'hui* (Paris, 1966). See also Arnold Van Gennep, *Manuel de folklore français contemporain* (Paris, 1938), vol. 4, 596-620. Little of this work, however, rises above the level of routine compilation and what the French call *la petite histoire,* and the struggle between authorized and unauthorized healers rarely receives systematic consideration. What is more, the archival sources that might illuminate relations between physicians and their rivals have not been fully exploited.

The local records on public health in the French *archives départementales* provide an unusual glimpse of unauthorized healers. For the 19th century, the materials on the regulation of medical practice are mostly in the "M" series. A few local studies have been based on these records: Jacques Nouvel, "L'Exercice illégal de la médecine dans la Marne de 1803 à 1868," *Mémoires de la Société d'Agriculture, Sciences et Arts de la Marne,* vol. 84 (1969), 109-68; and for the beginning of the century, Hérissay, "L'Exercice illégal de la médecine dans l'Eure," *Bulletin de la Société Francaise d'Histoire de la Médecine* (1932), 84-94, and François Forestier, "Vingt ans d'exercice de la médecine dans l'Yonne: 1790-1810," unpublished thesis, Paris Faculty of Medicine (1950, No. 296). A more extensive treatment appears in the forthcoming thesis (*thèse de doctorat d'état*) by Jacques Léonard on medical practice in western France in the 19th century. Jean-Pierre Goubert also discusses illegal medical practice at the end of the 18th century in *Malades et médecins en Bretagne: 1770-1790* (Paris, 1974). I am indebted to him for his assistance during my research in Paris.

2. On the public health tradition in the 18th century, see George Rosen, *A History of Public Health* (New York, 1958), chapter 5; and Alfons Fischer, *Geschichte des deutschen Gesundheitswesens* (Berlin, 1933), vol. 2. Cf. R. A. Dorwart, *The Prussian State before 1740* (Cambridge, Mass., 1971), part 5.

3. Archives Départementales du Bas-Rhin, 5 M 22, hereafter abbreviated as A.D.B.R. Unless otherwise indicated, all references to the archives of the Bas-Rhin are to this box.

4. Illich, *Medical Nemesis: The Expropriation of Health* (New York, 1976). Foucault has suggested the theory in *Madness and Civilization: A History of Insanity in the Age of Reason* (translated by Richard Howard, New York, 1965) and *The Birth of the Clinic: An Archeology of Medical Perception* (translated by A. M. Sheridan Smith, New York, 1973); he has developed the theme in his recent lectures at the Collège de France. "Le pouvoir médical" was also a topic in the seminar given by Jean-Pierre Peter at the Ecole des Hautes Etudes en Sciences Sociales during 1974-75.

5. The text appears in the *Bulletin des Lois,* 3rd series, vol. 7, 567-76. See also the article on medicine in Desire and Armand Dalloz, *Jurisprudence générale,* new edition, vol. 31 (Paris, 1854) 536-602. René Roland, *Les Médecins et la loi du 19 ventôse an XI* (Paris, 1883) gives an overview of the legislation and its effects. Jean Waquet of the Archives Nationales in Paris is preparing an article on this subject.

6. J. B. Treilhard, *Motifs du code d'instruction criminelle* (1808) 14, cited by Foucault, *Surveiller et punir: naissance de la prison* (Paris, 1975), 219. Foucault compares the Ancien Régime's treatment of the deviant to the expulsion of the leper from the community in the Middle Ages; and the new system of surveillance and control to the identification and isolation of plague victims in their homes in the early modern period. These models could apply to the treatment of quacks and popular healers.

7. Fernand L'Huillier, *Recherches sur l'Alsace napoleonienne* (N.p., 1947), 160-63; the quotations are from p. 162. On Lezay-Marnésia's career, see Egon von Westerholt, *Lezay-Marnésia, Sohn der Aufklärung und Präfekt Napoleons: 1769-1814* (Meisenheim-am-Glan, 1958).

8. Jacques Léonard, "L'Exemple d'une catégorie socio-professionnelle au XIXe siècle: les médecins français," in *Ordres et classes: colloque d'histoire sociale, Saint-Cloud, 1967* (Paris and The Hague, 1973), 226; P. Leuillot, *L'Alsace au début du XIXe siècle* (Paris, 1959-60), vol. 2; 18-20; and R. Boeglin, *L'Evolution historique de la pharmacie en Alsace* (Strasbourg, 1939) 139. Fischer, *Geschichte,* vol. II; 55-57, discusses the German *Physikus.*

9. Alfred Franklin, *La Vie privée d'autrefois,* vol. 11, *Les Médecins* (Paris, 1892), gives an anecdotal history of medical practitioners in the Ancien Régime; see also vol. 12, *Les Chirurgiens* (1893), and. vol. 14, *Variétés chirurgicales* (1894). Cf. Paul Delaunay, *Le Monde médical parisien au dix-huitième siècle* (Paris, 1906). The situation in the Bas-Rhin was not

entirely representative of France as a whole. Some traditional German medical institutions persisted there; barber-surgeons, for example, survived at a time when surgeons had achieved a higher status in many parts of France, and the number of "barbers" on the lists of illegal practitioners may therefore be unusually high. See Fischer, *Geschichte*, vol. II; 55-57, and Boeglin, *L'Evolution*, 98. Since German was the local idiom, a cultural distance separated the rural population and non-francophone healers from the official urban healers, who at least wrote French and were already set off from laymen by the symbolic use of Latin. See Michel de Certeau, Dominique Julia, and Jacques Revel, *Une Politique de la langue: la Révolution Francaise et les patois* (Paris, 1975) 275-83 relate to Alsace. Cf. Leuillot, *L'Alsace*, vol. 2, 318-19. The frequent passage of itinerants from the adjacent regions of Germany and from Switzerland must have contributed to the image of the quack as a foreigner, as well as hindered repressive action by local authorities.

This account, which draws on police records on medical practice, cannot give a complete picture of actual medical conditions in early 19th-century Alsace. For the demography of the region, see Leuillot, *L'Alsace*, vol. 2, chapter 1, and L'Huillier, *Recherches*, 556-66; on medicine in the Ancien Regime, Charles Hoffmann, *L'Alsace au XVIIIe siecle*, vol. 2 (Colmar, 1906), 194-98. We will of course be looking at popular healers through the eyes of their opponents. Modern folklore studies are a partial corrective, although I would suggest that a different bias may result from the form of the questions put by the ethnographic investigator, who is looking for "folkloric" activities just as much as the policeman is looking for illegal ones. See Van Gennep, *Manuel*, vol. 4, 605, and E. Linckenheld, *Quinze ans de folklore alsacien: 1918-1936* (Colmar, 1936), 106-11. Work on Alsatian folk medicine must be supplemented by studies of other provinces.

10. Boeglin, *L'Evolution*, 123, cites a report from Joseph Lambert at Wissembourg (1790) on Tyrolians and peddlers of orvietan (A.D.B.R., L 839). An 1834 circular to mayors notes that Tyrolians sell "Swiss pectoral tea" cheaply as a come-on and then sell harmful drugs at higher prices; one mixture contained sulfuric acid (A.D.B.R. No. 186, "Circulaire à MM. les Maires, relative au colportage de drogues ou remèdes secrets," 31 March 1834).

11. A.D.B.R., series "M," *Statistique Agricole* for 1814, Eckversheim, 1 March 1815, cited by Leuillot, *L'Alsace*, vol. 2, 21.

12. See Bouteiller, *Médecine populaire*, 23-24.

13. A.D.B.R. No. 12, decree of the subprefect of Wissembourg, 8 Thermidor year X (27 July 1802), sent with a report (No. 11) to the secretary general of the prefecture.

14. Archives Nationales, F[17] 8185, report of the prefect of the Roer to the Councillor of State for the First Arrondissement of the General Police, 16 November 1807. The law punished the use of a false title more severely than illegal medical practice alone. In 1836, Gangshoff, the cantonal physician at Stutzheim, reported three empirics who were barely literate but had usurped the title of medical doctor (A.D.B.R. No. 189, to prefect, 2 March 1836). On the relevant jurisprudence, see the article "Médecine" in Dalloz, *Jurisprudence généralé*, section 54, and note 96 below.

15. Archives Nationales, F[7] 8185, subprefect at Spire (Speyer) to prefect of Mont-Tonnerre, 25 October 1810.

16. A.D.B.R. No. 210, report of Jacobi, cantonal physician at Schiltigheim, to prefect, 23 March 1844.

17. A.D.B.R. No. 24, Aronsohn to prefect, 24 February 1811.

18. A.D.B.R. No. 23, mayor of Bergzabern to subprefect at Wissembourg.

19. A.D.B.R. No. 28, imperial prosecutor at Wissembourg to prefect, 24 March 1811.

20. A.D.B.R. No. 20, subprefect of Wissembourg to prefect, 19 September 1811; No. 26, Aronsohn to prefect, 24 February 1811, says Dr. Johann is from the environs of Strasbourg.

21. A.D.B.R. No. 42, Buchholtz, cantonal physician at Wissembourg to prefect, 28 June 1813; he also says that Dr. Johann is from Bergzabern.

22. A.D.B.R. No. 26 (cited in note 20); No. 22, cantonal physician at Wissembourg to subprefect, 14 August 1811; No. 28 (cited in note 19).

23. A.D.B.R. No. 42 (cited in note 21). Cf. below, pp. 000000.

24. A.D.B.R. No. 29, hearing at Wissembourg court, 11 March 1811; on the occupation, No. 42 (cited in note 21) and No. 49, list of empirics practicing in the arrondissement of Wissembourg, 1813; on the nickname, No. 40, report by Muller, cantonal physician at Brumath, 21 June 1813.

25. A.D.B.R. No. 31. Hoffmann gives a list of remedies he himself used, including a liquor of hartshorn.

26. A.D.B.R. No. 40 (cited in note 24).

27. A.D.B.R. No. 42 (cited in note 21).

28. A.D.B.R. No. 44, report of 10 June 1813.

29. A.D.B.R. No. 56, Ministry of the Interior, First Division, to subprefect of Wissembourg: No. 57, Lion, cantonal physician at Soultz-sous-Forêts, to prefect, 17 January 1820; No. 58, royal prosecutor at Wissembourg to prefect, 6 March 1820. Lion had already denounced Volk in 1813 (No. 35, 19 June, report to prefect).

30. A.D.B.R. No. 4, mayor of Strasbourg to prefect, 26 Thermidor year IX (14 July 1801); No. 5, mayor's report of 14 Prairial (3 May), with Dränkler's flyer ("Nachricht"), and a draft of the prefect's decree.

31. A.D.B.R. No. 9, interrogation of Barbe Richert, and No. 10, of Küchel; No. 8, report by Marchand, justice of the peace, 12 Messidor year VII (30 June 1799); and No. 18, Küchel's announcement. Küchel claimed that his method involved neither magnetism nor electricity nor sympathy.

32. Emile and Ernest Chouillier, "Pierre Richard, dit le saint de Savières," in *Annuaire de l'Aube pour 1881*, 75-97.

33. A.D.B.R. No. 53, directive from Ministry of the Interior, First Division; and No. 55, report to subprefect at Wissembourg, 4 May 1818.

34. A.D.B.R. No. 205, cantonal physician at Sélestat to subprefect, 23 May 1841; No. 204, subprefect to prefect, 24 May.

35. For an interesting discussion of forensic psychiatry in this period, see Michel Foucault (editor), *I Pierre Rivière, having slaughtered my mother, my sister, and my brother . . .: A Case of Parricide in the Nineteenth Century* (translated by Frank Jellinek, New York, 1975).

36. Archives Nationales, F^8 160, prefect of the Bas-Rhin to Minister of the Interior; he encloses Lion's report and suggests that the General Consistory be advised.

37. Freddy Raphaël, "Rites de naissance et médecine populaire dans le judaïsme rural d'Alsace," *Ethnologie Française,* new series, vol. I (1971), 83-94.

38. A.D.B.R. No. 61, subprefect of Wissembourg to prefect, 22 March 1820.

39. A.D.B.R. No. 15, "Note des personnes qui sans qualite' exercent la médecine à Strasbourg," Ventôse year XIII (February-March, 1805); No. 14, report of medical jury to imperial prosecutor (*tribunal de police correctionnelle*) 13 Ventôse year XIII (4 March 1805); No. 13, response of the deputy imperial prosecutor, 18 Ventôse (9 March).

40. This is the only attempt to prepare a detailed census of unauthorized healers that I have discovered for France at the beginning of the 19th century. It is not certain how many cantonal physicians responded; a little over a third of the cantons of the Bas-Rhin are represented in the surviving lists. The reports come from all four arrondissements of the department: Saverne, Sélestat (Schléstadt), Strasbourg, and Wissembourg. There is also a composite list for each arrondissement. In the case of Saverne, the reports of the individual cantonal physicians are missing. The list of empirics for the arrondissement (No. 48) includes the cantons of Brulingen and Petite-Pierre, out of seven cantons; it names 27 individuals in 21 communes. The majority (sixteen) were accused of illegal practice of midwifery — an offense about which the cantonal physicians in the other arrondissements complained, but usually without giving a detailed list. The Sélestat dossier covers ten cases; two cantons out of eight are represented (No. 47, list for the arrondissement; No. 39, canton of Benfeld, 7 November 1813; No. 43, canton of Marckolsheim). Half the empirics are barbers, if we include the daughter of a barber who performs phlebotomies, one of the traditional medical functions of that trade. The list for the arrondissement of Strasbourg (No. 45) includes the town of Strasbourg itself (which comprised four cantons) and two other cantons. The reports mention ten healers, not counting two apparently qualified surgeons who did not appear on the lists of authorized practitioners (No. 38, canton of Geispolsheim, 5 November 1813; No. 40, canton of Brumath, 21 June 1813). The cantonal reports for the arrondissement of Wissembourg are the most nearly complete; five out of ten cantons are represented (No. 49, list for the arrondissement; No. 35, canton of Soultz-sous-Forêts, 19 June 1813; No. 41, canton of Candel, 28 June 1813; No. 42, canton of Wissembourg, 28 June 1813; No. 44, canton of Woerth, 10 June 1813). To the seventeen individuals mentioned by name, including four barbers and three midwives, must be added five midwives who are identified only by the names of their communes.

41. Justin Breit, a "vagabond" no less dangerous than Dr. Hans, in the view of the cantonal physician at Soultz-sous-Forêts, usually lives with a farmer at Birlenbach. Breit, also known as "Justul," is a native of Wissembourg; he has no known trade other than quackery. (No. 35)

   A gardener of Strasbourg, living just outside the town, "makes frequent circuits in the communes of the [neighboring] canton of Oberhausbergen, to undertake the treatment of the most serious diseases," as does a fruitseller living within the town walls." (No. 45)

   In the arrondissement of Saverne, two persons coming from outside the region "enter the communes furtively and practice medicine and surgery." (No. 48) The cantonal physician of Soultz-sous-Forêts (Wissembourg) denounces "Tyrolians" and other vagabonds, peddlers of "very strong drugs." (No. 35)

   On Dr. Hans and Dr. Johann, see above, 000. Dr. Johann is mentioned in No. 42, Dr. Hans in Nos. 35, 40, 42 and 44 (see note 40).

42. The cantonal physician at Benfield (Selestat) reports three barbers. Dürr, sixty years old, practices medicine and surgery at Huttenheim "with extreme audacity." The inhabitants of the commune "have a blind confidence in this individual, despite the fact that he is under the influence of wine from the morning on, and that he dispatches a good many victims each year." Another barber, Wolff, about fifty years old, also practices surgery, but "since the inhabitants have no confidence in him, he is in no way dangerous to society." (No. 39)

At Stotzheim, in the same canton, two barbers are mentioned. Brenner, who practices medicine and surgery, "would be very enterprising if he enjoyed the confidence of the inhabitants;" while Hess, "extremely mild, in no way enterprising," limits himself to bleeding and applying vesicatories ordered by a physician or surgeon of the region. (No. 39)

The cantonal physician at Soultz-sous-Forêts cites four barbers, of whom the most offensive is a François Adam Birckbüchler ("Fraentzel") of Rittershoffen, who "practices medicine with unbelievable audacity." (Two other barbers practicing medicine actually deserve the title of *officier de santé,* according to the physician.) (No. 35)

43. A.D.B.R. No. 35. In Germany the executioner traditionally practiced veterinary medicine (Boeglin, *L'Evolution,* 100).

44. The two *sages-femmes* who practice medicine and surgery are a 65-year-old woman in the arrondissement of Strasbourg, who has worked in two cantons, and another in the same arrondissement, canton of Geispolsheim. (No. 45)

Among the women accused of practicing midwifery without a license are the *accoucheuses* of five communes in the canton of Woerth (Wissembourg) and three in the canton of Soultz-sous-Forêts, in the same arrondissement (No. 44, No. 35). In the arrondissement of Saverne, 16 accusations out of 27 are directed against unauthorized midwives, among them two anonymous "old women" and another in the commune of Adamswiller, whose mayor refuses to divulge her name. (No. 48)

45. A.D.B.R. No. 38 (Geispolsheim).

46. At Marckolsheim (Sélestat), a Catherine Lehmann, daughter of a barber and wife of a country policeman (*garde-champêtre*) performs surgical operations and sells drugs. According to the cantonal physician, "although bleedings are rarely indicated in our region, this woman would not hesitate to bleed an entire commune for six *sols.* " (No. 43)

In the canton of Brumath (Strasbourg), the wife of a dealer in rope and twine makes ointments and plasters and dabbles in surgery. "In spite of her lack of skill," the cantonal physician complains, "she knows how to win men's confidence." (No. 40)

Two women appear in the list for the arrondissement of Saverne: at Hambach, a married woman practices medicine and surgery, and at Burbach the mother of the Protestant pastor is an "oculist" (ocular surgeon). (If the midwives are included, two-thirds of the empirics on the list for Saverne are women.) No. 48

In the arrondissement of Wissembourg, the cantonal physician at Candel reports a certain Marie-Françoise Reinhard, a resident of Rheinzabern, who says that she has once been a nun. She sells remedies and visits patients in several communes of the canton. (No. 41)

All of the women are identified by association with a male, except the former nun; in that case the Church seems to stand for the husband.

47. The legislation of the year XI did not specifically bar them from practicing. See Dalloz, *Jurisprudence générale,* article "Médecine," section 37.

48. A certain Lettenberg, living at Haussen in Baden, practices medicine without authorization at Schoeneau (canton of Marckolsheim, Sélestat), "with extreme audacity." (No. 43) In the town of Brumath (arrondissement of Strasbourg), a "harmful quack" named Diebold practices medicine and surgery. (No. 40)

49. A.D.B.R. No. 38 (Geispolsheim) and No. 40 (Brumath).

50. A.D.B.R. No. 44.

51. At Brumath, arrondissement of Strasbourg, the cantonal physician cites a certain Stolz, a former priest living at Merzweiler, canton of Niederbronn (in the arrondissement of Wissembourg, more than 15 kilometers from Brumath). Stolz was denounced by the can-

tonal physicians of Brumath, Niederbronn and Haguenau at the time of an epidemic which raged at Bernoldsheim the previous year. The physician at Haguenau even made a collection of Stolz's recipes "in order to reveal this man's charlatanism." (A.D.B.R. No. 40) In the arrondissement of Saverne, a Protestant minister who took a course in medicine at the University of Heidelberg practices illegally. (No. 48)

52. A.D.B.R. No. 35.

53. Gasser, a shoemaker at Baldenheim, canton of Marckolsheim (Sélestat), sells amulettes to cure rheumatism. (No. 43)

At Ehenweyer, in the township of Müttersholz (Marckolsheim), a weaver named Eberlé "undertakes to cure everything, sometimes using mystical and sympathetic remedies, sometimes chemical drugs, according to the taste and choice of those who come to him." (No. 43)

The list of empirics in the arrondissement of Sélestat also includes the names of two wet-coopers at Rosheim. (No. 47)

The cantonal physician of Geispolsheim (arrondissement of Strasbourg) reports a Jean-Michel Fritsch, nicknamed "Pfiffenschnider" (*Pfeifenschneider*, or pipe carver), who "practices exorcism and other superstitious exercises and also abuses in various ways the confidence with which the lower class favors him." (No. 38)

In the town of Woerth (Wissembourg), a cartwright named Scheuk practices medicine; the cantonal physician adds that he is "adept in the magical arts and sorcery." (No. 44)

In the commune of Hoffen (canton of Soultz-sous-Forêts, Wissembourg), a former weaver, Jacques Vern, practices quack medicine. His sobriquet, "Weber Jackel," recalls his former occupation. (No. 35)

54. Similar cases appear in the records of petitions for approval of secret remedies, Archives Nationales, F[8] 149-67 and Académie Nationale de Médecine, mss. 14-15; for the 19th century, Académie Nationale de Médecine, register ms. 43.

55. See, for example, Van Gennep, *Le Folklore du Dauphiné* (Paris, 1932), vol. I, 60.

56. In contrast, a study of folk healers in Anjou carried out in 1961 showed that 60 per cent were *cultivateurs* (Bouteiller, *Médecine populaire,* 153)

57. A.D.B.R. No. 40.

58. A.D.B.R. No. 47.

59. A.D.B.R. No. 48.

60. In column two, "midwives" include regular practitioners as well as unauthorized *matrones;* the figure in column three refers only to cases of illegal midwifery. In column three, the same healer may appear in more than one category: the total therefore exceeds 71.

61. A.D.B.R. No. 35 (1813).

62. A.D.B.R. No. 210, Jacobi, cantonal physician, to prefect, 23 March 1844.

63. A.D.B.R. No. 42.

64. A.D.B.R. No. 55, report to subprefect at Wissembourg, 4 May 1818.

65. Buchholtz cites one trained *officier de santé,* an able man, a champion of the vaccination program, and the only surgeon in an area including seven communes (A.D.B.R. No. 42, 1813); in No. 40 we learn of a surgeon, formerly in the army, who says that his practice will not allow him to pay the examination fee.

66. Léonard, "Une catégorie socio-professionnelle," 226.

67. A.D.B.R. No. 22, cantonal physician at Wissembourg to subprefect, 14 August 1811.

68. A.D.B.R. No. 26, Aronsohn, cantonal physician at Sarre-Union, to prefect, 24 February 1811.

69. A.D.B.R. No. 43 (1813 report, canton of Marckolsheim).

70. A.D.B.R. No. 23, mayor of Bergzabern to subprefect at Wissembourg.

71. A.D.B.R. No. 31, Hoffmann's report, 12 January 1811. The cantonal physician, contradicting Hoffmann, found that the disease did not have a "dangerous character" (mentioned by Buchholtz in his 1813 report, No. 42).

72. A.D.B.R. No. 55, cantonal physician at Niederbronn to subprefect at Wissembourg, 4 May 1818.

73. A.D.B.R. No. 43, 1813 report.

74. A.D.B.R. No. 55 (cited in note 72).

75. A.D.B.R. No. 40 (1813 report).

76. A.D.B.R. No. 38 (1813 report).

77. A.D.B.R. No. 49, general list; No. 35, Lion's report.

78. A.D.B.R. No. 43, 1813 report, canton of Marckolsheim.

79. A.D.B.R. No. 50, 1813 report, canton of Benfold.

80. One of the best examples is a manuscript memoir in the archives of the Societe Royale de Médecine (at the Académie Nationale de Médecine, Paris) by Chifoliau, a physician at Saint-Malo: "Préjugés opposés aux sages précautions du gouvernement, aux efforts des ministres de la santé, et à la voix de la nature" (22 March 1780, box 124 of the archives). Jean-Pierre Peter kindly called my attention to this document. For a good general discussion of the Société Royale de Médecine, see Caroline C. Hannaway, "The Société Royale de Médecine and Epidemics in the Ancien Régime," *Bulletin of the History of Medicine,* vol. 46 (1972), 257-73.

81. See, for example, A. Richerand, *Des Erreurs populaires relatives a la medecine* (Paris, 1810) and the memoirs of the Académie Celtique. Natalie Davis discusses the tradition of writing on vulgar errors in "Proverbial Wisdom and Popular Errors," *Society and Culture in Early Modern France* (Stanford, 1975), 227-67. A good example of a report on medical folklore by a physician for the period considered here is a note by Lecourt de Cantilly on the treatment of "les hunes" in Brittany (Archives de la Société Médicale d'Emulation de Paris, 1827, Paris Faculty of Medicine ms. 2196, No. 6).

82. A.D.B.R. No. 30, notice from the secretary-general, for the prefect, 5 February 1811.

83. A.D.B.R. No. 51, "Art de guérir: mesures répressives contre les charlatans et les empiriques," 10 January 1817. Another circular was dated 20 April 1819.

84. A.D.B.R. No. 42.

85. A.D.B.R. No. 38.

86. A.D.B.R. No. 56, First Division to subprefect, February, 1820.

87. For example, A.D.B.R. No. 43 (1813 report, Marckolsheim).

88. A.D.B.R. No. 48.

89. See note 15.

90. See note 14.

91. For 1820, No. 57, Lion, cantonal physician at Soultz-sous-Forêts.

92. A.D.B.R. No. 44, 1813 report, canton of Woerth. Cf. a case from the Revolutionary period: Antoine Esslinger, a miller and mayor of Chatenois, who used a sympathetic powder (A.D.B.R. 1 L 838, No. 4).

93. A.D.B.R. No. 11, subprefect to secretary general of the prefecture.

94. E.g. Ritzinger, cantonal physician at Marckolsheim, denounces four practitioners who went unpunished in spite of his pleas in court (A.D.B.R. No. 43); the phrase "medical vandalism" is from No. 55, cantonal physician at Niederbronn to subprefect at Wissembourg, 4 May 1818.

95. A.D.B.R. No. 28, imperial prosecutor to prefect, 24 March 1811.

96. A.D.B.R. No. 29, sentence of the tribunal of the arrondissement of Wissembourg, 1 March 1811. The law of 19 Ventose prescribed a penalty of up to 1000 frances for offenders who took the title of physician, 500 francs for those who posed as *officiers de santé* but the legislator neglected to fix a fine for those who practiced illegally without usurpation of a title. In the 1830's and '40's, the courts established that the penalty could not exceed *une amende de simple police,* 1-15 francs. (Dalloz, *Jurisprudence générale,* vol. 31, 552). In practice, penalties varied widely during the first decades of the 19th century.

97. A.D.B.R. No. 42, Buchholtz, 1813 report.

98. A.D.B.R. No. 31, Hoffmann, 1811 report.

99. A.D.B.R. No. 42.

100. A.D.B.R. No. 19, prefect to subprefect at Wissembourg, 28 September 1811.

101. A.D.B.R. No. 26, Aronsohn, cantonal physician at Sarre-Union, to prefect, 24 February 1811. .

102. A.D.B.R. No. 23, mayor of Bergzabern to subprefect at Wissembourg.

103. A.D.B.R. No. 22, cantonal physician at Wissembourg to subprefect, 14 August 1811

104. A.D.B.R. No. 50, to the dean of the Faculty of Medicine of Strasbourg, 5 November 1816.

105. A.D.B.R. No. 57, to prefect, 17 January 1820.

106. A.D.B.R. No. 107, Third Division to prefect, 12 February 1822.

107. A.D.B.R. No. 42.

108. For example, C.-F.-E Dupin, *Statistique des Deux-Sèvres* (Paris, an IX). On the *Statistique des préfets* and popular culture, see M.-N. Bourguet, "Race et folklore: l'image officielle de la France en 1800, *Annales: E.S.C.,* vol. 31 (1976), 802-23.

109. Luc Boltanski, *Prime éducation et morale de classe* (Paris and The Hague, 1969).

110. On modernization and popular medicine, see Bouteiller, *Médecine populaire,* 112-21.

Jean-Pierre Goubert

THE EXTENT OF MEDICAL PRACTICE
IN FRANCE AROUND 1780

At the beginning of this study, two questions arise: It is known that urban concentration and medical concentration coincided in Anjou and Brittany at the end of the eighteenth century;[1] But this poses a problem: can we generalize from these regional examples to the whole of France?

Following this a related question: what were the actual number and density of practitioners in France around 1780 who were officially admitted for medical practice? What exactly was this rural "medical desert" denounced by the "enlightened" doctors of that period?[2]

An attempt to resolve these initial problems was made in the major administrative survey of 1786, which foreshadows the medical statistics following the laws of Year XI on medicine and pharmacy. Launched by the Controller general, Calonne and under the patronage of the Royal Society of Medicine, this survey was conducted during the last year in which the administrative machinery of the *intendances* was regularly working. In addition, a second survey, made at the end of 1790, was available.

These two surveys enable us to count the members of the medical community, doctors and surgeons, who were officially admitted for medical practice. However, the survey of 1786, because it was not centralized at that time, preserved, in whole or in part, only a third of the generalities in France at this period.[3] As for the survey of 1790, only a hundred replies were analyzed, after being concentrated in Paris.[4] It was originated by the *Comité de Salubrité* (of the Constituent Assembly), and its object was to describe "the practice of surgery" in the kingdom. In order to do this it was addressed to the official representatives of the surgeons, the Lieutenants of the Royal First Surgeon.

The 1786 survey allows us to count the doctors and surgeons of the time, while the 1790 survey allows us to count the surgeons only. This applies to the cities as well as to the towns and rural areas. The two surveys were conducted under different administrative systems – in one case that of the sub-delegation, in the other that of the Lieutenancy of the First Surgeon of the King (that is, the court of the royal bailiff).

It was also necessary to calculate the total population of a *généralité*, both rural and urban, in order to determine the different rates of medical density. This proved to be a delicate task, because, as the chevalier des Pommelles wrote in 1789, ". . . there does not exist and has never existed any general census in the Kingdom."[5] Hence, it was necessary to use estimates proposed by statisticians of the protostatistical era[6] and to make use of the various works of present day demographers and historians.[7] At the same time, as a control or when necessity dictated, I used figures from the survey of 1809 on the total population.[8] Finally, of course, various historical works on certain regions and cities of 18th Century France were examined.

As a result, the population figures and rates of medical density which will be proposed merely constitute standard of comparison. For two groups, however, the established statistics are of a greater precision: i.e., the *généralités* of Rennes and Soissons. In these two cases, an effort was made in three different directions:

1) to get medical statistics, as reliable as possible, while attempting to overcome the pitfalls inherent to any such endeavor;[9]

2) to choose population estimates based on widespread documentation (such as data from the population survey ordered by Abbot Terray) and, if possible, also based on studies of historical demography;

3) to set up lists by parish and by sub-delegation which would result in as reliable as possible a cartographic diagram.[10]

By way of example, here are some of the problems which arose on this occasion. Counting the same practitioner in two different parishes[11] falsifies the calculated rates, even if it reveals a social reality which is far more important; that is, the fact that the geographical area within which a practitioner works, even if small because he travels by horseback, cannot be confused with a parish, nor even with the limits of a sub-delegation or a *généralité*![12] Another difficulty arises: the level of activity of a practitioner is highly variable. Thus, "the Messeurs Beraud, Gallet and Mortier are all three members of the *Communauté* from Bourg, and this is the reason why they are included in its list; but they no longer practise."[13] Likewise, in the sub-delegation of Loudun, out of 24 practitioners that have been recorded, one "has stopped practising;" five practise only "a little" or "very little" either because they don't enjoy "public confidence" or owing to their age; finally two don't work any more as a result of their physical disability.[14] Yet, the sub-delegate rarely took the trouble to make note of these details, so that the statistics inevitably lack precision.

Another problem we had to solve involved practitioners who, although holding diplomas, did not present themselves before the college of doctors or the association of surgeons, either due to lack of time — because in 1786 their establishment had just recently been set up — or because of their unwillingness to appear. Thus the sub-delegate of Châteaugiron noted in his observation that: "We have only an imperfect knowledge of surgeons dispersed throughout the countryside. There are many who practice without having been accepted (by the association of surgeons).[15] Finally, I decided to retain all those I knew held a title sanctioning an official medical education.[16] But if this solution seemed at first glance to have the merit of clarity, it raised in its turn another problem, that of the gap between legal medicine and the so called discount medicine, between learned medicine and "popular medicine." In fact, according to the replies given in 1790 by several Lieutenants of the First Surgeon to the King, some country surgeons were only celebrated charlatans. Thus, the Lieutenant of Montdidier pointed at: "... a dangerous charlatan admitted by the previous surgeon in 1761 ..., and three bone setters improperly admitted a long time ago. ...."[17] Likewise, the members of the Intermediate Commission of Alsace wrote in 1788: "Our greatest fault is the excessive multiplication of admissions of surgeons in the Province. These excesses have reached such a point that there is no community of any size which does not have several surgeons with some sort of title and often others without any at all ...."[18] Or again, the sub-delegate on his own account excluded surgeons who do not enjoy "... a certain reputation."[19]

As a result, the calculated rate of *official* medicalization are dependent on the degree of severity or laxity with which a particular college or community was willing to admit colleagues, particularly as in the case of admission of country surgeons. Consequently, inasmuch as the country surgeons are by far the most numerous the rates of medicalization that have been calculated are more interesting at the socio-cultural level than at the purely statistical one. They actually reflect the image of official medicine projected by the representatives of the royal power (the sub-delegates), or the Lieutenants of the First Surgeon of the King, in a particular region or city of France on the eve of the revolution.

Because of gaps in the archives, the rates of "medicalization" could be analyzed for only six *généralités,* all situated in northern France. In this geographical area, the average rate of density comes to 4.54 practitioners (i.e., doctors and surgeons) per 10,000 inhabitants (cf. table 1); however, excluding Brittany, the rate rises to 5.9.

Regional distinctions are to be made however: the northeastern *généralités* (Amiens, Dijon, Soissons) reached/or exceeded a rate of 7 for 10,000; on the other hand, the western *généralités* had lower rates: 5.5 in the *généralité* of Caen, 4.8 in the *généralité* of Tours, only 2.4 in the *généralité* of Rennes. As a result, the total rates in the 6 *généralités,* combined seem relatively high, even when compared with rates dating from the First Empire.[20] All the more so, since even in the west particular areas, such as the county of Nantes and Upper Brittany, frequently reached a rate of 4 for 10,000, whereas Anjou shows a rate of 7.6.

Besides this overall impression and the regional disparities just noted, a third statistical fact is clear. Whether it be in absolute or relative figures (the rate of "medicalization"), the doctors are four to ten times fewer than the surgeons. Yet, here too, regional disparities are in evidence. Thus, the *généralités* of Caen and Dijon seem the best provided with doctors, with a respective rate of 1.7 and 1.4 for 10,000 inhabitants. In contrast, the *généralités* of Amiens, Rennes, Tours, and Soissons had a rate of approximately 0.5 to 0.6 for 10,000.

However, the distribution between doctors and surgeons per *généralité* was far from uniform. Thus, for the *généralités* of Amiens, Soissons, and even in the case of Tours, the figures showed a below average proportion of doctors; on the contrary, the *généralité* of Caen, which had the highest proportion of doctors, has only a relatively low proportion of surgeons.

How can such disparities be explained? First we would need a long examination, aided by numerous local studies, in order to determine the validity of the medical statistics used. Next, we would need to refine our knowledge of the medical community and its settlement. Finally, we would have to achieve a better understanding of the society and urban network of a particular region;[21] for, the demand for health personnel emanates — in large part — from the social elite. Thus the above-average rate of medicalization of the areas under the influence of Caen, Angers or Rennes can be explained in part by the activities of a city, and especially by the presence of a Faculty of Medicine or School of Surgery.

But the real problem emerges in counting the country surgeons, who obtained a mastery of "limited skill." Assuredly the most numerous and the least trained group, they were scorned by their more socially favored colleagues; to such an extent that certain sub-delegates commented in their regard: "There are some other surgeons in the country parishes but one dare neither trust them nor inspire the confidence of others on their behalf."[22] The sub-delegate of Villers-Cotterets, for his part, wrote: "It is an unquestionable truth that in the rural areas three quarters of the people who become seriously ill die through the ineptitude of the surgeons treating them . . ."[23] And the sub-delegate of Seurre denounced the "fatal ignorance" of surgeons, and more particularly one of them "who was little more than a public assasin, having the right to kill the sick with impunity . . . ."[24]

Another example: for the city of Caen, at the time of the survey of 1786, the intendancy considered only the licensed members of the College of Doctors who were authorized to build up a clientele, and it excluded university professors who did not practice in the city; likewise, it rejected those surgeons who did not satisfactorily complete qualifying examinations.[25] Then, if the same rule were applied to the entire généralité of Caen, one can explain, on the one hand, the small number of surgeons counted in the 1786 survey, on the other hand the relatively low rate of "medicalization" based by the number of country surgeons (3.16 for 10,000). One can as a result advance the following hypothesis: a large number of country surgeons, of unequal quality and more or less in line with existing legislation, have escaped, the calculations of the historian, dependent as he is on his sources.

To be sure, two other complicating factors blur the statistical image of medical practice at the end of the 18th century: first, the heterogeneity of replies to the survey; second, the heterogeneity of the medical community. It remains that the "medical desert" of the countryside is not in fact a void. This belief arises from the "enlightened" judgment of a minority of the medical community, who perceive a desert wherever the most learned medicine is absent. It also stems and one must keep this in mind, from the institutional organization of medicine and surgery on the eve of the revolution, an organization which condemns the countryside to the ranks of the least educated, the least *scholarly* elements of the medical community, which is not necessarily the most inept!

The opposition between city and countryside, between urban doctors and rural surgeons are very obvious in the discourse of the medical elite at the end of the 18th century that may constitute polarities which should be softened.

Certainly, rates of medicalization calculated for the urban world and the rural world present some difficulties. The first difficulty involves the separation

nto two juridicial categories of medical practitioners who in everyday medical-
zed a particular area or small region *together.* A second disadvantage involved
eparating completely a city from its surrounding countryside, whereas on the
•ve of the revolution a particular city preserved many rural aspects, *altered* the
urrounding rural life, and indeed lived off its surrounding countryside.

However, despite these problems, calculating the rates of medicalization
'or the urban and rural sectors, and for doctors and surgeons, was of definite
nterest. First, it allowed us to qualify the assertion of an exclusively urban
•stablishment made by doctors of medicine. In three *généralités* out of six, the
aumber of doctors residing in the rural areas proved to be extremely low: 1 in
he *généralité* of Soissons, 2 in the *généralité* of Amiens, 5 in the *généralité* of
Rennes. In contrast, 18 doctors were established in the towns and countryside of
he *généralité* of Tours, 39 in the *généralité* of Caen, and 44 in the *généralité* of
Dijon. This distortion may be explained in part by the legal definition of a city
under the Old Regime. In Brittany, a number of small groups had city status,
vhile this was not so often the case in Normandy or Burgundy.

Furthermore, calculating the different rates of "medicalization" facilitated a
omparative analysis. Thus the two *généralités* of Amiens and Rennes, which
howed the same rate of urbanization (17%), had very similar urban rates of
medicalization: 8.2 for 10,000 in Picardy, 7.7 in Brittany. Yet their rural
medical rates turn out very different: 7.2 for 10,000 in Picardy, 1.3 in Brittany.
Such a sizable difference cannot be accounted for merely by the heterogeneity
•f the documentation used. But where Picardy is concerned, only a regional
uistorical study would enable us to grasp the reasons for such intensive medical
•ctivity at the rural level.

We observe the same phenomenon when we compare the medicalization by
urgeons in the cities and in the rural areas of Picardy and Brittany. Thus the
ities of Picardy and Brittany show a rather similar rate for surgeons: 5.4 and
4.7, respectively. But the difference is striking when we compare the rate for
urgeons established in the countryside: 7.2 for 10,000 in Picardy, as against
..27 in Brittany.

This brief comparison suggests two comments:

1) there appears to be, as one would expect, a certain correlation between
he rate of urbanization and rate of medicalization of the cities, within these two
eneralities.

2) the overall medicalization rates, that is, those valid for the aggregates
'ormed by the cities and rural areas together, can conceal, from one *généralité* to
he other, important differences which have to be disclosed, if not explained.

Medical Activity in the Country

For the six *généralités* considered, the average global rate of medical activity
eaches 3.51 for 10,000, or one practitioner for 2,857 rural inhabitants. But if
ve exclude from this sample the Breton countryside which accounted for more
han half, the average overall rate comes to 4.85 for 10,000, or one practitioner
'or 2,061 country-people.

Therefore, in a general sense the "medical desert" of the countryside does not
:orrespond to a socio-historical reality. All the more so because, even if this is an

infrequent occurrence, the city practitioners travel out to the country; as, for example, when they were summoned by the orders of the intendancy, during an epidemic.

In the second place, in 90 to 99% of the cases medical treatment in the countryside is provided by the surgeons, in conformity with the regulations of the 1707 Edict of Marly (cf. table 2C). Unfortunately, the distinction drawn by the Edict of Marly among three types of master surgeons did not show up in the replies to the 1786 survey, except rarely. Thus, the subdelegate of Valognes, alone among his colleagues of the *généralité* of Caen, made this distinction, when he noted "5 surgeons admitted for *(grand chef-d'oeuvre)* . . . 5 second-order surgeons . . . (and) 21 third-order surgeons admitted with limited skill . . ."[26] Nevertheless, although we don't have overall statistics on this point, there is little doubt that the great majority of master surgeons established in the towns and countryside had gained mastery of "limited skill",[27] according to the pattern of the Edict of Marly provided.

The calculated rates for the rural areas vary somewhat from one *généralité* to the next. The overall rate in fact varies along a "scale" running from 1 to 7, while the mode is located at about 4.5 practitioners for 10,000 country-people.

The rates for country doctors in the rural areas are noticeably weak. Nonetheless they present an extremely wide range, running from 1 to 80; regional distinctions thus appear as we extend the territory included in the survey.

"Medicalization" in the cities

Generally speaking, the average overall rate for the cities is three times higher than that of the countryside (cf. table 1). The overall rates for the cities range from 7.7 for 10,000 in Brittany up to 18.3 in Burgundy. Therefore they move along a relatively narrow range falling between 1 to 2.25. Moreover they are distributed around two modes, one 8, the other 14 for 10,000.

As to the division between doctors and surgeons, the surgeons predominated half as much as their fellow doctors (cf. table 1). The rates for doctors and surgeons vary along an analogous scale, from 1 to 2.7 and from 1 to 2 respectively.

On the whole, the medical framework observed for the cities consists of 38.5% doctors and 61.5% surgeons. In all, 383 doctors out of 491, or 78%, reside in the city, according to the legal definition of this term at the end of the Old Regime. In contrast, barely 26% of the surgeons, or 611 out of 2,356, live in the city. As a result, the "cliche" which opposes the city doctor with the country surgeon must be corrected.[28] In fact medicalization in the cities is mainly provided by surgeons, but by surgeons of the first or second order; surgeons of the first order, if the city contains a community of surgeons; surgeons of the second order, if the city does not.

In the second place, "medicalization" in the cities is due to the work of the doctors of medicine: 383, for an urban population estimated at some 900,000 inhabitants. As a result, there were two kinds of practitioners in the cities and the rural areas. The first category included doctors of medicine plus first- or second-order master surgeons, admitted for practice in the cities. The second type consisted in third-order surgeons admitted for practice in the villages and country. This gap can be confirmed by examining the share of head taxes paid by doctors and surgeons in the cities of Anjou and Brittany, as well as in Lyon.[29]

The medicalization of the cities offers a final characteristic. In general, the smaller the city the higher its rate of medicalization (cf. table 3 and cf. graph 1). For a city containing between 1,500 and 5,000 inhabitants, the rate varied with very abrupt changes due to its small number of practitioners: that is between 10 and 35 for 10,000. Cities numbering from 5,000 to 10,000 inhabitants showed a rate ranging from 10 to 25 for 10,000. Larger cities numbering from 10,000 to 20,000 inhabitants showed a rate from 7 to 15. Finally, populations of 20,000 to 80,000 inhabitants had a rate running from 5 to 10 for 10,000. Therefore, the large and medium-sized cities had the lowest rate, with only a few exceptions, even if they involved the largest number of practitioners. The paradox is only an apparent one. In fact, in the 18th century the potential or real clientele of urban practitioners did not vary as a direct function of the population of the city where they lived, because at this time there was no system of health-insurance! As a result, the urban practitioner's clientele depended mainly on the importance of the fraction of the population which called him to its bedside and which was able to pay him, whether this clientele lived in the city, or in the countryside.[30] One may add that the visit of a practitioner was only within the financial reach of a minority. Several replies to the 1786 survey clearly indicated as much. Thus, the *intendant* of the *généralité* of Soissons commented: "... it is only the rich who call for doctors in case of illness...." In any case, the fee demanded by surgeons was generally lower, except in the case of major operations. "They are the doctors of the people," insisted the *intendant* of Soissons, because "... they are very numerous, they almost all practice medicine... , the people who find them within reach call upon them for all kinds of illnesses...." It is an established custom. In many circumstances necessity even makes it a law, because of the lack of funds of most sick people."[31] On this subject the testimony was unanimous and the parish priests were not the last to express their concern. Thus the priest of Sartes wrote: "We have neither doctors nor surgeons in my parish .... The rich send for them once or twice, never more. The poor, bereft of all support, are already too wretched, without adding doctors' bills." [32] Yet even the country surgeons' fee was too high for many sick people: "Most poor parishioners ... don't dare turn to the surgeons, who charge too much for their travel and remedies. I see sick people visited five times and treated with some ordinary remedies, for which surgeons living just a league away are paid forty-four pounds."[33] Indeed, besides the cost of the visit, the country residents must pay the practitioners travel expenses. Thus the visit of a doctor *in a city,* like Saint-Brieuc, in 1783 cost about one pound.[34] But the visit of a *surgeon* in the region of Loudéac, around 1775-1779, was in total as expensive, if not more so, due to the travel costs, to say nothing of the medicines prescribed, which amounted to half of the total bill. This is why, from 1776 to 1778, about 20% of the fees owed this surgeon were still unpaid.[35]

Generally speaking, the average global rate for the cities is three times as high as the rate for the country (cf. table 1). The global rates for the cities range from 7.7 for 10,000 in Brittany up to 18.3 in Burgundy. Therefore they move along a relatively straight scale running from 1 to 2.25. Moreover they are distributed around two modes, one 8 the other 14 for 10,000.

As concerns the distribution between doctors and surgeons, the surgeons predominate, more numerous by half as their fellow doctors (cf. table 1). The rates for doctors and surgeons vary along an analogous scale, from 1 to 2.7 and from 1 to 2 respectively.

On the whole, from a global perspective, the medical environment observed for the cities splits into 38.5% doctors and 61.5% surgeons. In all, 383 doctors out of 491, or 78%, reside in the city, according to the legal definition of this term at the end of the Old Regime. In contrast, barely 26% of the surgeons, or 611 out of 2,356, live in the city. As a result, the "cliche" which opposes the city doctor with the country surgeon must be corrected (28). In fact, medical treatment in the cities is mainly provided by surgeons, but by surgeons of the first or second order; surgeons of the first order, if the city contains an association of surgeons, medialization, however, it moved into second place for rate of doctors.

On the other hand, the *généralité* of Dijon, which occupied second-to-last place for its urbanization rate (13.7%), was in first place for overall rate of medicalization and rate of doctors, while it took second place for rate of surgeons. Thus neither the overall figure nor the urban population ratio governs the rates of medicalization; so that two cities of such different size as Ham and Guise (1500 and 3000 residents), for example, had the same number of established practitioners: one doctor and four surgeons. Which is not to say that the professional activity of these practitioners was the same, too!

It would be hazardous and undoubtedly rather futile to proceed with a comparative analysis of rates of urbanization and rates of medicalization. In fact, neither the urban phenomenon nor the medical phenomenon can be reduced to a statistical description. Moreover, there are technical difficulties: the absence of a census for the decennial 1780, the legal definition of the cities, and the inconsistent value of medical statistics.

On the other hand this study suggests the need for in-depth research at the local or regional level. The only way for us to gain a sufficient awareness of the scope of medicalization, and to measure regional differences, if necessary, is to examine a range of documents large enough to encompass the medical activity of French practitioners at the end of the 18th century.

It is therefore advisable to give priority (although not exclusively) to professional documents, such as memoranda-books and nosological observations, which are still available two centuries later. And from this perspective, it is also fitting that we appreciate the economic vitality, the literacy level, and collective behavior regarding the body and health.

Thus the research we have presented raises more problems than it solves. However, it enables us to state two certitudes and to envision a general hypothesis.

First, the superposition of the medical network and the urban network proves to be general, at least for northern France (with southern France and Alsace still to be checked). It is based upon the institutional organization of medicine and surgery, an organization which operates from the city, and is charged with distributing the men who compose and surround it.

In the second place, regional diversity, as seen in the above medical rates, cannot rest solely on the heterogeneity of replies to the 1786 survey. It thus poses the problem, on the regional level, of the unequal medicalization in the French society at the end of the Old Regime.

Finally, a general hypothesis: would not a high rate of medicalization — extending even into certain rural areas — indicate for certain French regions the diffusion of urban culture? More particularly, of a learned, secularized culture, with greater confidence in the knowledge and ability of doctors.

Ecole des Hautes Etudes en Jean-Pierre GOUBERT
Sciences Sociales (Paris)

FOOTNOTES

1. Cf. J.-P. GOUBERT and F. LEBRUN, "Médecins et chirurgiens dans la société française du XVIIIe siécle", in *Annales Cisalpines d'Histoire sociale,* no. 4 (1973) 126 and table I 133.

2. Cf. J.-P. PETER, "Une enquête de la Société royale de Médecine (1774-1794). Malades et maladies à la fin du XVIIIe siècle", in *Annales E.S.C.* (1967) 711-751.

3. This survey is preserved in Series C of the *Archives Departementales.* I chose to analyze it for the six *généralités* where the replies to the survey were the best preserved.

4. These replies to the survey of 1790 are found in the Archives Nationales under the classification no. F^{15} 226 to 228 (2) and F ^{17} 2276.

5. Chevalier des Pommelles, *Tableau de la population de toutes les provinces du royaume,* Paris (1789) 45.

6. I am referring in particular to the works of Expilly, Orry, Hesseln, Messance, Necker and Calonne.

7. I am thinking in particular about the works of Marcel Reinhard on the French population and French cities at the time of the revolution and of the empire.

8. Cf. R. LE MEE, "Population agglomérée, population éparse au début du XIXe siècle", in *Annales de Démographie historique,* (1971) 455-510. I wish to thank L. Bergeron and J. Mallet for letting me consult the statistical documentation which forms the basis of the census of 1806 and of surveys said to be for 1000 and 2000 people.

9. Cf. J. LEONARD, *Les médecins de l'Ouest au XIXe siècle,* state doctoral examination in Contemporary History, Paris, 1975 (ex. typewritten), vol. I, p. 14 and following.

10. I wish to express my gratitude to G. ARBELLOT and J. MALLET for their aid and valuable collaboration. The medical statistics could not be cartographed on the subdelegation level, for lack of an available fund for cartographic work.

11. I could verify this fact for certain cases in the *généralités* of Soissons and the *généralité* of Tours.

12. The annals indicate the area within which doctors and surgeons practice in the diocese of Toulouse in 1786: for each community without its own established practitioners, they designate the doctor (rarely) and the surgeon(s) (most often) whom the residents summon

for medical treatment. Archives Départementales [hereafter referred to as A.D.] Haute-Garonne, C. 59.

13. A.D. Côte d'Or, C.367, 1786, Bourg-en Bresse.

14. A.D. Indre-et-Loire, C. 404, Loudun, November 15, 1784.

15. Ibid., C. 354, Châteaugiron, 1786.

16. On this basis I must exclude, for Carhaix, three ex-students or assistant surgeons from the army "practising all aspects of medicine without qualifications and without taking a prerequisite examination." A.D. Finistere, 10 L 162, Carhaix, March 6, 1791. In certain provinces, a considerable number of army and marine surgeons practise "illegally."

17. Archives Nationales, F 15 228 2, document 3, Montdidier, November 30, 1790. In this regard, cf. J.-P. GOUBERT, "Médecine savante et médecine populaire en France en 1790", article to appear in a forthcoming Cahier des Annales.

18. A.D. Bas-Rhin, C. 399, Strasbourg, February 14, 1788.

19. A.D. Ille-et-Vilaine, C 1325, Redon, 1786.

20. Thus the rate for Brittany reaches 2.4 for 10,000 in 1786 and about 3.4 for 10,000 in 1801-1803, in western France, as this region is defined by Jacques Léonard (i.e., the region comprising the five breton departments and Mayenne). For the medical statistics from Year XI, cf. the article by Mme Antoine and J. Waquet. "La medicine civile en France a l'epoque napoleonienne et le legs du XVIII siecle . . . ", in Revue de L'Institut Napoleon no. 132, 1976, 67-90.

21. Cf. J. MEYER, "Quelques vues sur l'histoire des villes à l'époque moderne", in Annales E.S.C., (Nov.-Dec. 1974) no. 6, 1551-1568.

22. A.D. Marne, C. 367, Château-Porcien, March 15, 1786.

23. A.D. Aisne, C 19, Villers-Cotterests March 18, 1786.

24. A.D. Côte d'Or, C 367, Seurre March 27, 1786.

25. Information provided by Jean-Claude Perrot. Concerning doctors and medicine in Caen, cf. J.-Cl. PERROT, Genèse d'une ville moderne. Caen au XVIIIe siècle (Paris-La Haye, 1975) vol. II; 882 and following.

26. A.D. Calvados, C 925, 1786.

27. Thus the court of the bailiff of Auxerre in 1786 numbers 9 first-order masters of surgery who constitute the association of Auxerre; 38 second-order masters for cities without an association; and 50 third-order masters for the towns and rural areas. A.D. Yonne, C 4.

28. As regards this "cliche," cf. J.-E. GILBERT, L'anarchie medicinale Neufchâtel, 1772, vol. 17: "Travel the world over, and count the titled doctors: what will you find? 1) In the most civilized countries, there are doctors only in the alrge cities. 2) Almost all the rural areas are covered by surgeons, dressers, marshals and charlatans."

29. On this point, cf. J. MEYER, "L'enquéte de l'Académie de médecine sur less épidémies, 1774-1794", in Etudes rurales, no. 34, 1969, p. 27 and 28. Cf. F. LEBRUN, Les hommes et la mort en Anjou aux XVIIe et XVIIIe siècles . . . , (Paris-La Haye, 1971) 219 and following. Cf. M. GARDEN, Lyon et les lyonnais au XVIIIe siècle (Paris, 1970) 190; 738-739.

30. Dr. Lavergne in Lamballe at the end of the 18th century, and Dr. Cornudet in La

Roche-Bernard during the first half of the 19th century, have a sizable rural clientele (examples taken from J. P. GOUBERT *op. cit.* and J. LEONARD, *op. cit.*).

31. A.D. Aisne, C 19, Soissons, October 1, 1786. .

32. A.D. Vosges, 1 C 43, subdelegation of Neufchâteau, 1786. .

33. A.D. Cher, C 146, document 139, observation by Allée, the priest of Murlin, in the Charité election, 1783. This comment is found at the bottom of the account of baptisms, marriages, and burials for the year 1783, an account established in accordance with instructions for the survey launched by Abbot Terray. Document communicated by Jacky Gelis.

34. J.-P. GOUBERT, *op. cit.*, 154.

35. Notebook (1775-1779) of the surgeon Louis Lavergne, private fund A. Rouaült de la Vigne.

36. Cf. R. LE MEE, article cited, in *Annales de démographie historique* (1971) 494.

Aggregate 1806		Sample (6 *généralités*, 1786) (provisionally)
Paris	10.4%	absent
Lyon	1.8%	1.8%
50,000 – 99,999 residents	9.3%	18.7%
20,000 – 49,999 residents	14.4%	25.8%
10,000 – 19,999 residents	14.1%	5.6%
2,000 – 9,999 residents	50%	14.8%

TABLE 1

THE AVERAGE MEDICAL DENSITY IN SIX FRENCH GÉNÉRALITÉS IN 1786

(Amiens, Caen, Dijon, Rennes, Soissons, Tours)

	Population		Doctors and surgeons		Doctors		Surgeons	
	Number	%	Number	Rate for 10,000	Number	Rate for 10,000	Number	Rate for 10,000
Cities and countryside	6,260,000	100	2847	4,54	491	0,78	2356	3,76
Cities	903,000	14,4	383	11,03	383	4,24	611	6,76
Countryside	5,257,000	85,6	1853	3,51	108	0,20	1745	3,31

TABLE 2
REGIONAL DISPARITIES IN MEDICAL ACTIVITY

A. Global disparities (cities and countryside)

Généralité	Population	Doctors and surgeons Number	Rate for 10,000	Doctors Number	Rate for 10,000	Surgeons Number	Rate for 10,000
Amiens	520,000	384	7,38	29	0,56	355	6,82
Caen	620,000	343	5,53	106	1,71	237	3,82
Dijon	1,000,000	711	7,11	145	1,45	566	5,66
Rennes	2,300,000	509	2,21	104	0,45	405	1,76
Soissons	420,000	294	7	27	0,65	267	6,35
Tours	1,300,000	627	4,82	79	0,60	548	4,22

B. Medical density in the cities

Généralité	Urban Population	% of Urb. Pop.	Doctors and surgeons Number	Rate for 10,000	Doctors Number	Rate for 10,000	Surgeons Number	Rate for 10,000
Amiens	95,000	17	78	7,99	27	2,63	51	5,36
Caen	130,000	21	149	11,45	67	5,15	82	6,30
Dijon	137,000	13,7	251	18,31	102	7,44	149	10,87
Rennes	333,000	14,4	257	7,70	99	2,97	158	4,73
Soissons	63,000	15	96	15,23	27	4,28	69	10,95
Tours	145,000	11,2	163	11,23	61	4,20	102	7,03

C. Medical density in the countryside

Généralités	Urban Population	% of Rur. Pop.	Doctors and surgeons Number	Rate for 10,000	Doctors Number	Rate for 10,000	Surgeons Number	Rate for 10,000
Amiens	425,000	83	306	7,19	2	0,04	304	7,15
Caen	490,000	79	194	3,95	39	0,79	155	3,16
Dijon	863,000	86,3	450	5,20	43	0,49	407	4,71
Rennes	1,967,000	85,6	252	1,27	5	0,02	247	1,25
Soissons	357,000	85	199	5,56	1	0,02	198	5,54
Tours	1,155,000	88,8	452	3,9	18	0,15	434	3,75

TABLE 3
HIERARCHY OF CITIES AND MEDICAL DENSITY
(in the six généralités)

A. CITIES WITH 2,000 TO 5,000 RESIDENTS:

		Rate of doctors	Rate of surgeons
1. *Average global rate* (doctors + surgeons) for 60 cities		(for 10,000)	(for 10,000)
	15.95	5.78	10.17
2. *Rate per généralité*			
Amiens (3 cities)	20.1	7.6	12.5
Caen (3 cities)	20.8	9.8	11
Dijon (15 cities)	21.6	8.9	12.7
Rennes (21 cities)	12.6	3.6	9
Soissons (9 cities)	14.6	4.1	10.5
Tours (9 cities)	15.3	5.3	10

B. CITIES WITH 5,000 TO 10,000 RESIDENTS:

		Rate of doctors	Rate of surgeons
1. *Average global rate* (doctors + surgeons) for 32 cities	12.3	5	7.3
2. *Rate per généralité*			
Amiens (1 city)	8.6	3.7	4.9
Caen (6 cities)	8	6	2
Dijon (6 cities)	15.6	7.1	8.5
Rennes (11 cities)	9.1	3.7	5.4
Soissons (3 cities)	13.8	6.1	7.7
Tours (5 cities)	13.2	3.2	10

C. CITIES WITH 10,000 TO 20,000 RESIDENTS:

		Rate of doctors	Rate of surgeons
Average global rate (for 8 cities)	9.96	3.65	6.01

D. CITIES WITH 20,000 TO 40,000 RESIDENTS:

		Rate of doctors	Rate of surgeons
Average global rate (for 17 cities)	9.74	4.14	5.6

E. CITIES WITH 40,000 TO 80,000 RESIDENTS:

		Rate of doctors	Rate of surgeons
Average global rate (for 2 cities)	10.1	4.2	6

F. CITIES WITH 80,000 TO 160,000 RESIDENTS:

Average global rate (for 4 cities)	7.6	1.7	5.8

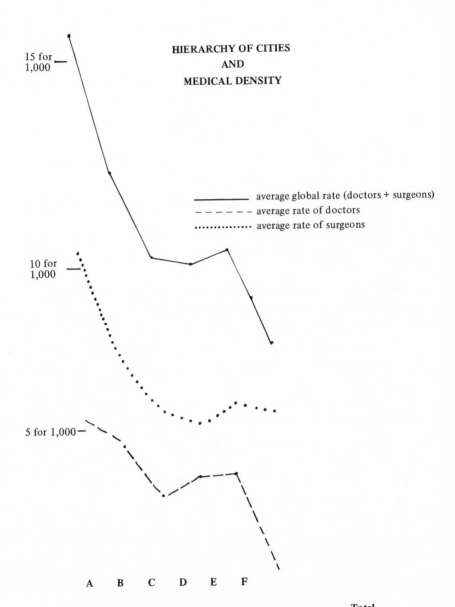

HIERARCHY OF CITIES
AND
MEDICAL DENSITY

——————— average global rate (doctors + surgeons)
– – – – – – average rate of doctors
················· average rate of surgeons

			Total
A	:	cities with 2,000 to 5,000 residents (59 cities)	195,000
B	:	cities with 5,000 to 10,000 residents (39 cities)	221,000
C	:	cities with 10,000 to 20,000 residents (10 cities)	134,200
D	:	cities with 20,000 to 40,000 residents (17 cities)	532,000
E	:	cities with 40,000 to 80,000 residents (2 cities)	112,000
F	:	cities with 80,000 to 160,000 residents (4 cities)	468,000

STATISTICS USED
for Graph 1

A. **Cities with 2,000 to 5,000 residents (59 cities):**

Total urban population	:	195,500
Average global rate (doctors + surgeons)	:	15.95 for 10,000
Average rate of doctors	:	5.78 for 10,000
Average rate of surgeons	:	10.17 for 10,000

B. **Cities with 5,000 to 10,000 residents (29 cities):**

Total urban population	:	221,000
Average global rate (doctors + surgeons)	:	12.3 for 10,000
Average rate of doctors	:	5 for 10,000
Average rate of surgeons	:	7.3 for 10,000

C. **Cities with 10,000 to 20,000 residents (10 cities):**

Total urban population	:	134,200
Average global rate (doctors + surgeons)	:	9.9 for 10,000
Average rate of doctors	:	3.5 for 10,000
Average rate of surgeons	:	6.3 for 10,000

D. **Cities with 20,000 to 40,000 residents (17 cities):**

Total urban population	:	532,000
Average global rate (doctors + surgeons)	:	9.7 for 10,000
Average rate of doctors	:	4.1 for 10,000
Average rate of surgeons	:	5.6 for 10,000

E. **Cities with 40,000 to 80,000 residents (2 cities):**

Total urban population	:	112,000
Average global rate (doctors + surgeons)	:	10.1 for 10,000
Average rate of doctors	:	4.2 for 10,000
Average rate of surgeons	:	5.9 for 10,000

F. **Cities with 80,000 to 160,000 residents (4 cities):**

Total urban population	:	468,000 residents
Average global rate (doctors + surgeons)	:	7.6 for 10,000
Average rate of doctors	:	1.7 for 10,000
Average rate of surgeons	:	5.8 for 10,000.

RATES OF MEDICAL ACTIVITY IN THE CITIES
(for 10,000 residents)

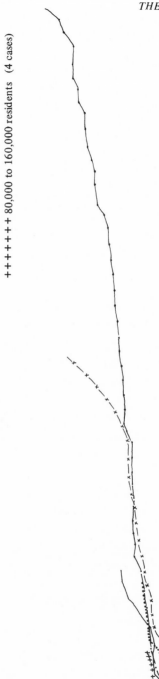

–·–·–·–	2,000 to	5,000 residents (59 cases)
x–x–x–x–x	5,000 to	10,000 residents (29 cases)
——	10,000 to	20,000 residents (10 cases)
·········	20,000 to	80,000 residents (9 cases)
+ + + + + +	80,000 to	160,000 residents (4 cases)

STATISTICS USED FOR GRAPH 2

Rates of medical activity for cities with 2,000 to 5,000 inhabitants (for 10,000):

3,2	16,1
7,1	16,2
7,6	17
8,5	17,3
8,8	17,3
9	17,6
9,3	18,1
9,7	18,1
10	18,5
10,2	18,7
10,7	19,3
12,1	21,2
12,2	21,4
12,5	21,7
12,5	21,8
12,7	22,5
12,8	23,6
12,8	23,8
13,1	24,2
13,1	24,6
13,7	25,9
14,2	26
14,8	26,9
14,8	26,9
14,8	27
15	29,1
15,3	30
15,6	33,3
16,1	40
16,1	

STATISTICS USED FOR GRAPH 2

Rates of medical activity for cities with 5,000 to 10,000 inhabitants (for 10,000):

3,6	12
5,2	12,5
5,2	13
5,4	13,1
6,6	13,2
8	13,4
8,1	13,7
8,3	15,1
8,6	16,3
10	17,7
10,2	19,6
10,6	21,5
11,4	24,3
11,6	27,4
11,8	

Rates of medical activity for cities with 10,000 to 20,000 inhabitants (for 10,000):

5,2	10,7
7,3	12,5
7,6	14
7,7	14,9
8	15,2

Rates of medical activity for cities with 20,000 to 80,000 inhabitants (for 10,000):

4	9,3
4,3	9,4
6,4	10,2
6,7	10,4
8,5	

Rates of medical activity for cities with 80,000 to 160,000 inhabitants (for 10,000):

5,7
7,5
8
9,5

Edna Hindie Lemay

THOMAS HÉRIER.
A COUNTRY SURGEON OUTSIDE ANGOULÊME
AT THE END OF THE XVIIIth CENTURY: A CONTRIBUTION
TO SOCIAL HISTORY

Surgeons composed two-thirds of the French medical corps in 1786. Very little is known of those living in the provinces and even less of those living in the countryside, because historians have tended to devote their time only to the important names in the history of medicine. Thus, when the departmental archives of Angoulême[1] signaled the existence of a country surgeon's account book and journal, we decided, with the advice and help of Jean-Pierre Goubert[2] to make a thorough study of this manuscript.[3]

Thomas Hérier, born and died in St. Christophe-de-Chalais, 1754-1809, was the oldest child of Jacques Hérier[4] and Jeanne Chambaudie[5], parents of four children. He is found on enough official lists, even as late as 1816, seven years after his death,[6] to guarantee that he was an officially recognized surgeon in the village of St. Christophe-de-Chalais, 46 kilometers south of Angoulême. Nevertheless, when at forty-four years of age and after seventeen years of practice, he went to register the death of his tenth and last child, a son, ten months old, his profession was listed as "cultivateur" or farmer. This little fact shows the importance of what appeared to be his chief livelihood in the eyes of the parish priest. The village community knew very well that he was a master surgeon since he had, as such, been elected one of their deputies at the General Assembly of March 1789, presided over by Germain Desages, the lawyer-judge who had signed the official registration of Herier's "livre-journal" on April 28, 1777.

It was in Angoulême, three weeks earlier, that Thomas Hérier received his surgeon's diploma. He must, therefore, have been apprenticed during the preceding years, roughly when he was between 19 and 23 years of age. True, his name did not appear on the list of apprenticeships registered during 1763-1776 by the city of Angoulême.[7] However, since he was apprenticed most probably after 1772, when rules became much laxer and community surgeons were free to teach at a professional level,[8] he very probably followed the courses of one or the other of the seventeen master surgeons working there.[9]

Based on the Edict of Marly of March 1707, and its successive amendments, the procedure of becoming a master surgeon was uniform throughout the whole of France. Candidates had to be Roman Catholic and had to undergo at least two consecutive years of apprenticeship followed by three years of practical experience. This latter experience was especially required for those seeking to practice in Angoulême, many of whom had worked in Paris, Bordeaux or even the West Indies. In the earlier contracts, the average sum paid by parents or sponsors for a two-year apprenticeship has been 300 pounds, as well as providing the tools of work and covering the laundry bills. As of April 2, 1772, a royal decree allowed students to complete only one year of apprenticeship, and from that time on, most of the contracts no longer indicated the length of time or the sum to be paid. Who sought apprenticeship to surgeons? In an analysis made of 68 contracts during the period 1763-1776, two-thirds of the fathers' professions are known and they appear to cover a rather large group of smaller officials, employees, artisans. About one-sixth of the sample were sons of town or village surgeons, about one-seventh were sons of minor judicial officials, such as bailiff *(huissier)*, public attorney *(procureur)* and notary. And finally one-third (or fourteen candidates) were sons of artisans, an innkeeper and village tradesmen. (Cf. Appendix I) Thus the wide range of backgrounds from which aspirants came to medicine and surgery assures us that this profession was thought to be an honourable one.

Like all candidates from Angoulême and the surrounding countryside, Hérier obtained his diploma from that city's Community of Master Surgeons. Three types of diplomas were granted: the first one allowed the candidate to practice after passing nine examinations given by five different surgeons over a period of four months. (Cf. Appendix II) This diploma cost about two thousand pounds. The second diploma involved two examinations on two consecutive days or in two consecutive sessions of the same day. It allowed the candidate to practice in a smaller city of his choice outside of Angoulême (such as LaRochefoucauld, LaValette, Ruffec, Jarnac...), but not in Angoulême itself. He was first examined on anatomy, fractures and luxations; and then on bloodletting, wounds, ulcers and medicines. Finally, the last type of diploma involved the passing of one examination on the principles of surgery, bloodletting, tumors, wounds and medicines; it cost about seventy pounds and allowed the candidate to practice only in the village of his choice.[10] Such surgeons even had to take an oath not to undertake any operation on their own without previously consulting a master surgeon from Angoulême. This was the diploma Hérier obtained after undergoing an apprenticeship which, as stated above, probably cost him about 300 pounds for two years.

Thomas Hérier lived at Le Bosquet (St. Christophe-de-Chalais), a property consisting of a house, several outbuildings, a stable, gardens and land composed of fertile fields and vineyards. At his death the property was estimated at 9800 francs yielding a yearly income of 490 francs, a sum which constituted half of the capital set up by the terms of the marriage contract, dated December 10, 1777, and signed in the presence of the notary Brisson, between Thomas Hérier and Jeanne Mioulle, minor daughter of Jean Mioulle, royal notary. The wedding took place in 1778 at Châtignac, where Jeanne's brother, Mathieu, practiced as a master surgeon. Married thirty-one years, the surgeon and his wife had ten children born during the first eighteen years of their marriage, or roughly a child every eighteen months. It is interesting to note that at Hérier's death in 1809 only five of his children were still alive, all of these survivors being, with one exception, children of the first eleven years of marriage. All four born between 1790 and 1796 died in their early years. Hérier's patients lived in an area of about ten kilometers around St. Christophe-de-Chalais. A village of some 550-600 inhabitants in 1789,[11] it was only a kilometer from Chalais, a more important small town of some thousand inhabitants, located above the Tude river. Of a total population of about 5,000 persons at the most, Hérier took care of some 300 families or roughly one thousand persons during his lifetime.[12] That is to say that one out of every five persons called upon him for medical care from 1776 to 1809. His patients were scattered throughout ninety rural communities, many with no more than fifteen to twenty inhabitants. (Cf. Appendix III.) Since he did not always indicate their profession or trade, the origins of only fifty-five persons (or a little less than 1/5 of the total) are known. They are as follows:

	Total No.	Percentages
CRAFTSMEN, including 4 tailors, 1 hatmaker, 2 shoemakers, 1 carder, 1 haberdasher, 1 joiner, 1 stone-cutter, 1 navvy (digger or "terrassier"), 1 gardener, 1 blacksmith, 1 cutler, 1 locksmith, 3 carpenters, 1 weaver	20	36.4%
TRADESMEN, including 1 grocer and 1 tanner	2	3.6%
LIVE OFF AGRICULTURE, including 18 farmers ("metayers"), 6 tenant-farmers ("colons"), 2 very small tenant farmers ("bordiers"), 2 ploughmen	28	51.0%
ECCLESIASTICAL, including 1 parish priest and 1 sacristan	2	3.6%
Gendarme	1	1.8%
Count	1	1.8%
Intendant	1	1.8%
	55	100%

Roughly one half (28) of these patients were farm workers and one third (20) craftsmen. These percentages are comparable to those found in a similar table of persons present at the General Assembly of St. Christophe-de Chalais in March 1789, when only forty inhabitants attended. Of these about one half lived off agriculture and a little less than one third off various small crafts, as follows:

	Total No.	Percentage
Men of LAW and JUSTICE, including 1 lawyer judge, 1 court clerk, 1 police officer	3	7.5%
TRADESMEN, MERCHANTS, including 1 tradesman, 1 tradesman tanner, 1 flour merchant, 1 merchant	4	10.0%
CRAFTSMEN, including 4 makers of sabots, 2 carpenters, 2 weavers, 1 blacksmith, 1 hatmaker, 1 tailor	11	27.5%
LIVE OFF AGRICULTURE, including 10 day labourers, 9 ploughmen	19	45.5%
SURGEONS	2	5.0%
PROFESSION UNKNOWN	1	2.5%
	40	100%

It is true that Thomas Hérier was never called on by the lawyer judge, Germain Desages, who registered his Journal and presided over the General Assembly, but he had a count and an intendant among his patients.

Besides the number and social standing of the families he visited, Hérier's Journal allows one to measure the intensity of his medical career. Thanks to a careful chronological analysis of the Journal, it is possible to distinguish the busy seasons from those less busy, the active from the less active years.

At first, over the four years extending from 1777 to 1780, the number of Hérier's patients slowly increased from four families to some twenty families, but then in the next five years there was a very noticeable decline which is hard to explain as epidemics were common. The decline in the number of medical visits continued throughout the years 1789 to 1795 when, during this latter year, only three families were visited four times on four different days. Several explanations may perhaps account for this rather important drop in Thomas Hérier's medical practice over a period of fourteen years from 1781 to 1795. In the first place, he was perhaps too busy as heir of Le Bosquet and devoted the early years of his marriage to the most efficient management of the property. Then also the gift of money received from his uncle probably at the time of his setting up as surgeon, may have helped him during those years. Perhaps also the arrival of other surgeons in the neighbourhood drew many patients, especially if his own were not too satisfied. But most probably rival colleagues were less significant a hindrance to Hérier's medical practice than were his own interest in his farm and the difficulties of the years immediately before and during the Revolution when people may have thought twice before summoning a doctor or surgeon.

At the turn of the century, however, there was to be a noticeable increase in the number of Thomas Hérier's patients, perhaps because of new public health measures and propaganda as well as the more stable political situation. It was then, on 29 messidor, year 11 (July 15, 1803),[13] when he was almost fifty years old, that his surgical diploma of the Old Regime was recognized by the new authorities at the Tribunal of Barbézieux. An analysis of the last three years of his career shows he visited an average of ninety families yearly and that there was a very noticeable decline of bloodletting in comparison with earlier years. It is also evident that medicine was something of a seasonal profession for it was at the end of winter or spring and autumn which were the busiest periods for the country surgeon: these months coincided with the seasonal morbidity generally observed.

It is difficult to find out how much Hérier made in his medical practice. He often wrote "paid" at the end of a page in his Journal (for 240 families from a total of 300) when the family settled its account, but for only 115 families did he give the sum paid, as a global amount, not specifying what services it really covered. Tentatively, one can state that, at the beginning of his career (1777-1780), he charged 1.50 francs a visit, and roughly 2 to 3 francs towards the end (1800-1809). In Paris at the end of the 18th century, the price of a medical consultation was from three to six pounds.[14] By adding up all the money, 2805 francs, Hérier claims as earned from the 115 families who paid, and supposing that the 285 other families finally paid off, one can rougly estimate that he earned three times as much or a total of 8415 francs during his thirty-two year medical career, an average of 263 francs annually, less than a franc a day. It remains clear that no matter how devoted to his profession he was, Hérier could not support a family on these earnings.

What diseases did Thomas Hérier try to cure during his years of medical practice? This is the subject about which his journal is the most deficient because he never described what his patients were suffering from, being satisfied to record only the treatments they underwent. Since his primary role seems to have been that of "cultivateur," he was much more accustomed to keeping strict accounts than a journal of medical observation. He did, however, sometimes note the price for remedies he prescribed.

In an attempt to describe the treatments offered by our country surgeon during his years of service, we have broken down the entire list into various sections, each time indicating the first and last years in which each treatment or medicine was prescribed. It is worth noting that, with few exceptions, Hérier was very faithful during the last years of his career to the treatments and medicines he prescribed during the earlier years. The very moment he began to practice (and in two cases, even during the year before), he prescribed:

Aspiet oil	1777 - 1779	3 times
Baselicum ointment	1777 - 1808	21 "
Emetics	1777 - 1809	195 "
Gargle	1777 - 1804	5 "
Ointments:		
Delamere ointment	1777 - 1808	73 "
White ointment	1777 - 1808	3 "
Phlebotomy	1776 - 1808	131 "
Plaster	1777 - 1808	26 "
Simple digestive	1777 - 1808	29 "
Vesicatory	1777 - 1808	111 "
Vulnerary	1777 - 1808	33 "
White of whale	1776 - 1807	10 "

Except for Aspiet oil, ordered only three times in three years, and the gargle, which he did not order after 1804, all the other items on the above list run through Hérier's career. The most commonly given can be picked out at once: in thirty-two years emetics were prescribed 195 times or about an average of six a year, and blood was let 131 times or an average of about four times a year. We should remind ourselves here, however, that phlebotomies were far more common at the beginning than at the end of Hérier's career, a point of some significance for the history of medical treatment at this time. In thirty-one years, the vesicatory was used 111 times (ca. three and a half times a year), and Delamere ointment was prescribed 73 times.

During the next several years, 1778-1779, Herier's arsenal of medical per-scriptions almost doubled:

Anti-worm medicine	1779-1807	11 times
Apozeme	1778-1807	9 "
Camphor	1779-1808	28 "
Citrine pomade	1778-1808	5 "
Dessicative powder	1779-1808	5 "
Enema (rectal injection)	1778-1808	57 "
Extract of Sion water	1779	1 "
Infusion of Tamarind water	1779-1808	15 "
Laxatives	1779-1807	19 "
Lemonade	1779-1780	5 "
Martial tablets	1779-1806	5 "
Ointments:		
Dalthea	1778-1808	19 "
Divine	1778-1808	8 "
Quinquina	1779-1806	12 "
Rhubarb	1778-1808	19 "
Sirop	1779-1806	29 "
Sirop of white poppies	Dec. 4, 1778	1 "
Theriac	Feb. 1778	1 "

Three products were tried only once: extract of Sion water, sirop of white poppies, and theriac. Lemonade was prescribed five times but only during the years 1779-1780. Most of the remaining products were used off and on until the end of Hérier's career, but rather rarely. For example, in 27 to 30 years, camphor was prescribed 28 times, citrine pomade 23 times, Dalthea ointment 19 times, quinquina 12 times, rhubarb 30 times, and laxatives 19 times. By far the most common treatment on this list is the enema given 57 times in 30 years or roughly an average of twice a year.

During the following twenty years of his career, 1780-1799, only twenty new products treatments were used to enlarge Hérier's range of action, which corresponds to the decline in the number of his patients during this period. Thirteen of these items were prescribed less than ten times. Four others were used somewhat more often, such as: ipecacuanha, diuretic infusions, ulcer dressings and "hydrogogue" wine. Sweet almonds and oriental safran were employed 42 and 32 times respectively during Hérier's whole career. But the product to beat all records in this list was that of saltpetre (*sel de nitre*) prescribed 200 times. (Cf. Appendix IV)

It was during the last years of his career, however, that Hérier's repertoire attained its maximum with the addition of 75 new products or treatments not prescribed before the year 1800. (Cf. Appendix V) The outstanding figure in this list is the number of times that various waters or lotions were prescribed: 225 during the short period of 1802-1808. One may certainly conclude that they were new to a country surgeon's repertoire and wonder where they came from. Did the country surgeon learn of them in Angoulême where he might have gone to replenish his stock or was there a sort of publicity in the countryside for new products made available?

Behind the waters in frequency, a special capillary sirop was prescribed 113 times in seven years, marshmallow flowers 76 times during the same period, and epispastic pomade 65 times. Suppurative ointment was given 40 times during a brief period of five years and a variety of infusions 39 times in three years and, surprisingly enough, not sooner. One can continue down the list, in diminishing numbers all the time, but it is certain that, unlike the present author, a person with medical training could draw many more useful conclusions. It is interesting to point out, however, that there were 37 treatments prescribed only once or twice in these last years of Hérier's career and that they covered such odd items as Spanish flies (cantharides flies), an orange, Glauber's salt, Cod-sirop, sugar, tea, wine and a laxative. Between these extremes one also notes the moderate use of liquorice (twenty-five times in six years) and creamed rice (fifteen times in three years). Last, but not least, Thomas Hérier finally pulled out a dozen teeth in the last two years of his career, a minor operation he probably was not allowed to perform sooner. However, there is no indication in his Journal of his ever having taken care of a woman in childbirth, which leads one to surmise that St. Christophe-de-Chalais had its midwives.

On the whole, the impression derived from this inventory of Hérier's medical remedies is that they were closely related to the botanical world of flowers and fruits, such as camomile, hyacinth, camphor, lemons, peaches, etc. and also to the mineral world of nitric salt and mineral water which he prescribed so many times. As one would expect, such common practices as giving enemas, emetics and bleeding abounded.

Thomas Hérier died at fifty-five, a little later in life than his father had, at the very peak of his medical career when he had to travel more extensively to visit his patients. We know that he could not live off his medical art and that it was as a farmer or proprietor of a *metairie* that this father of ten children was able to survive. What induced him when young to turn to surgery? Was there more to his choice than a way of supplementing his agricultural income? Unlike the city surgeon, who often belonged to medical families dating back one or more generations, or families who sought official posts (such as demonstrator of child-delivery) as a way of increasing their earnings, the country surgeon perhaps chose this career for sincerely humane or vocational reasons. The city surgeon formed part of the urban middle class who could afford the much higher costs of obtaining the full surgeon's diploma after years of apprenticeship, practical experience and months of examinations. The country surgeon had to live in a modest way unless he owned some other means of livelihood by inheritance or by marriage. His patients were limited in numbers and in wealth, and he himself faced the problem of competing with colleagues in neighbouring villages. Nonetheless, his position was, in a minor way, an enviable one since, as we have seen in the apprenticeship contracts, the profession was well-considered and it was as master surgeon that Thomas Hérier was elected one of the deputies of his village in 1789. Also although he learned nothing directly from Paris or any other important medical centre, and probably had very little theoretical learning at all, his medical repertoire increased enormously during his lifetime. It would be interesting to discover many other country surgeons' or doctors' journals throughout France in order to measure to what extent progress in scientific knowledge at the Paris level descended the pyramid of a centralized bureaucracy and educational system to reach all the minor local practitioners at the turn of the 18th and 19th centuries. Such a survey would also allow one to trace the gradual emergence of the surgeon or doctor of medicine in the village life of France at the beginning of the 19th century as compared to the already long-established importance of the doctor of law.

Centre de Recherches Historiques   Edna Hindie Lemay
Ecole des Hautes Etudes en Sciences Sociales
Paris

FOOTNOTES

All the documents cited below are to be found in the Departmental Archives at Angoulême, except for those indicated as being at the Archives Nationales in Paris.

1. Acknowledgement is hereby made of the very kind collaboration of Mme. Ducluzeau, Director of the Departmental Archives, Angoulême, who answered our many letters, and her assistants, Mme. Breteché and Mlle. Cogulet who assisted me during my short stay there in April 1976.

2. This study has been conducted within the framework of the much vaster survey "La Medecine et les medecins en France depuis deux siecles," undertaken by J.P. Aron, J.P. Goubert and J.P. Peter. See *Société de Démographie historique, Bulletin d'Information,* 11 (Jan., 1974).

3. Livre Journal pour servir a Thomas Hérier, Maître Chirurgien de La Paroisse de St. Christophe-de-Chalis, J446.

4. Jacques Hérier died at the age of 47 or 48 on June 27, 1777, shortly after his son Thomas became a surgeon.

5. Jeanne Chambaudie died at the age of 72 on Oct. 1, 1792, which means that she was ten years older than her deceased husband. (3E330-1, *Régistre d'Etat civil*).

6. Medical personnel of Angoulême, 1803-1847, M786. Cf. also J. Léonard, *Les médecins de l'Ouest au XIXe siècle* (typed thesis, vol. I, 14 Paris, 1975) for his remarks concerning official lists.

7. Register of newly licensed Masters of Surgery in Angoulême, 1763-1776 (J119).

8. Pierre Rambaud "L'enseignement de la chirurgie à Poitiers avant le XIXe siècle," *Janus,* 21 (1916)

9. Surgeons and others, 1765-1789, HH3.

10. Cf. also, J.P. Goubert, *Malades et Médecins en Bretagne, 1770-1790,* (Paris Klinck-sieck 1974), 136. Mme. Pichevin-Chatelin, *Contribution à l'étude de la chirurgie de l'Ouest au XVIIIe siecle et principalment à Rennes d'après les travaux du professeur P. Hardouin* (medical thesis, Rennes, 1957).

11. P. Boissonnade, *Cahiers de doléances de la sénéchausee d'Angoulême* (Paris, 1907).

12. Cf. J. Leonard, *op. cit.,* vol. II, 523, who has made a similar study.

13. Archives Nationales, BBI-205.

14. J.P. Goubert and François Lebrun, "Médecins et chirurgiens dans la Société française du XVIIIe siècle", in *Annales Cisalpines d'Histoire sociale, 4 (1973), 133. Cf. also J. Leonard,* op. cit., II, 513.

APPENDIX I: J119

Social Background of Apprentices, 1763-1776, Whose Contracts were Registered by the Community of Master Surgeons of Angoulême

Profession of the Father or Sponsor	Quantity
Intendant to the Count, living in the castle	1
Administrator-general of the Marquisate	1
Employee in the royal public works	1
Bailiffs (of taxes, at the	
"Eaux et Forets" administration,	
at the Presidial of Angoumois)	3
Public attorney *(procureur d'office)*	1
Notary	2
Master surgeon of a town	3
Master surgeon of a village	4
Innkeeper	2
Craftsmen (Wigmaker, baker, caterer)	3
Tradesmen	9
Farmers	2
Bourgeois	6
Parish priest	4
	42
Profession unknown	26
TOTAL:	68

APPENDIX II: J119

The Procedure Followed by Antoine Lafond to
Obtain His Mastery in Surgery

Date	Procedure
1763	
12 April	1st written request asking to be dispensed of a certificate of apprenticeship and to be admitted as candidate.
23 April	General brief exam: admitted & matriculated
21 May	First exam
	Principles of Surgery, tumors, wounds, ulcers.
21 May	2nd written request to begin the Six Exams of three weeks: granted
21 July	Osteology exam
	head, chest, spine and limbs
23 July	Diseases exam
	bones, fractures, dislocations, bandages & various medical apparatuses
25 July	Anatomy exam
	main parts of the body
29 July	Surgical operations exam
	cure of tumors, wounds, amputations, lithotomy, trepanation, cancer, treatment of stones, punctures, hernia, opening of abcesses, fistuals.
2 August	Bloodletting exam
	theory and practice, especially how to open the vein & how to make a ligature; bandages, aneurism, bloodletting accidents. . .
5 August	Exam on medicines
	simple and compound, emollients, resolvents, plasters, cataplasms, flatulency, various oils, simple and compound balsams.
5 August	Third written request to pass the last exam: granted
13 August	Final Exam, "Examen de rigueur": admitted
	replied satisfactorily and was accepted into the Community as sworn master surgeon.

APPENDIX III-1

List of More Important Places Where Hérier's Patients Lived.

	Approximative No. of Kms. from St. Christophe-de-Chalais	No. of Inhabitants (when known)$_X$	No. of families visited	No. of visits
Bazac	5		3	40
Chalais	1	1000	41	510
Courlac	,4	300	16	166
Curac	4		4	16
Le Colombier	0.5		3	56
Chenaud	8.5	500	1	2
Farzioux	1.0		8	264
Godinaud	1.5		1	9
Le Mas	1.0		2	21
Medillac	5 to 6		3	38
Orival & surroundings	1 to 3	450	43	750
Rioux-Martin	5		10	80
Rouffiac	3.5	210	6	49
Saint Avit	3.0		8	136
St. Christophe & surroundings	0 to 1	475	42	774
Ste Marie & surroundings	1.75 to 6.25		40	413
St. Quentin & surroundings	2 to 6	860	45	531
St. Romain (Limoges en. . .)	9		2	6
St. Vallier	8		2	34
Sauvignac	8			136
Serignac	2 to 3		2	29
Various places			17	172
Totals		3795	300	4132

P. Boissonnade, *Cahiers de doléances de la sénéchaussee d'Angoulême* (Paris, 1907).

APPENDIX IV: J446

List of Medicines or Treatments Which Entered Hérier's Repertoire During the Period 1780-1799

	Period when prescribed	No. of times prescribed
"Argent vif" (mercury?)	May 1780	1
Belt for gall bladder	1785-1806	3
Chicory sirop	1781-1806	4
Dessicative		
pomade	1781-1804	6
water	1781-1802	3
Diuretic infusions	1780-1808	14

APPENDIX IV: J446

	Period when prescribed	No. of times prescribed
Dressing for wounds	1783-1807	7
Dressings for abcesses & tumors	1783-1802	3
Dressings for ulcers	1780-1806	10
Ipecacuanha	1783-1804	12
Lama origanum	1780	1
Lunar caustic	1780-1806	6
Ointments		
Deachillont	1780-1803	2
Gar-gale	1780-1808	5
Oriental safran	1786-1808	32
Saltpetre	1783-1809	200
Silver balsam	1786-1804	3
Sudorific infusion	1797	2
Sweet almonds (oil milk)	1780-1807	42
Wine *(hydrogogue)*	1781-1808	11

APPENDIX V: J446

List of Medicines or Treatments Which Entered Hérier's Repertoire During the Period 1800 - 1808

	Period when prescribed	No. of times prescribed
Anise oil	1804	1
Antispastic	1806, Feb.	2
	1807, Nov.	
Arsenic	1807, June	1
Balsam		
Tranquil balsam	1804-1806	3
Commander balsam	1806-1807	5
Belloste pills	1807	1
Camomile flowers	1803-1807	8
Cantharide flies (Spanish Flies)	1808	1
Carminative potion	1802-1808	15
Cassia water	1803-1808	14
Cataplasm	1803-1808	14
"Cecilia"	1807	2
Cerate	1803-1808	26
Cinnamon	1804-1807	4
Cucumber	1804-1805	2
Diuretic roots	1807, Feb. & March	2
Domestic opiate *(opiat menager)*	1804	1
Elder *(sureau)*	*1802 & 1808*	*2*
Epispastic pomade	1802-1808	65
Febrifuge		
pills	1803	2
opiate	1803-1805	10
Flowers		
Hyacinth	1806-1808	7
Melilot	1803-1807	3
Peach	1804-1808	6
Marshmallow	1802-1808	76
Mallow	1806-1807	7
Furuncle on the leg	1804-1806	4
Glauber's salt	1808	1

APPENDIX V: J446

Hemp	1807	1
Infusions		
(Lime-blossoms, sudorofic,		
laxative, diuretic, astringent,		
emmenagogue, *"leidoriphique"*)	1806-1808	39
Lavender oil	1804	1
Laxative	1808, Jan.	1
Lemons	1803-1808	8
Liniment	1806-1808	12
Liquorice	1803-1808	25
Long life (*Longue-vie*)		
pills or sirop	1804-1808	4
Manna	1803-1807	2
Mineral Cristal	1808	1
Ointments		
Populeum	1804-1808	3
Black	1806-1807	14
Grey	1803-1808	12
Suppurative	1804-1808	40
Orange	1806	1
Olive oil	1806	1
Pessary	1804	1
Powders		
Tulia	1806, Oct.	1
Eye	1806, Feb.	1
Quince jelly	1803-1807	16
Rice, creamed	1804-1806	15
Sea Moss	1804	1
Sedative (Julep potion)	1807, Nov.	1
Setting of an arm luxation (dislocation)	1804-1808	6
Sleeping-draught	1804-1807	2
Soothing emulsion (*looch*)	1806-1808	10
Soups		
pectoral	1802-1807	12
chicken	1803-1808	5
Squillitic Oxymel	1807, May & June	4
Sugar	1808, Jan.	1
Syrups		
Capillary	1802-1808	113
Cod	1806, Oct.	1
Buckthorn	1807, March	2
Tartar		
Cream of	1806 & 1807	5
Emetic	1808	1
Folliculous earth of	1807, March	3
Tea	1807, May	1

APPENDIX V: J446

Tooth extraction	1807-1808	12
Topical remedy	1803	2
Truss (*bandage herniaire*)	1806	1
Turpentine of Venice	1807, Jan.	1
Vaccination	1804	2
Vermifuge		
tablets and potion	1803-1807	10
Waters		
Goulard, Orange Flower, Morel,		
Cologne, Vegetable, Mineral,		
Camphor, Benzoin (*Virginal*)	1802-1808	225
Wine		
White	1804-1805	2
Alicante	1804	1
Wood-louse (crustacean, *cloportes*)	1804 & 1807	2

Olivier Faure

PHYSICIANS IN LYON DURING THE NINETEENTH CENTURY: AN EXTRAORDINARY SOCIAL SUCCESS*

In scarcely a century, the physicians of Lyon improved their social status from one of relative mediocrity to a ranking of the first order. Two features made their success unusual. First, this change was the result of a number of steps consciously taken by the physicians themselves. Second, the classic pattern of social ascendency was paralleled in this case by an equally vigorous rise through the power structure. Such a double movement on the part of the physicians was highly unique. Indeed, at the same time that the physicians were establishing themselves as a veritable "corps" or community, in terms that would have been understood during the *Ancien Régime,* this particular mode of social organization was gradually disappearing from society in general.[1]

I A Pivotal Period

By 1805, a strong minority of the Lyon medical corps was composed of those who had entered the profession before 1789. Better established and more dynamic than their younger colleagues, they transform the doctors whole group in "gens a talent" as it existed at the end of the *Ancien Regime.*[2] In addition, modest beginnings and intellectual boldness were generally shared by the doctors of Lyon. In the context of the new conditions imposed by the Revolution, these characteristics helped stimulate changes in the attitude and demeanor of the physicians of Lyon.

1. The Requirements of Medical Science

As was the case at the end of the 18th Century, medical science in Lyon in the years 1790-1810 sought to discover a single method of treatment beneficial for all maladies. In the writings of the time, a strong interest was shown in medical "systems," in particular "Vitalism," but also "Mechanicalism" and treatment by hypnosis.[3] Vitalism, characterized by a "wait and see" approach to medicine and by the utilization of a single remedy, quinine, was practiced by a significant number of physicians.[4] It would have been a sign of rigidity had any one of these theories become predominant. However, the competition among these various systems attested to the vitality of the medical community.

From this singular scientific debate, medical practice in Lyon was about to move towards public health issues, in the manner described by J. P. Peter.[5] Physicians of the time discovered that organs constitute a whole. Illnesses were no longer described and classified as separate entities, but instead were always considered in relationship to the patient. This change in attitude was very marked, to the extent that one way to categorize diseases at that time was according to the type of patient.[6] Placing the patient at the focal point of medical inquiry inevitably meant that medicine acquired "a social dimension."[7] Consequently, the circumstances which gave rise to disease were investigated. As in the 18th Century, the influence of the atmosphere was in particular the object of medical research.[8]

One direct effect of these studies was an appeal by increasing numbers of doctors for public health measures. From 1790 to 1800, a group of physicians belonging to The Society of Medical Colleagues[9] published a medical journal[10] which tried to alert the informed segment of the populace – and only that – about hygiene matters. The impact of the quality of the air on an individual's well being was of primary concern.

The collaboration of Lyonnais physicians in writing medical dictionaries also helped disseminate a certain medical knowledge among the elite classes.[11] After 1800, concern with public health was more generally shared by the physicians, so that the subsequent demands of doctors were more effective than they had previously been. The medical society created in 1800,[12] for instance, included in its membership half of the doctors in the *département* and a majority of the physicians of Lyon. This society examined specific cases, such as the unhealthy conditions of the Perrache Swamp[13] and the fevers of 1812.[14] The physicians did not publish leaflets intended for the general public. Instead, they directly confronted the authorities in order to obtain concrete results, in particular the creation of an Office of Public Relief.[15]

Despite the lack of success of these first steps, the fact that the medical corps appealed to local officials reveals a common interest of the two groups. Parallel to the activities of the doctors, local authorities began as early as 1780 to pass health related legislation. Among the measures adopted were the creation of a board of wet nurses,[16] the hiring of prison doctors, and the establishment of a medical grand jury.[17]

2. Enlightenment Intellectuals

This concern with public health revealed a point of view and feeling shared by physicians and officials alike. The most visible aspect of this convergence of interests was the active participation of a substantial minority of doctors in the philosophical movement of the Enlightenment.

Of the 77 physicians practicing in the *département* in 1805, one out of five had been a member of the Lyon Academy[18] and one out of ten belonged to the agricultural society. Both groups were strongly influenced by Enlightenment thought. Also during the year 1805, one of every seven members of the Lyon Academy was a physician. A doctor wrote the annual report of the Academy and four others contributed to other reports. One of the Lyonnais physicians was not only associated with the Polish experiment of benevolent despotism, but was also invited into the salon of the future Madame Roland and was in addition a Free-Mason.[19]

Such interest in the intellectual movements of the time derived above all from the physicians' attitude with regard to society: Their determination to "measure everything by the yardstick of current rationalistic norms"[20] was linked to a great sensitivity to human misery. The rationalism of the Lyon physicians was evident in their desire to classify everything. This concern with classification was inherited from the tradition of nosography [21] and promoted the keeping of medical statistics. Their interest was also reinforced by the practice of botany,[22] a science which was at the forefront in the ordering of human knowledge.[23] The preoccupation of Lyonnais doctors with classification was brought to bear on the analysis of society at the very moment that social issues assumed a great importance in the practice of medicine itself.

Socially-oriented medicine drew attention to the poor state of health of the urban lower classes. Because of their devotion to order, doctors ascribed this undesirable situation to the dissolute lifestyle of the poor. In order to remedy this health problem, the physicians proposed the creation of an Office of Public Relief.

Local officials were equally enamored of classification, as well as being convinced of the benefits of rational order. These factors — as well as a naissant fear of the lower classes — led the officials to grant at this same time stronger and more generalized regulatory powers to the wealthy over the poor.[24] This convergence of interests between physicians and the elite classes gave birth to two parallel and quite independent enterprises. However, frustrated socially and wanting to have closer ties to the more influential members of society, the physicians subordinated their proposal for a relief agency to the wider ranging plans of local officials.

3. Rejection of the Status Quo and Social Mediocrity

The dissatisfaction of the physicians with their social status derived from the disparity between their intellectual sophistication, which was like that of the elite classes, and their social standing, which was quite different. This similarity of intellect made the doctors' stated hostility for the authorities impractical. Little by little, social status would have to become more consistent with parity in intellectual matters.

The relative poverty and modest social origins of the doctors characterize rather well the gap which existed between the medical corps and the elite classes. If we apply the classification proposed by Pierre Léon[25] to the estates which were left by Lyon physicians and officially recorded between 1810 and 1830, we find that three-fourths of the doctors left inheritances in the lower-middle or middle-middle class range.[26] This estimate, based on somewhat insufficient data, seems, if anything, to be excessively high. In 1817, only 65% of the doctors paid the voting tax (300 francs) and nearly half of them came close to being disqualified altogether from voting.[27] The practice of medicine in Lyon was attractive only to the less privileged classes since medical careers were financially disappointing. Hospitals recruited very few doctors and physicians had to wait between twelve and twenty years following completion of their dissertation before obtaining such a position. A small number of craftsmen and merchants from Lyon encouraged their sons to become doctors. Otherwise, physicians came from moderately well off rural families living in generally the poorest areas adjacent to Lyon, such as Bugey. Doctors also tended to be sons of low ranking officers, retired merchants living on investments, and especially surgeons (this was the case of 30% of all doctors practicing in 1805). With the exception of surgeons, most physicians and their daughters married within these same social milieux. Likewise, sons of physicians were generally drawn to these same professions.

This unpromising state of affairs was not tolerated for long. Physicians soon chose to marry within the social milieu of their birth, rather than within their professional milieu. They dissuaded their children from also becoming doctors, at least after such time that legal restraints were imposed on incorporation. In addition, the social disruption caused by the Revolution did not always have positive consequences. For one thing, the warfare associated with the Revolution attracted large numbers of men to the field of medicine. Upon return to civilian life, these individuals only aggravated the problem of insufficient job opportunities for physicians.[28]

It is interesting to note that, even though few in number, those physicians actively involved in the Revolution — both for idealistic reasons and because of bitterness over their social status — supported either the Girondin or Feuillant factions. Since these became in time the parties of post-Revolutionary leading citizens,[29] such support demonstrates the obvious incapacity of the physicians to dispel their own fascination for the socially and politically prominent.

Around 1820, Lyonnais physicians took very serious measures to safeguard their future. They managed to encounter the local authorities more and more frequently in the salons and to join them in political activity. Sometimes physicians even succeeded in marrying into the important families.[30] But this fact is of only minor significance. The key to the eventual success of the medical community was professional in nature. Motivated by the same ideals as were the elite classes, physicians needed only to become associated with the many regulatory agencies and thus improve their status by succeeding professionally.

II The Socially Prominent Physician

In this vast process of acculturation which was completed during the 19th Century, physicians made great progress and were able to become indispensable to society. They acquired wealth and prestige and very rapidly gave proof of their own uniqueness.

1. The Means: Uniform Health Standards

The fight to impose uniform health standards took place on two fronts, within "charitable" institutions which became more and more health related, and also within the ever improving system of medical facilities *per se.*

Between 1800 and 1850, so-called charitable institutions both multiplied and improved. Increasingly, these institutions became more closely associated with the medical community. Around 1850, in fact, they were being directed by physicians themselves. In addition to the Office of the Public Relief, created was in 1800,[31] the Dispensary[32] and the Council on Public Health (which was particularly effective, since it provided for neighborhood committees)[33] were established in 1818 and 1822, respectively. The Public Health Administration,[34] whose influence reached beyond the city limits, existed only briefly, although its local committees in Tarare[35] and La Guillotière were maintained, as was its vaccination department.

This type of regulatory activity became more and more complete and permanent as it extended to larger geographical areas. At first, the poor were to be safeguarded in matters of health, then in the domain of housing. Wider ranging but still discontinuous regulations were instituted in 1822. These dealt with the regulation of conditions in public places and in manufacturing plants and they became more permanent after the creation of a standing Committee on Cowpox.[36]

Having at the outset assumed a minor role in these official agencies, physicians in time made their mark, aided by a number of circumstances, especially during the menacing cholera epidemic in 1831 and 1832. With the creation of the Dispensary in 1818, the doctor for the first time entered *ex officio* the domicile of his patients. After 1830, there was an increase in the aid to the hospitalization of the Office of Public Relief. This growing emphasis on medical issues enhanced the role of physicians in these agencies. By 1830, municipal authorities recognized the preeminent role of doctors in social service agencies.[37]

In addition to the lower classes, whose health needs required government safeguards, were other social groups more explicitly aware of the necessity of maintaining health standards. Physicians had only to respond to such concerns and, if possible, capitalize on this interest in medical care. To this end, private doctors' offices were set up. As at every other level, this improvement in medical services did not occur simultaneously in both urban and rural settings.

At the beginning of the century, the network of doctors' offices was better established in the cities than in the surrounding countryside. However, even within city limits, the number of these facilities varied depending on the neighborhood. Most physicians lived in the center of town, moving little by little to wealthy outlying areas and finally to the poorer outskirts. This new geographic distribution transformed the doctor-patient relationship. The neighborhood physician who personally knew and carefully watched over the needs of his patients appeared in the wealthier parts of town after 1825 and in poorer sections after 1845.

In rural areas, the number of private doctors increased even more rapidly, but in a disorderly fashion, with one village enjoying the services of several physicians, while other areas did not have any private medical facilities at all. This unequal distribution created financial hardships for those doctors so that they had to frequently change the location of their medical practice. Between 1825 and 1845, however, the number of "surplus" physicians decreased, gaps in medical services disappeared, and a certain balance between medical supply and demand was achieved.

The goals of this double network of public and private medical facilities conformed precisely to the wishes of the ruling classes. Medical documents written about these improvements in health services have revealing titles.[38] In all of these endeavors, it was constantly a matter of repressing the excesses of the lower classes and raising their moral standards. And, in point of fact, nothing contradicts this interpretation of these developments: Physicians not only collaborated with the authorities in maintaining public order by making public health inspections, but they also relied on local officials for deciding whether or not to hospitalize indigent patients.[39]

2. Acceptance Into the Social Elite

Participation in official agencies clearly aided the physicians in their desire for social ascendency. Both their prestige and, indirectly, their incomes benefited from efforts in this domain. As far as the lower classes were concerned, respect for physicians was certainly tainted by hostility.[40] The growing influence of the medical profession was more immediately beneficial in terms of relationships with the upper classes. Recruitment of new doctors, for instance, widened until it extended to the entire area around Lyon and even beyond. The social background of members of the medical profession also became more varied and prestigious: In the generation of 1825, there were four to five times more doctors from the independently wealthy *rentier* classes than in the preceding generation. Since careers in medicine seemed attractive, physicians also gained an enviable social position: One fourth of the doctors accepted into the profession between 1805 and 1825 were from independently wealthy families, and one third of these individuals married into families from either the wealthy *rentier* or judiciary milieux.

This rise up the social ladder had a pronounced effect on the already increasing wealth of physicians, a process which had been initiated when the practice of medicine itself became more profitable. Financial gains made directly from the profession should of course be judged only according to the income of the individual doctors, and not according to the estates left by physicians. An individual's estate may naturally include inherited wealth as well as wealth acquired through the practice of medicine. The approximate incomes of doctors are known thanks to voting tax records. From 1827 to 1845, the percentage of physicians who were eligible to vote remained constant, but these chosen few were in less and less danger of being struck from the voting lists.[41]

There was, consequently, only minor improvement of income levels in terms of immediate professional earnings. This modest increase corresponds to the salaries paid by medical institutions[42] at those times — which were more and more frequent, yet still irregular — when the services of a physician were required. This view of the financial status of the medical profession is corroborated by the monetary differences existing between country and city doctors. Just as was the case in terms of professional opportunities, physicians located in rural areas were less well off economically than their urban colleagues. There were fewer registered voters among doctors practicing in the country and the total amount of taxes paid by them was always low. Their situation in 1845 corresponded to that of physicians living in Lyon twenty years earlier. If we next consider total wealth, we have a strong impression that the improvement of the financial status of physicians was rapid. Starting with the decade 1840-1850, half of the estates of physicians which were officially recorded were in the upper-middle and upper-upper middle-class range. Professional activity seems thus to be quite secondary in the financial betterment of doctors, especially when compared to the impact of wealth acquired through either inheritance or marriage. As a result, physicians were able to obtain a solid position in socially and politically prominent circles. The management of family inheritances reinforces this impression. The importance of real estate holdings increased in proportion to the total declared value of the inheritance. More and more frequently, real estate holdings in rural areas seem to be voluntary investments by doctors, rather than properties that had been inherited by the physician.[43]

In time, the attitude and life style of physicians became similar to those of the ruling classes in every respect, and not just in terms of their shared outlook on society.

Like the elite, doctors were drawn *en masse* to political careers. Nearly one rural doctor in three occupied an elective position between 1815 and 1848.

In Lyon under the July Monarchy, the municipal council always included four or five doctors. Half of these men held their posts for longer than ten years, a very long mandate which was similar to that of upper class political figures. Similarly, several physicians represented an urban district and a rural area at the same time, a type of political plurality which was characteristic of upper class officials who maintained two residences. Allegiance to a specific political party was relatively unimportant to the political careers of physicians, who merely had to play a role in politics which was befitting their position in society. In fact, certain doctors continued their political careers undisturbed during four different national administrations.

Overwhelming support by physicians for the July Monarchy, a regime which was ideologically neutral, is equally indicative of the attitude of the medical profession. Only the government or party which made the greatest concession to the medical community received support. In order to satisfy their hunger for responsibility, physicians formulated their political positions according to the political tendencies of the community: In Vaise or La Guillotière, doctors were democratic, whereas in the highly Catholic western sections of Lyon they tended to be ultra-royalists. The political position of the physician corresponded rather precisely to his social status. In rural areas with fewer and less affluent physicians, the doctor tended to be only a minor official, serving as mayor or member of the municipal council of a village. In contrast, in Lyon, which had a great many wealthy doctors, responsibility for both the city government and for much of the deputies of the *département* was assumed by physicians on a continuing basis.

Physicians did not renounce their previous intellectual tendencies, but rather added a certain witty coloration to them. Philosophy, Ethics, and History were the chief extra-medical preoccupations of physicians, with the result being a constant glorification of the predominant moral standards, support for classical notions of culture, and the primacy of Ethics over Science. Their contempt for specialization also reached its apogee: membership in non-medical societies was more frequent than in medical associations, and, on average, one doctor in ten wrote at least three works devoted to non-medical subjects.

3. Unforeseen Success

The assimilation of physicians into the ranks of the socially and politically prominent, first, a highly desirable yet in fact merely accidental strategy, became in time practically a process of osmosis. Paradoxically, the mechanism which explains this intermingling of classes was also the source of a growing awareness of the uniqueness of the medical profession.

As uniform health regulations were imposed on a wider scale, professional activities became proportionately more important in the personal life of doctors. Medical practitioners not only earned greater income from their profession,[44] but also became increasingly concerned with specific issues, such as the first campaigns against unlicensed physicians, the institution of competitive exams for the recruitment of doctors for public and private hospitals,[45] and the rivalry for university positions in the new School of Medicine.[46] Each of these matters provided a new outlet for the dynamism of the medical community.

The growing role of physicians in medical institutions was consistent with this pattern. Since they were aware of their unique position, physicians were anxious to augment their influence beyond their immediate area of expertise. Such attempts were made especially in the field of child welfare, first through published writings[47] and then through the creation of specific agencies for the regulation of child welfare.[48]

Physicians also participated in endeavors designed to "aid" those segments of the poorer class which had so far been neglected (workers and the unemployed), as well as individuals living on the margin of society (prisoners, prostitutes, unwed mothers, etc.).[49] In every social agency devoted to such groups, doctors constituted a separate and distinct administrative structure: medical committees operated within the Office of Public Relief, for instance.[50]

A similar radial shift in the position of medicine had also begun to occur in terms of social status. No longer shunned as it had been, the profession began to attract first the sons of famous physicians who had begun to practice between 1805 and 1825, and then an entire third of the offspring of doctors who had entered medicine from 1825 to 1845. Just as it was during the *Ancien Régime,* the practice of medicine became once again a hereditary affair. This tradition of several generations of doctors in the same family had been briefly interrupted after the Revolution. Before 1789, this custom had been simply tolerated by the sons of physicians, but now this tradition became a matter of choice as well as being a sign of the increased professional pride which existed among doctors of the time.

The final manifestation of incipient professional solidarity was the desire of physicians to guide public officials. Doctors served as the intermediary, for instance, between officials and criminals who were ill.[51]

III A Distinctive Group

Professional solidarity and a greater sense of hierarchy characterize the medical community after 1850. After a momentary crisis, which temporarily masked the clear cut success of the profession, the new status of the medical community became obvious.

1. Opportunities

Just as during the critical period 1780-1800, the years 1850-1880 represented a turning point for physicians. During this time, new professional conditions caused changes in the make-up of the medical community.

Physicians wanted to reduce as rapidly as possible resistance to the existing system of medical care. The greater this opposition, the greater were the hardships suffered by individual physicians. As a consequence of popular resistance to medicine, doctors experienced financial difficulties between 1850 and 1870.[52] This situation produced two reactions on the part of the profession. First, there was a readjustment in the total number of physicians: This number remained constant between 1845 and 1865, while at the same time there was an increase in the overall population. Health care facilities seemed to correspond better to the needs of the populace after this period, and in retrospect, there seems to have been a surfeit of doctors in 1845. Simultaneously, these professional hardships brought to the fore the solidarity of physicians, a factor which had been slowly growing in importance during the preceding period. The Association of Physicians of the Rhone Département[53] was formed in order to fight unlicensed doctors and also patients who refused to pay doctors' fees. Physicians in every professional specialty belonged to this group, which was not disbanded after the immediate crisis had passed. The Association helped maintain the monopoly of the medical community over public health agencies and medical services.[54]

These difficulties alone do not explain the increasing tough mindedness in the outlook of physicians. Other, more permanent professional changes seem to play a greater role in this modification. Although not yet developed to their fullest, health regulations affected all social groups by 1850. Once the patients were put at the disposition of doctors, the second phase in the process of consolidating the position of the medical profession could begin. Focusing on the human body itself, health care became more specialized and more elaborate, and no longer treated the body as a coherent whole. This phase required that doctors specialize in the study of specific illnesses[55] or parts of the body.[56] Due to lack of consistent refunding for health care as well as gaps in the network of medical facilities, physicians having a specialty were led to accept only those patients who were well off and convinced of the need for specialized health care. In fact, this select group of patients demanded a new kind of medical practice. Frequent, regular office hours replaced visits by the physician to the home of the patient.[57] Nursing homes and private clinics appeared at this time.[58]

Little by little, a new type of doctor-patient relationship became frequent, one which was more contractual in nature and in which money played a more significant role. This second phase in the process of consolidating the position of the medical profession meant that poor patients were temporarily neglected. However, the support of local authorities, whose role in medical issues was declining, was no longer needed in order for this phase to succeed.

Without a doubt, these changes in the medical profession hinged in part on the desire for increased wealth which physicians had developed through contact with the elite classes. This goal was quickly realized: The number of impoverished doctors diminished, with the majority of physicians being quite well off, judging by the size of the estates they left. Indeed, a third of all doctors belonged to the highest ranks of the bourgeoisie according to these figures.

2. An Influential Group

Unified, wealthy, and independent in the conduct of their profession, physicians started to maintain a new social profile. Inexorably, professional solidarity expanded beyond its original framework, influencing the lifestyle of doctors more and more as the profession itself gained in status.

Doctors grew increasingly isolated from other social groups, resigning *en masse* from learned societies,[59] for instance, while maintaining membership in the expanding number of medical societies. Restricting their social contacts to the company of other physicians also meant that doctors no longer married outside of their own milieu. This sort of ostracism was equally imposed on the offspring of physicians. Seventy percent of the doctors who started a medical practice during the last third of the century married either the daughters or the sisters of colleagues. In addition, 30 to 40 % of the sons of physicians followed in their father's footsteps. This insularity did not indicate that the interest of physicians in the wealthy and powerful had entirely disappeared, owing to the more influential social position of doctors.[60]

This impression of withdrawal from society as a whole, which is created by rather incomplete statistical data, is directly confirmed by the doctors themselves. Their writings at this time invariably served their professional interests. Three out of four works authored by physicians were directly related to medicine, and the remainder had an indirect link to the field. The scientific areas which had the most immediate impact on medicine[61] were still of interest to doctors, however. The few literary works written by physicians were aimed at justifying medicine and doctors: Medicine was chosen as the subject of stories, and even served as the inspiration for poetry. . . .

This increasing interest in medicine for its own sake did not signal a withdrawal by doctors from providing health care for the masses. On the contrary, this concern was strengthened during this period. Physicians took over positions on public health agencies which had been vacated by other officials. Doctors even succeeded in patterning public health care services, which were paid for by the community as a whole, after their private practice. Notable changes included the fact that physicians began to distribute medicines to patients,[62] that office appointments replaced visits by doctors to the home of the patient, and that free consultations for individuals outside the medical community were eliminated.[63] The most resistant social groups were thus gradually forced to accept the same kind of medical care which the least resistant patients enjoyed.

This strengthened role in public health agencies stimulated the physicians' desire for power. They wanted to serve other social agencies in their professional capacity as doctors. To this end, their interest in education and childhood was established, first through various writings, and then through the membership of physicians in societies which were involved in these two issues.[64]

With the same goal of increasing their personal power uppermost in importance, physicians also reinforced their previous role on the political scene. Under the Second Empire, most political figures from the elite classes – including some physicians – lost their influence. Such politicians were poorly suited to face universal suffrage and had little stomach for the official populist stance of the government. Consequently, these political figures abandoned the political arena, in many cases, for good. However, most physicians could not fill the resultant gap in the power structure, since the Second Empire represented a period of uncertainty for the medical community, as we have already discussed in part. The lack of participation by physicians in the political activity of the period is more the result of this loss of influence rather than of planned political opposition. From 1860 to the end of the century, the majority of doctors supported Radicalism, which was somewhat inconsistent on their part. This political position was manifestly in contradiction to both the social status of doctors as well as to the attitude of the medical community toward the poor. Nonetheless, support for Radicalism corresponded rather well to certain initiatives taken until then by the medical profession, which were designed to aid the rise of physicians to the highest ranks of society. Support for Radicalism was not merely a matter of political astuteness. Instinctively, physicians realized that, under an oligarchy, their influence would remain secondary. With the elimination of the traditional ruling elite in a democratic government, however, the social prominence of physicians would bring them to the apex of power. Such political activity was of course without risk to the physicians, given the large degree of control which doctors were able to exercise over the masses during this period.

Nor was there anything truly revolutionary in the verbal radicalism of the physicians who had been elected as députés from the Rhone Département. These officials were devoted to the so-called "sinistrisme." During this period French politicians moved towards the political right when growing older; concurrently their statement of policy became more and more to the left. This double demeanor was named "sinistrisme" by French politicians. That such a leftist stance should have been practically unanimous among these physicians is not surprising: the solidarity of the medical community along other fronts and the similarity of their reactions to other issues adequately explain this political solidarity. Such political activism was well rewarded: one out of every ten doctors held at least one elective office at this time. This situation was justified by the popularity of the political stance chosen by physicians[65] and also by the overall influence of doctors on society. That influence was quickly strengthened by the elimination of other elite groups from the political arena.[66] If the political standing of physicians is examined in greater detail, it can be noted that the higher the elective office is, the higher the physicians' success. At the very top echelon, the role of doctors is running the Lyon city government and in representing the Département in the Chambre des Députés was indeed enormous. This was especially true considering the small total number of medical practitioners at the time.[67]

3. A Microcosm of Society?

Exclusive, unified, and fortunate in all its undertakings, the medical community was however less monolithic than ever. Increasing specialization caused a division to be established within the profession itself.

In addition to a minority of eminent physicians, who monopolized hospital and university positions as well as the management of private clinics, there was a mass of doctors of low rank. This distinction between doctors could also be measured in terms of wealth, although the range in the financial worth of physicians was surely greater than would be indicated by an analysis of extant wills. A similar divergence appeared in other domains. Only the wealthy elite group of doctors was attracted to literature or occupied the most prestigious elective posts. Compared with this elite, most doctors scarcely appeared in the records of the time, and we can describe the mass of physicians in negative terms only.

These professional differences were not only integrated into the socio-professional superstructure of the medical community, but in fact contributed to the strength of that superstructure. In this regard, professional solidarity, for the least successful physicians, consisted of mere mimetism of the elite. Curiously, the more influential physicians never claimed any title other than "physician," despite all of their activity. Were they also caught up in the illusion of professional solidarity, or did they want their less fortunate colleagues to overlook their cumulative success? It must be admitted, at any rate, that the medical, literary, or political renown of the elite in fact reflected favorably on the entire medical community. Being sensitive to this last fact, the majority of doctors unconsciously adopted — on a reduced scale, one might say — the attitudes of the elite.

The medical community constituted a microcosm of society, in which the wealthy set the example in all matters. Many specific cases, ranging from the management of wealth to political careers, can be cited in which this pattern is duplicated.

Real estate investments became less important for the wealthiest physicians before 1860, for instance, but it was not until ten years later that this was true for middle class doctors and only after 1880 for the poorest. Similarly, the first bank accounts were included in the wills of the richest physicians between 1860 and 1870, a practice which was adopted by other doctors only twenty years later.

In effect, new types of investments always seemed to have been made according to this same pattern. The most well off made the initial investments, and then similar investments were made in succession by progressively less wealthy physicians.

This pattern of mimetism is perhaps not very conclusive, since it was also found throughout French society, although with greater variation and with less regularity. Other behaviors which were characteristic of Lyonnais physicians in particular also give evidence of this pattern. Only the most famous physicians wrote about childhood or education.[68] Concurrently however, other doctors demonstrated their real, though lesser, interest in these same subjects by joining the Education Commission or the Commission for the Protection of Childhood.

All things considered, the political career of country doctors essentially duplicated that of their urban colleagues. In both cases, there was a similar support for Radicalism, a similar predilection for offices in municipal government, and a similar tradition of holding political office. The only real difference was that the offices held by rural physicians were not as prestigious as those to which their colleagues were elected.

The medical community of Lyon succeeded at the end of the century in assimilating external interests into its own ranks. The convergence of politics and religion represents one such external concern which was able to be formally enunciated within the group of doctors. Although the majority of physicians supported Radicalism, this support was not unanimous. Certain doctors were Bonapartists; others were clericalism supporters and conservatives. This divergence of political interests which existed among doctors remained restricted to the medical group.

At the end of the century, three medical societies having partly professional and partly religious goals were eatablished. The existence of the Society of Hospital Vigil-Keepers, the Society of St. Come and St. Damian, and the Association for the Development of Medical Studies[69] proved that, for physicians, all issues were considered above all in relationship to one's profession and one's professional affiliation.

Physicians in Lyon seem thus to have succeeded in constructing a society in miniature, complete with its hierarchy of jobs, its few impoverished members and many wealthy ones, its leftists and its conservatives, its writers, and its political representatives. Numerous sub-groups and societies existed within the profession which were concerned with all the special interests of medical personnel. These societies permitted each doctor not only to feel at ease, but also to want to sustain the solidarity of his profession. The only organization lacking in this social edifice, which was otherwise totally coherent and independent, was a judicial system, and even this gap was to be filled eventually.

The outline of the social ascendence of physicians which has been proposed in this paper is somewhat oversimplified and so it does a certain injustice to the unique social reality which existed in Lyon.[70]

The history of this professional group is, in some respects, unique in relationship to the general evolution of society. If physicians participated in the vast movement which resulted in an increased observation and regulation of the individual, and if they became more and more like the bourgeoisie, at least doctors did so according to their own timetable.

The idea physicians had of their profession and the progress they made in medical science are two mental phenomena which were largely autonomous of the overall patterns of social evolution. Yet these phenomena seem nevertheless to have played a primary role in the progressive changes that were experienced by the medical community during the 19th Century.

Center for Economic and Social History   Olivier Faure
University of Lyon II

FOOTNOTES

*Translated by J. R. Antos, Carnegie Mellon University

1. This article is taken from a Master's thesis defended in 1975 which will be substantially reprinted by the Centre d'Histoire Economique et Sociale de la Region Klonnaise in a subsequent publication devoted to health problems in the Lyonnais region during the 19th Century.

2. Pierre Goubert, *L'Ancien Regime* (Paris: Colin, 1969), i, 232.

3. Louis Trenard, "Les idées medicales de Barthez à Récamier," *numéro spécial de la Revue Lyonnaise de Médecine,* 1958.

4. Pariset, *Eloge de Vitet* (Lyon: 1809).

5. Jean-Pierre Peter, "Malades et maladies á la fin du XVIIIe siècle," *Annales Economies, societes, civilisations,* 4 (July-August, 1967), 711-751.

6. ,Nichet, *Notes et observations sur les maladies des femmes et des enfants.* Brachet, *Traite pratique des maladies de l'enfance.* Beamers, *Les maladies des fammes en coucnes.*

Beaumers, *Les maladies des femmes en couches.*

7. Peter, 711-751 speaks of "Médecine de l'espace social."

8. Girard, *La santé peut elle êntre altérée pas les exhalaisons qui sortent des cimétieres.* Ballay, *Météorologie médicale.* Willermoz, *Influence des miasmes des lieux où l'on pratique le rouissage du chanvre.*

9. Martin, *Eloge de Parat* (Lyon, 1839).

10. Trenard, op. cit.

11. Sante-Marie, Formulaire medical et pharmaceutique Bottex, in *Dictionnaire encyclopedique de Sciences Medicales.*

12. Archives Municipales de Lyon, sous-série 5 1_2 (commissions sanitaires).

13. Ibid.

14. Richard de Laprade, *Monographie sur les fièvres graves de 1812.*

15. Archives Municipales de Lyon, serie I 5_2 (seance du 22 thermidor an IX).

16. Maurice Garden, *Lyon et les Lyonnais* (Paris, 1975), 82-84.

17. Archives Municipales de Lyon, série I 5, sous-série 4 (Police médicale).

18. Maurice Garden, op. cit., 300.

19. Sante-Marie, *le Docteur Jean Emmanuel Gilibert* (Lyon 1814).

20. "Tout mesurer à l'aune des normes rationalistes à la mode" in the words of Jean Meyer "Le Personnel médical en Bretagne à la fin du XVIIIe siècle," *Medecins, climats et épidémies à la fin du XVIIIe siècle* (Paris, 1972), 4, 1973-224.

21. Nosography, the methodical description and classification of illnesses (translator's note).

22. One physician out of five or six was a member of a botanical society at the beginning of the century.

23. Richard Harrisson Shryock, *Histoire de la médecine moderne, facteur scientifique, facteur social* (Paris, 1956), 31.

24. In the month of Frimaire, year X, local officials created Offices of Public Relief which were to regulate the poor in matters not necessarily related to health.

25. Pierre Leon, *Géographie de la Fortune et structures sociales à Lyon au XIXe (1815-1914)* (Lyon, 1974), 37-39.

26. Estates valued between 5,000 and 10,000 Francs.

27. Forty-five percent of physicians who were registered to vote paid a poll tax of between 300 and 400 Francs.

28. From this point on, the doctorate was obtained only after some delay (according to the fichier Drivon, collection de biographies médicales, Musée des Hospices Civils, Lyon).

29. The three doctors who had started a political career in 1789 broke with the Revolution during the siege of Lyon which was conducted by the revolutionary army (August 9-October 9, 1793).

30. Archives Départementales du Rhône, Fonds Frecon (Généalogies des familles lyonnaise célèbres), Familles non consulaires, tomes VIII, X, XII, XVI.

31. Archives Municipales de Lyon, Bureaux de bienfaisance de Lyon (sous-série Q I) de la Guillotière (sous-serie Q I des Archives de la Guillotière, dossiers 1-3).

32. Archives Municipales de Lyon, série I, sous-série I_6 I_7.

33. Archives Municipales de Lyon, série I, sous-série I_2, I_8.

34. Archives Municipales de Lyon, série I, sous-série I_5 (dossiers 8, 9).

35. Archives Départementales du Rhone, série Z, versement de 1931, liasse 124.

36. Ibid.

37. Archives Municipales de Lyon, série I, sous-série 5, dossier 2.

38. Theodore Perri, *Sur la mendicite et les moyens de la reprimer* (Lyon, 1854); Ibid., *La morale tiree de la physiologie;* Ibid. *L'ame, source do resistance vitale.* Deray, *La medecine morale* (Lyon, 1861).

39. Archives Municipales de Lyon, serie Q, sub-sorie 10, Archives de la Guillotiere.

40. Monique Engrand and Charles Engrand "Le choléra à Lille en 1832," *L'homme, la vie et la mort dans le Nord au XIXe,* ed. Marcel Gillet (Paris, 1972).

41. Thirty-seven percent of the doctors who were registered to vote paid between 200 and 400 Francs in tax, as compared with forty-five percent 17 years earlier.

42. Since 1832, Archives Municipales de Lyon, sous-serie I_5, dossier 6.

43. In contrast to the previous period, the real estate tax which appeared in the voting lists was very rarely imposed in the physician's place of birth.

44. In the voting lists, the percentage of doctors duly licensed increased from 27% to 69%. Real estate taxes, for those who were obliged to pay them, ranged from 200 to 600 Francs, one part in four, 6 to 10, 17%.

45. Archives Municipales de Lyon, sous-série Q I des archives de la Guillotière.

46. Alain Horvilleur, *L'enseignement médical à Lyon de 1789 à 1821, naissance de l'école secondaire de medecine* (Lyon, 1965) medicine thesis.

47. J. F. Terme and I. de Poliniere, *Les enfants abandonnés* (the most famous of these).

48. Mougin Rusand, *Annuaire de Lyon* (1863).

49. Archives Municipales de Lyon, sous-série Q I, dossier 2.

50. Archives municipales de Lyon, sous-série I$_5$, dossier 7 (dispensaire général, comptes rendus).

51. Bottex, *Médecine légale et législation criminelle.*

52. Between 35% and 50% of the estates which were declared upon death were valued at less than 20,000 Francs, or at less than 50,000 Francs after 1860.

53. Anonymous, *L'Association des Médecins du Rhone.*

54. Ibid., *Assemblées générales de 1869 et 1879.*

55. Mental illness: see the works of Faivre, Lacour, Arthaud, and Brached. The importance of "Antiquaille" hospital, then by Bron, hospitals reserved for the mentally ill. Treatments mentally ill. Treatments for veneral disease: see the many works by Baumes, Gauthier, and especially Diday.

56. Gayet was the first to practice ophthalmology in Lyon. He held the first chair of ophthalmology at the Faculté de Lyon.

57. Archives Municipales de Lyon, sous-série, I$_5$ dossier 6.

58. The nursing home established by Dr. Binet. St. Joseph's Hospital.

59. Only one doctor in 20 was retained, in the group practicing medicine in 1885.

60. Manufacturers replaced merchants; high governmental officials replaced *rentiers.*

61. Natural sciences.

62. Archives Municipales de Lyon, sous-séries, I$_5$, dossier 6 (règlement de 1861 du service médical du dispensaire).

63. Labaume, *Indicateur de Lyon* (1865).

64. One non-medical work in three. One membership in a non-medical society in four.

65. Ten doctors were elected in 1874, 16 in 1881, and 23 in 1892. There is a correlation between radical tendencies and the number of doctors elected.

66. Physicians participated actively in this movement. Two of them even terminated the political careers of the Marquis d'Albon and the Marquis de Fenoyl, who were typical examples of old style political figures.

67. Out of 59 elections for *députés* between 1876 and 1900, a physician was elected 11 times. During this period, only 450 doctors were practicing medicine in total in the *département.*

68. Especially the works of Maurice Cazeneuve.

69. Concerning these societies: Archives Départementales du Rhone, sous-série 4 M, associations professionnelles, liasse 1.

70. See the paper being written by Michel Boyer for the "Centre d'Histoire Economique" on the establishment of the medical corps in the Ardèche département.

Nancy M. Frieden

THE RUSSIAN CHOLERA EPIDEMIC, 1892-93, AND MEDICAL PROFESSIONALIZATION

Cholera epidemics of the 19th century produced disaster and devastation and also valuable historical evidence. The disarray of cholera crises affords the historian unusual opportunities to scrutinize critical and sensitive facets of society — cultural lag or progress, social well-being or discontent, the resilience of political and administrative institutions, and the comparative development of medical professions. Deepseated, unresolved problems surfaced during cholera epidemics, exposing conditions that might otherwise have remained inaccessible to the historian. Thus in his pioneering work, Louis Chevalier reasoned that the cholera disorders of the 1830s magnified endemic social tensions. Charles E. Rosenberg has investigated the cholera epidemics of 19th-century America from a slightly different angle, using them as a type of historical litmus paper to test the vitality and responsiveness of political institutions and the effectiveness of public opinion.[1] In studying Russia's first encounter with cholera, Roderick E. McGrew evaluated Russia's degree of modernity, her "medical facilities, training and methods, . . . administrative techniques, . . . (and) the social reactions which cholera produced."[2] All of these modes of analysis can profitably be applied to Russia's numerous epidemics in the 19th century to examine the festering problems of poverty, illiteracy, the strains of industrialization and urbanization, and to assess the capacities of the local self-governments and of the central administration. This paper will focus particularly on the impact of the Russian cholera crisis of 1892-93 on physicians' corporate consciousness and on medical professionalization.

I

The professional development of physicians in Russia's bureaucratized and stratified society followed an entirely different course than medical professionalization in the West. Just as the terms "feudalism" and "estates" require particular definition when applied to Russia, so too must the term "profession" be used advisedly. In most Western lands medical professions were "free professions" in law as well as name, existing as autonomous corporate groups with specified rights and privileges. In addition to providing a means for sharing scientific interests, medical professions in the West regulated their members' ethics and performance, controlled medical training, and in the 19th century acquired increasing influence over public policy.[3] The amount of autonomy varied from country to country, existing to a lesser extent, perhaps, the further

East one traveled, but nevertheless autonomy remained a salient and fundamental feature of medical professions in the West. In Russia, on the other hand,
physicians did not possess the rights and privileges that one customarily associ-
ates with professional identity. They worked as mere cogs in the governmental
machinery.

The Russian state created the Russian medical profession. In the 18th century
the few physicians in Russia were primarily from the West, but the expansion of
medical schools in the early 19th century stimulated the training of native-born
medical personnel.[4] The state sponsored all medical education, was the sole
dispenser of medical licenses and the primary employer of physicians. From the
moment they enrolled in medical training, Russia's future physicians were "no
longer ordinary citizens but state officials,"[5] entering a lifelong career of state
service. Their role as bureaucrats set them apart from most physicians in the
West. The anomaly arose from Russia's special needs, the severe shortage of
trained personnel in all fields that compelled the state to establish and maintain
educational institutions for the express purpose of grooming future state servants.[6] The medical faculties, in particular, granted generous scholarship aid in
order to attract and support students, many of whom could not otherwise have
pursued higher education. When many physicians graduated, the state then
claimed their services in return for financing their education: they were obli-
gated to work for the government — usually in a hardship post — serving one or
two years for each year of the five year medical course.[7] Ten years as a prison
physician in Siberia or as a medical inspector in a desolate backwoods town
might be the price the physician paid for his medical diploma. One cannot
exaggerate the extent of the state's control over Russian-trained physicians,
beginning with their education and then encompassing their professional lives.

Russian physicians' employment situation determined their self-image and
social status. Work within the bureaucracy, and especially in military service,
placed the average physician in conflict with non-medical officers. Recalling life
as a regimental physician in the 1860s, one memorist wrote that the "primary,
persistent problem for the junior physician was the haughty mistreatment of him
by all the commanding officers, who were accustomed to regard him as an
unfeeling machine."[8] Another wrote of the officers in his regiment: "I felt my
dependence on them at every step. The junior physician was the last person in
the regiment and was usually subordinate to any ensign."[9] Although education
in Russia did open careers to talent, it could not efface social disdain nor
non-medical officials' demeaning treatment of physicians. The disabilities of
government employment were particularly acute because Russian physicians had
few career alternatives. Professional life outside of civilian and military service
had little attraction: most private practitioners could not make a living wage.[10]
Moreover, during their years of obligatory service physicians gained modest rank
and pension rights that they would relinquish on leaving government work, and
therefore reluctantly sought employment elsewhere. Unsatisfactory as government service may have been, it remained the matrix of their professional
activity.

In addition to Russia's institutional setting, another factor determined physicians' status: undistinguished social origins characterized a large proportion of the profession. Granted that in the West physicians did not always have the prestige they have recently acquired, they rarely came from so humble origins as did Russian physicians. Very few members of the upper classes enrolled in medical training, deeming such work unbecoming to their social rank. Instead, medical students were drawn from the clergy – a generally impoverished group with limited social status – or from families of pharmacists, barber surgeons *(feldshers)*, physicians, lowly bureaucrats, soldiers, and even from the Moscow foundling home and the peasantry.[11] In 1861, an article in the liberal journal, *The Contemporary,* remarked on the unprestigious social origins of most physicians, and the attitude of the upper classes toward the profession:

> We wish that our youth with independent means would not shy away from nor disdain the study of medical science. Archeology, history, literature, music, painting and engraving have among us their representatives belonging in origin to the wealthy classes; in medicine there are no such flattering examples, and physicians comprise a separate caste.[12]

The St. Petersburg census of 1864 grouped physicians with artisans *(remesleniki),* listing them midway between "porters, piano tuners and pianists on one side, and typesetters on the other."[13] The stigma of lower class origins, combined with physicians' typical role as low ranking bureaucrats, formed a complex set of characteristics that denied them the prestige and influence experienced by their counterparts abroad.

In the years after the Crimean War (1853-56), the Great Reforms altered Russia's institutions and stimulated a lively intellectual climate among the educated elite. The reformed medical administration had a profound impact on the dependent relationship of physicians to the state. The stimulating intellectual atmosphere produced a sharp rise in physicians' corporate consciousness; they began to reassess their role, review their lack of social status and unpleasant working conditions, the disrespectful attitudes of their non-medical superiors. With increasing stridency physicians analyzed their employment position, questioned the validity of laws imposing various obligations on them, and began to offer serious suggestions of means to improve their professional role.[14] Central to their discontents was their extreme reliance on the state. State service, the linchpin of their professional role, was also the major impediment to their development as autonomous professionals on the Western model. Medical professionalization in Russia, therefore, took a special tack: autonomy could be won only by freeing physicians from the inordinate powers of the state. The interplay and tensions between the government and physicians became the fulcrum of the battle for professional rights.[15]

II

The intellectual and psychological forces of the Reform Era would, for the next half-century, continue to ferment within the medical profession and stimulate physicians' strivings for autonomy. Some progress occurred, such as greater financial support for medical students, the addition of suitable insignia and epaulettes to uniforms, and improvement in some salaries and pensions.[16] But in conformity with Russia's pattern of reform from above, the state granted these benefits; the improvements merely ameliorated, but did not change, the basic configuration of state control over physicians' professional lives. However, one small, seemingly insignificant, institutional change did have long range ramifications. In 1864, the newly constituted institutions of local self-government *(zemstvos)* were introduced into Russia's thirty-four central provinces and received jurisdiction over some local welfare functions. The zemstvos' competence included the supervision of hospitals and rudimentary health programs for the peasantry.[17] Initially the zemstvos did very little in the field of public health because in each province the governor and the provincial medical inspector controlled important medical matters. Gradually, however, zemstvo medical personnel proved to be far more efficient than the gubernatorial officials in administering hospitals, vaccination programs, and in dealing with epidemics. By the end of the 1870s the zemstvos had established an innovative program of free rural health protection, "zemstvo medicine," and had been entrusted with expanded jurisdiction over public health.[18] The zemstvos also provided a different institutional setting for physicians, the possibility of a viable alternative to their dependent position in the bureaucracy. As such, zemstvo medicine gradually became one major focus of medical professionalization: the program offered a means to place a wedge between physicians and the state.

In the early years of zemstvo medicine, physicians did not find that zemstvo work differed radically from government employment. As originally developed, the program evolved out of the activities of elected zemstvo assemblies that voted on medical programs, and the powerful zemstvo boards of five or six members that supervised most zemstvo work. The elected representatives and the board members were primarily local landlords, for property holding was a requirement for participation. Zemstvo physicians, who rarely owned land and therefore could not serve as zemstvo representatives, had little influence over the planning and funding of their medical programs. They frequently complained that in their subordinate position they were forced to work "in a passive role, dependent on the zemstvo establishment, as hired men and unable to do anything for public health."[19] They deeply resented a situation where "even intelligent segments of society oppose the physician," where they must work under the "arbitrary rule of non-medical administrators," and accept overburdening responsibilities imposed by "incompetent people."[20] Physicians claimed a right to authority by virtue of their medical expertise, while the zemstvo representatives resisted the "pretensions" embodied in physicians' activities that seemed to infringe on their powers as elected agents. Underlying social antagonisms obviously compounded conflicts between zemstvo authorities – the politically powerful "superiors" – and their "inferiors" – the often better-educated physicians whom they employed.[21] The most common and also most critical disagreements between physicians and zemstvo representatives arose over the issue of preventive medicine. Zemstvo officials often reacted with hostility to physicians' efforts to expand health care beyond curative medicine by introducing programs that empowered them to act as educators and public health officers. One critic wrote that "if a physician wishes to prevent disease, there is only one way – to cease to be a physician and to occupy himself with the improvement of the economic, material and moral structure of our life."[22] Zemstvo physicians, on the other hand, considered preventive medicine essential for their work. Through hygiene education and extensive sanitary regulations, they sought to make basic changes in the unhealthy fabric of rural life. During a cholera epidemic, for example, they instructed the populace to observe strict cleanliness, boil drinking water, avoid fresh vegetables and to register cholera patients immediately, so that they could be isolated and the infection localized. Of course, such an education program could not be implemented without the cooperation of the zemstvo authorities.

Great variation characterized zemstvo medicine, for each district in the thirty-four zemstvo provinces independently legislated and administered its public health programs. Most areas progressed slowly, but in a few provinces such as Moscow and Kherson, the zemstvo developed outstanding medical organizations. Moscow, in particular, had resolved the difficult issue of physicians' powers and the conflict over the principle of preventive medicine. A medical bureau organized in the 1870s, and revamped in 1885, gave the Moscow zemstvo physicians an integral role in planning and supervising the province's medical program.[23] Zemstvo physicians in Moscow received dignified treatment and coordinated their public health measures in yearly medical meetings. Moscow, however, had an exceptional zemstvo organization, influenced no doubt by the public service tradition of the Moscow gentry and stimulated by contacts with Moscow University.[24] Moscow zemstvo medicine became an admired model that physicians sought to imitate wherever they worked. But only one-third of the zemstvos had medical bureaus in 1889, and very few of those duplicated the Moscow pattern that gave physicians adequate authority to work effectively.[25] Nevertheless, with a tangible example of success, zemstvo physicians elsewhere were encouraged to pressure their own zemstvo institutions to adopt the methods used in Moscow province. The cholera epidemic of the early 1890s would serve as convincing evidence of the validity of their arguments. That crisis forced the state to recognize and ratify – at least temporarily – physicians' autonomous role in conjunction with the zemstvos, or, in some instances, with local medical societies.

III

Cholera – the disease of the poor and hungry, the ignorant and superstitious, the symbol of backwardness – invaded Russia anew in 1892. The medical profession knew of the advances achieved in the West that could minimize the impact of cholera, knew what they must do to duplicate such methods, and they knew as well that Russia's administrative apparatus could not cope with the situation.[26] Unable to act effectively in most areas, because of inadequate bureaucratic institutions and because they lacked the political power and social status, Russian physicians waited in dread anticipation as cholera appeared.

During the famine of 1891 many physicians spoke out to demand a role in treating the sick and starving. Professor M. Ia. Kapustin of the Kazan Medical School stated bluntly that because of the known medical consequences of malnutrition, famine relief must not be left to mere administrators: "the physicians should be the most important advisors and co-workers in the struggle with the disasters of famine."[27] Medical leaders warned that epidemics would appear in the wake of famine and agitated for greater powers to institute preventive measures against such famine-related diseases as typhus, typhoid fever, and cholera. The devastating famine and the anticipation of epidemics precipitated numerous conflicts over zemstvo medicine and public health in general. It was, after all, the zemstvo physicians and medical volunteers who would shoulder the burden of cholera relief and suffer some of the consequences of the inadequacies of local public health programs. Under the circumstances, these physicians felt justified in voicing their discontents and pressing for improvements to facilitate their work.

A zemstvo physician in Saratov province reported his observations of the unsanitary conditions of the peasantry and the consequent high mortality rates. The terrible suffering from diseases, he argued, resulted from the zemstvos' failures to institute preventive medicine. The biweekly, *The Zemstvo Physician,* carried numerous commentaries and editorials on this article that concurred with its basic premise. One comment summarized the attitude: "The zemstvos were charged with the honorable mission of caring for the people's health in the broadest meaning of the word, but restrict their efforts to curative medicine and are frozen in indecision before a wide sea of sanitary measures."[28] Despite physicians' warnings, few zemstvos implemented preventive measures. In Saratov province the situation deteriorated rapidly during 1891. Whenever an epidemic threatened, Saratov province had a critical significance, for it was located on the Volga River, a major route for communicable diseases and for the social unrest that frequently accompanied epidemics. In the early 1890s the province was particularly vulnerable: it had suffered severely during the famine and its debilitated population would be easy prey to famine-related diseases. Further complicating the situation, its public health administration had been seriously weakened by a dispute between the zemstvo and its medical employees. The issue centered on the status of physicians in the Saratov district medical bureau. When introduced in 1887, the bureau followed the Moscow pattern, including both physicians and zemstvo representatives. The medical bureau reviewed physicians' reports and recommendations, formulated public health programs, and then submitted proposals to the zemstvo board, which in turn guided those proposals through the zemstvo assembly. In 1891, a newly elected body of representatives to the zemstvo assembly drastically reorganized the medical bureau. As reconstituted, the bureau eliminated the active participation of physicians; they might attend a meeting if invited by the zemstvo representatives who alone comprised the new bureau, but they were expressly barred from voting on its decisions. The unpleasant consequences of this loss of power became manifest early in 1892, when the chairman of the zemstvo board, in a particularly arbitrary action, demonstrated his contempt for the physicians' right to control their medical work. Contrary to the accepted practice of allowing zemstvo physicians to choose their assistant personnel, the chairman insisted that a physician accept a poorly trained medical assistant. When the zemstvo board ignored convincing proof that the assistant lacked the qualifications for the job, all eleven zemstvo physicians of the district resigned in protest. Explaining their action in a letter in the medical press, they described the situation and concluded that "our medical organization has been demolished with one blow, our personal and professional dignity trampled."[29] The incident dramatized physicians' difficulties in the zemstvos, where they labored under social inequalities, lacked power to formulate medical policies, and met frequent interference from their employers.

In only a few exceptional places did physicians succeed in implementing preventive techniques. In Kherson province, zemstvo physicians had tried for many years to set up medical-food supply stations for migrant workers, who presented a serious health hazard to the local population. Finally, in 1891, they received permission to introduce the program, a vital source of famine relief and a means to check the spread of famine-related diseases. In Moscow province, with its highly developed system of zemstvo medicine, there was little concern about the onslaught of cholera, for medical personnel had been adequately trained and the population was accustomed to working cooperatively with the zemstvo physicians. The standard precaution, however, was for governors of provinces vulnerable to disease and lacking adequate numbers of medical personnel to request that the Ministry of the Interior send "cholera physicians" to those hardship posts.[30] Although preparations varied, the epidemic took no one by surprise. But few anticipated the degree of social disarray that erupted in 1892.

Physicians' reports and the current medical press provide vivid eyewitness descriptions of the cholera crisis. At one level, medical personnel expressed sheer despair in confronting suffering and death. "There is one unhappy picture," a physician wrote,

> ... I shall never be able to forget. In a cottage lay the bodies of a mother who had died of cholera and of her three-month old infant, who had died of hunger, his body still warm. Outside lay the cholera-infected father and two frightened, starving, five- or six-year old children. There was no one else around.[31]

Early in the course of events one emotion predominated: fear. The cholera epidemic triggered popular riots of such dimensions that medical work became extremely hazardous. The serious threat of infection paled in comparison with the dangers posed by the irrational and even murderous actions that the populace directed against medical personnel.

The cholera epidemic struck first in the city of Astrakhan at the mouth of the Volga River, bearing its usual frightening characteristics of rapid spread, ghastly physical manifestations, and also an unusually high mortality rate.[32] Not only the clinical aspect of the disease created havoc, but cholera induced as well a wave of terror. Mass hysteria amidst Russia's backward conditions may have been unavoidable. Cholera terrified the populace because it moved with seemingly strange designs, striking the lower classes with extra force. The uneducated people referred to cholera as *"ona"* (she) as if the mere pronunciation of the name created danger.[33] Fear of the virulent scourge soon turned to rage. A frenzied mob invaded the cholera barracks, attacked the medical personnel, "rescued" the patients and burned down the buildings. Fleeing from the disease, the riots, and the troops sent to enforce the quarantine and to quell the disorders, crowds of migrant workers hurried north along the Volga River, spreading the news and rumors of the affliction among the thousands of workers who joined them in their flight.[34]

The cholera "terror" soon erupted elsewhere as the epidemic traveled up the Volga River. Full reports appeared in the popular weekly newsletter, *The Physician (Vrach)*. In one town in Astrakhan province, a medical assistant and a pharmacist were killed, the village policeman maimed, and a priest who tried to mollify the crowd was harried out of town. Peasants in Saratov district killed a student who tried to reason with a crowd, dragged the cholera patients into the street and burned down the cholera barracks. Migrant laborers on a ship entering Saratov harbor refused to submit to medical examinations and threatened to throw the captain overboard if he obeyed the quarantine; the city militia forcibly ended the disturbance. In Saratov itself, crowds of rioters raided the homes of six physicians, the police chief, a city council member, and of a music teacher suspected of hiding a physician.[35]

The frenzied reaction to the cholera crisis reached a peak with a grisly act of violence in the town of Khvalynsk, Saratov province. Dr. A. M. Molchanov, employed as a temporary cholera physician, had begun to supervise the preparation of the cholera barracks and to inform the populace of the necessary preventive measures. For several days the town authorities and Molchanov tried to calm the growing agitation and to dispel malicious rumors. They failed to reassure and pacify the people. *The Physician* reported the dire consequences:

> Tuesday, June 30, the rumors and rumblings among the people intensified.... A crowd of ruffians gathered, shouting and attacking the homes of members of the Sanitary Commission and the City Council, searching for these people and for physicians.... Part of the gang headed for the barracks to find Molchanov. But he had galloped off on horseback.... Finding the riot at its height he stopped at the home of Count B. Apparently the street urchins told the crowd of his refuge and the mob headed for Count B's home, arriving just as Molchanov came out. The mob hurled itself at him; ... beat and dragged him, raised him in the air and threw him on the roadway; seizing his feet they beat his head on the ground and trampled him.... Having butchered him beyond recognition, ... the murderers tossed him aside and left to menace others, leaving around the corpse several persons who would not allow the body to be moved or covered. Ruffians jeered at the corpse and peasant women spit in the face of the deceased and railed at his imagined crimes, rejoicing that the poisoner had received proper retribution.... Panic reigned in the city.[36]

The press and public followed such reports in horror and dismay, equating the occurrences with "a chapter from an African adventure of Livingstone or Stanley ... with a whole tribe of absolutely wild people."[37]

Reviewing the medical literature, one finds that the medical profession had a clear and sensitive understanding of the relationship between such irrational behavior and the clinical peculiarities of cholera. Strange and macabre physical characteristics frequently accompanied the disease. Physicians reported that "with cholera the living patients look like the dead and the dead like the living;"[38] on rare occasions it was difficult to make a diagnosis and patients had erroneously been pronounced dead on the basis of their deathly facial pallor and skin tone. Moreover, a disconcerting, eerie manifestation occurred after some cholera patients died: the corpse moved! Post-mortem muscle spasms of fingers and feet, appearing up to forty minutes after death, terrified onlookers and understandably created "a strong impression on the uneducated crowds and resulted in tales of people being buried alive."[39]

It was not entirely unrealistic for the "ragged working class" to fear a disease that seemed to have some strange predilection for the poor. Cholera statistics invariably showed that workers and peasants far outnumbered victims from the educated upper classes, suggesting that "the epidemic might in truth be called 'cholera of the poor' because without a doubt the educated people fulfilled all preventive measures, unlike the simple folk."[40] A virulent disease with gruesome manifestations that singled out the poor for its victims, cholera struck terror in the lower classes. They sought some explanation for the fearful scourge, and with what now appears to be a pattern of mass reaction during famine and epidemics,[41] misinterpreted the evidence.

Of the variety of myths and legends used to explain the appearance of the "dreaded guest," one gained particular currency: the government had willfully produced the epidemic for the specific purpose of killing a given number of people. The writer N. G. Korolenko (1853-1921) investigated and tried to explain the cholera disorders. His description of the rigid naval quarantine in the Astrakhan harbor shows how a frightened, uneducated populace could distort the facts into a tale of the government's sinister designs. At the beginning of the epidemic in 1892, the government halted hundreds of ships with thousands of passengers in the harbor. There they waited for many days to be cleared at a woefully understaffed medical examining station. Food and water became scarce, but at last a government vessel came into sight, raising hopes of relief. But, as Korolenko reported,

> When the steamship approached the quarantined ships, it seems that it bore neither a supply of fresh water nor bread for those detained. . . . Instead of all this, the steamship brought — coffins. The implication that it gave to the crowd was unusually clear: it had been decreed to kill as many people as there were coffins.[42]

To the superstitious, uneducated masses, this signified that the government had marked them for destruction.

Administrative actions further aggravated suspicions. Decrees that limited large religious gatherings and hazardous burial practices infringed upon traditions and challenged popular beliefs. Many believed that cholera was a mark of God's displeasure with worldly sinners, and some rural priests encouraged their parishioners to resist measures designed to alleviate the epidemic. "This was the stone in my garden," remarked one cholera volunteer who tried to teach the powers of clean hands and boiled water, while the local priest taught that God inflicted cholera in retribution for one's sins and warned his parishioners not to yield to "those young people who are seized with arrogance and who, in their blindness, seek to overcome cholera."[43] Preaching that God's wrath must be averted by special services, some priests organized large processionals of icon-carrying worshippers. A physician who had worked in Simbirsk during the epidemic reported the effects of a typical religious ritual designed to ward off the disease: Prayers began at 7 A.M. on July 12, an extremely hot day, and continued until 4 P.M. A large crowd followed the icons around the city limits, many of them succumbing to the heat, many drinking water directly from wells and the river. After July 12, the number of cholera victims rapidly increased, and the city was forced to open temporary cholera barracks; "but the passage of crowds of worshippers with icons from one house to another, often from sick to well, somehow failed to deliver the city from infection!"[44] The limitation of such gatherings had an adverse psychological effect, as did the rigid regulation of funerals and burials. Restrictions forbade the ritual bathing of the body and also funeral services inside the church. Victims were buried undressed or merely covered with a lime-soaked sheet, often without the services of a priest, who might be unavailable or unwilling to travel to the distant "cholera" cemetery.[45] One physician commented that "the disrespectful attitude toward the bodies of those who had died of cholera, and the absence of rites for the dead deeply affected even the educated."[46]

The innumerable difficulties in dealing with the cholera epidemic might have been amenable to control, had not the central administration perpetuated an atmosphere of terror and violence. Force, arbitrariness, and harsh treatment — these were the government's methods. Compulsory hospitalization in the dreaded cholera barracks, confiscation of cholera patients' possessions, and disinfection of their homes provoked severe reactions. When cholera riots erupted, government troops quelled them with predictable severity — mass arrests, death sentences and punishments of hard labor.[47] A report to Alexander III on the Astrakhan disorders elicited his opinion that "corporal punishment was the sole means of ending these rumblings," and the Ministry of the Interior instructed the governors to jail the leaders and "birch" the other offenders.[48] Contemporary observers believed that the government's harsh measures gave credence to popular superstitions and exacerbated the disturbances.[49] The chaos and suffering of the famine and epidemic years created massive problems for the state, shocked the numerous volunteers who assisted the poor, sick and starving, and left the countryside demoralized and enervated. The ordeal produced an emotional trauma that pervades physicians' memoirs and medical reports. The experience also served as a powerful catalyst for the growth of physicians' corporate consciousness.

IV

Paradoxically, the cholera crisis that brought physicians distress and tragedy, also gave them an opportunity to shed their old, unenviable position in society. Before the 1890s physicians had achieved relatively little in their efforts to exchange the stigma of the bureaucrat for the independence and dignity of a member of a free profession. The attempt to establish a new role in the zemstvos, in contrast to the subservient one in the central bureaucracy, had only slight success in all but a few provinces. Working under the acute hardships that confronted them in 1892, however, physicians developed greater consciousness of the need for change. Writing at the end of that year one physician expressed the rising hostility toward many zemstvo organizations:

> The zemstvos regard as useless the qualities of independence and initiative. . . . They want only simple workers who will be subordinate to the zemstvo board, whose positions are insecure and in some areas, such as Saratov, even deplorable.[50]

The medical press rang with embitterment bordering on despair. "The poor Russian physicians!" decried a popular medical weekly newsletter:

Honorably fulfilling their duties, they have not spared their strength against typhus, dysentery, scurvy, etc., have sickened and died by the dozens; and yet the blind masses hurl at them such insults and vile absurdities, and finally slaughter them, their most true and honorable servants. What a disgrace at the end of the 19th century and what a graphic lesson in the need for more light and learning. [51]

Although the cholera rioters' ignorance and violence caused grave concern, physicians viewed the popular reaction as only a symptom of pervasive, fundamental public health problems. They became convinced that if the medical profession had wielded adequate power and responsibility, the epidemic would not have been so dreadful. The cholera disaster thus stimulated physicians to reassess their professional role, the bitter consequences of their limited participation in health planning and lack of control over their professional lives. Reviewing their experiences, and focusing on their success in introducing makeshift measures when they had been given temporary emergency powers, they carefully analyzed the means to secure positive and lasting benefits that would improve their professional position.

Cholera physicians exhibited an acute interest in the mechanism of the deep popular distrust of medical personnel. Anyone and anything associated with the government, they found, created fears and could trigger violence. The cholera barracks, temporary buildings erected for contagious patients, aroused considerable alarm. "Many patients who recovered," reported a physician,

... told me of the terror they felt when they entered the cholera barracks, from which they thought there was only one exit – the grave. They had heard that some sort of *sanitaire* in leather gloves with an iron hook roamed the streets; if he saw someone who looked sick – or just a bit drunk – he would seize the unfortunate one with the hook, throw him like a dog into a cart, and carry him to the cholera hospital. There they would shower him with lime, cram it into his mouth, eyes and ears ... throw his bare body into a pitch coffin, nail down the lid, and without confession or Holy Communion throw him into a grave quite disrespectfully. And they would not even place a cross over the grave, so that no one would know where the unfortunate martyr was buried. [52]

The cholera barracks' reputation resulted from their association with the government's traditional use of force. The typical barrack

... was located in an area crowded with unskilled workers; therefore as a precaution against disorders there was a permanent guard of six militia under the supervision of the police and a cossack. But such a show of force could not be especially successful in convincing the workers of the advantage of the barracks. [53]

Physicians observing such popular reactions concluded that their role as government employees invited the wrath of cholera rioters. Rumors circulated that physicians were accomplices of the government's supposed intrigues against the poor: they allegedly poisoned the wells, forced the healthy into cholera barracks to contaminate or kill them, carted off wagons full of writhing bodies to be buried alive; and they committed these crimes under bureaucratic orders, to earn their salaries and also to create jobs for their colleagues whom they invited to assist them in their deadly work[54] One physician later recalled that his wife had asked some peasants why, in contrast to their former distrust of physicians, they had learned to trust her husband during the cholera epidemic. "But he is a free *(vol'nyi),* not a government physician," they answered; "What interest does he have in killing people?"[55]

Many physicians found that in order to gain the trust of the populace, they must dissociate themselves from the hated bureaucracy. Addressing the Kazan Medical Society, Professor Kapustin explicitly cautioned his colleagues to efface their image as "police officers introducing various constraints and prohibitions," and instead to project themselves as "public servants and friends of the sick."[56] Despite the ingrained popular distrust, many physicians managed to establish close and effective relationships with the troubled populace. One significant change occurred. Physicians who had long labored under obstacles imposed by poor central planning of public health and by the dissensions in the zemstvos, suddenly received emergency powers they needed to work effectively. Then, like experimenters in some gigantic laboratory, they could demonstrate their scientific expertise. Afterwards, physicians perceived these unusual developments as a type of controlled study, an opportunity to prove the profession's competence in contrast to the inept health administration by non-medical bureaucrats and zemstvo representatives.

The medical reports reveal a sense of satisfaction, even exhilaration, of physicians able to help during the emergency. Anton Chekhov put aside his writing to assist the cholera relief work and in a letter dated August 1, 1892, he commented on the vigor and effectiveness of medical activity: "Now all are at work. Fiercely they work. At the fair in Nizhnii they perform miracles that would force even Tolstoy to respect medicine and the contribution of cultured people to popular life."[57] V. Veresaev, a physician who had participated in epidemic work, portrayed the situation rather dramatically in a story published in 1895. The hero, a cholera physician who had finally gained the confidence of the local populace, mused:

> It's great to be alive! It's great to see lively work seething about you, to see that your efforts are successful, that not in vain have you worked, and to recognize – I won't be modest – that you are not a superfluous person and that you are able to work.[58]

In Simbirsk, physicians carefully adjusted their relief work to counteract prevalent rumors. They prohibited forced admission into the cholera hospitals; to forestall fears that patients were being buried alive, they changed hospital regulations so that cholera victims remained on view for several hours after death. In deference to popular feelings about the curtailment of religious ceremonies for the dead, physicians permitted the ritual washing under close supervision, and conventional burial in shrouds. To overcome the notion that the government had decreed a given number of deaths, coffins were neither made in advance nor "transported through the city"; instead carpenters built coffins in the hospital as needed.[59] In Nizhnii Novgorod, some physicians made home visits only at night, to overcome fears that the police would be notifed and the patients sent to the cholera barracks. There also, the authorities relaxed regulations so that people could be buried "like their fathers and grandfathers, not like cattle."[60]

Physicians gleaned several important insights during the cholera crisis. They found that they could manage the extremely delicate situations when the populace blamed its troubles on the government and turned against its agents, the medical personnel who appeared so suspiciously at the same time as the epidemic.[61] To gain the trust of the uneducated populace, they learned to efface the bureaucratic image, to be sensitive to common fears, and to construct their programs accordingly. On a broader spectrum the cholera crisis proved that where physicians supervised relief measures through local medical organizations, rampant epidemics could be controlled. A month after the Astrakhan riots and Molchanov's murder, Chekhov predicted that in his district of Moscow province neither an epidemic nor any "terror" would occur. Moscow zemstvo medicine, he observed, gave the populace confidence in local medical personnel and also "entrusted physicians with the wide powers" needed for effective action.[62] And, in fact, Moscow province suffered only slightly in 1892, a persuasive argument that Moscow's public health procedures should be adopted elsewhere.[63]

In 1892, physicians gained a heightened awareness of their disadvantaged position and also witnessed the beginnings of a more prestigious phase in their professional development. Previously consigned to a subservient role in their relationships with local and central administrators, they suddenly gained some leverage; their opinions and services became highly valued and eagerly sought.[64] They had acquired a new public image as humanitarians and even martyrs, receiving accolades and formal protestations of gratitude from all levels of society, from illiterate peasants, local officials, zemstvo representatives, and many governors.[65] The tsar decreed that every cholera physician should receive a document of recognition, still a highly prized symbol of dignity and worth.[66] Nor were these merely empty marks of praise, signifying a transient stage of influence. On the contrary, emergency decrees and new legislation encouraged physicians to believe that they would retain their newly acquired role.

Concrete changes in the organization of health administration had occurred. The parallel authorities of the gubernatorial office and the zemstvo institutions had, before 1892, undefined and conflicting lines of command that hindered action during medical emergencies — an invitation to duplication or more often, inaction, with each organ relying on the other to do the job. The Ministry of the Interior overcame this defect in 1893: in every province threatened by cholera, it established a coordinating body, a Sanitary Executive Commission composed of local administrators, zemstvo and city representatives, and numerous physicians.[67] The Sanitary Commissions instituted to supervise epidemic work projected physicians into positions of great authority. Invested with primary responsibility for local sanitation and cholera relief work, physicians introduced both short- and long-range prophylactic measures and much-needed programs of hygiene education, usually following the example of the Moscow zemstvo.[68]

An atypical, almost unprecedented move indicated the government's increased reliance on the medical profession. At the end of 1892, the Minister of the Interior convened in Petersburg a conference of medical professors, zemstvo representatives, local administrators, and many physicians experienced in cholera relief work.[69] Although its purpose of setting guidelines for future epidemic controls may not seem unusual, the action created a stir, for the state rarely called upon extra-governmental individuals for advice. But the government had been forced to acknowledge its failure, "the weakness of quarantines and the absence of a modern sanitary structure,"[70] and to seek assistance from the zemstvos and the private sector. The conference participants reviewed the past year's record, and knowing from experience that cholera epidemics increased in severity during their second year, suggested stringent measures.[71]

What may seem but a simple bureaucratic reshuffling of medical functions constituted, in fact, a radical shift. Armed with government support, physicians and local organizations redoubled their efforts in anticipation of another crisis in 1893. In Kherson province a seven day conference attended by zemstvo representatives and physicians employed in factories, zemstvos, and the armed forces, planned medical services and increased the work of the medical-food supply stations that had been opened during the famine of 1891-92.[72] Elsewhere similar meetings of zemstvo physicians and medical societies focused on emergency measures and attempted to overcome the handicap of years of inattention to preventive measures. After years of resistance, therefore, and with the active support of the central administration, the medical profession finally convinced local authorities of the urgent need for preventive medicine and proceeded to implement such programs.

By the end of 1893, abundant evidence showed that the medical profession, either in cooperation with the local self-governments or through local medical organizations, had performed effectively. Contrary to all expectations and the pattern of earlier epidemics, cholera claimed far fewer victims during its second year. *The Physician* reported 38,922 cholera deaths in 1893, a striking contrast to the 215,157 deaths estimated for 1892.[73] Many factors caused the radical improvement, but the medical profession and the zemstvos gladly took the credit.[74] The general press turned from sensational reports of mob violence to examine records of successful epidemic work. In a district in Kherson, for example, three "sanitary squadrons," each composed of a physician and six assistants, had traveled through many villages and taught peasants to boil drinking water, disinfect houses, and detect and care for cholera victims. Elsewhere physicians, who had organized educational programs and instituted various preventive measures, reported that they had achieved exceptional results.[75] The epidemic had presented the profession an unusual opportunity: having received broad emergency powers, it had proved its capabilities and transformed its role. Physicians lost no time in capitalizing on their sudden advantage, using the situation to legitimize and maintain their newly gained influence.

V

The cholera emergency produced a heightened sense of corporate consciousness among Russian physicians. The professional strivings that had developed since mid-century had crystallized by the mid-1890s. After the cholera crisis physicians looked back with pride of accomplishment and forward with the expectation of a better professional life. A changed intellectual climate could not, of course, alone guarantee a transformation of physicians' role; but in the years immediately after the cholera epidemic several innovations suggested that such a change could, indeed, occur. Physicians' concerted activities for the public welfare, closer cooperation through their professional organizations, and greater responsibilities in the zemstvo institutions seemed to presage a new era of prestige and independence.

As the cholera crisis passed and physicians began to assess the emergency's impact on their lives, they focused initially on the issue of popular violence. With public opinion aroused by the cholera disturbances, medical societies found the times propitious to solicit support for hygiene education programs. Such educational efforts had been attempted in the past as an integral part of preventive medicine programs, but had achieved very little success because of the resistance and lethargy of local authorities and the central government's distrust of *intelligentsia* seeking close contact with the lower classes.[76] But after the cholera riots the press kept the issue before the public with frequent references to Russia's cultural lag. In Tomsk, six villagers stood trial for murdering a woman they had believed to be "cholera"; they had rushed into town after the deed, shouting "Give thanks unto God! We have killed cholera, dressed as a woman above, but underneath a man."[77] Veresaev's fictionalized version of his own experience emphasized the ignorance of the common folk: "An old man with dysentery received carbolic acid to disinfect the outhouse; 'Why use medicine in such a place?' he mused, drank it and by evening lay 'under the icon'."[78] The national medical society, the Pirogov Society, resolved to establish a commission for the hygiene education of the populace "to restore the honor and good name of the physicians, who were discredited by the cholera risings," as well as to control disease by shedding "the light of learning and understanding on the impenetrably dark realm of the popular masses."[79] After 1894, the campaign to spread hygiene education gained momentum, receiving wide cooperation and financial support from physicians and becoming one of the profession's major contributions to the general welfare.

The Pirogov Society's initiative and industry in directing hygiene education revealed a dramatic growth in corporate consciousness. The Society, founded in 1883, had been only a loose affiliation that met every two or three years, but in 1892 it received permission to publish a journal and to adopt a new charter that strengthened its structure. In the succeeding decade the Pirogov Society expanded its activities, delving into such problems as the medical consequences of corporal punishment, reform of urban and rural health programs, medical ethics, the reorganization of Russia's hospital system, and the distribution of famine relief.[80] Through this Society Russian physicians perceived their potential strength as members of an autonomous corporate group.

But what of that central factor — state control — that had determined the structure of the Russian medical profession since its infancy? Even this seemed to change, suggesting the possibility of a new relationship of physicians to the state. The Zemstvo Statute of 1890, although considered a "counter-reform" in respect to some aspects of zemstvo governance, measurably improved the position of zemstvo physicians. Several articles of the Statute specified stronger powers for medical experts and set the legal basis for specialized bureaus in charge of technical issues such as sanitation. In practice, this encouraged the zemstvos to reorganize the Sanitary Executive Commissions established during the cholera emergency; they became the core of permanent medical bureaus patterned on the Moscow model.[81] In subsequent years zemstvo medical bureaus developed rapidly, providing professional support for physicians, mediating their relations with the zemstvo representatives, and sometimes shielding them from the interference of the central government. Thus the zemstvo institutions had in actuality realized earlier hopes that in the local government physicians might forge a more independent professional role. Only fifteen percent of all Russian physicians worked in the zemstvos at a given time, but most considered zemstvo medicine and the medical bureaus as models for their professional organization.[82] In hospitals, urban medical councils, factories and mines, physicians began to pressure for similar bureaus for their professional protection. Success within the zemstvos seemed to symbolize physicians' improved position vis-à-vis the state.

The medical profession appeared to be progressing toward its goals. The changes, however, rested on an exceedingly insubstantial foundation: autocratic power. The Pirogov Society's new powers and physicians' more responsible role had been instituted by statute and could as easily be removed. Indeed, in the period of repression after 1900, the central government perceived that its release of functions to independent technical experts in the zemstvos constituted an infringement of autocratic power. Privileges granted to zemstvo physicians and to the Pirogov Society were summarily rescinded. The state reasserted its control over physicians, declaring, in effect, their perpetual dependence as servants of the state.[83] The appearance of physicians' gains had been empty symbols after all.

The cholera epidemic of 1892-93 exposed and magnified the Russian medical profession's peculiar position within its social and institutional milieu. Profoundly affected by the crisis, physicians remained essentially powerless to protect themselves against similar tragedies in the future. In Russia, medical professionalization — in the sense of establishing a protective mechanism for physicians — could be achieved only through eliminating physicians' dependence on the state. But this dependence constituted the intrinsic and historic foundations of the Russian medical profession: the state had nurtured the profession, preserved its prerogatives over it, and perceived corporate autonomy as contrary to the mandate of the autocracy. Under the tsars, Russian physicians did not attain the status of members of an independent corporate group as did their counterparts abroad. Their predicament suggests that professional autonomy may be an unattainable goal in societies with entrenched autocratic institutions.

Mount Holyoke College   Nancy M. Frieden

FOOTNOTES

For research and travel support the author wishes to thank the National Library of Medicine (NIH Grant 1 RO1 LM 02590), the International Research and Exchanges Board, and the Ministry of Higher and Specialized Education of the U.S.S.R. Special thanks are due to the personnel of the Central State Historical Archives of the U.S.S.R. in Leningrad for access to unpublished materials, and to the administrators and bibliographers of the Central State Medical-Scientific Library in Moscow.

1. Louis Chevalier, *Le choléra: La première épidémie du XIXᵉ siècle* (La Roche-sur-Yon,

1958); Charles E. Rosenberg, *The Cholera Years: The United States in 1832, 1849, and 1866* (Chicago, 1962). See also Asa Briggs, "Cholera and Society in the 19th Century," *Past and Present* 19 (April, 1961) 76-96.

2. Roderick E. McGrew, *Russia and the Cholera, 1823-1832* (Madison and Milwaukee, 1965) 16.

3. Toby Gelfand, "From Guild to Profession: The Surgeons of France in the 18th Century," *Texas Reports on Biology and Medicine: The Humanities and Medicine* 32 no. 1 (Spring 1974) 121-34; Jeanne L. Brand, *Doctors and the State: The British Medical Profession and Government Action in Public Health,* 1870-1912 (Baltimore, 1965); William G. Rothstein, *American Physicians in the 19th Century: From Sects to Science* (Baltimore, 1972); Jeanne M. Peterson, "Kinship, Status and Social Mobility in the Mid-Victorian Medical Profession" (Ph.D. dissertation, University of California, Berkeley, 1972; to be published by University of California Press).

4. John T. Alexander, "Medical Developments in Petrine Russia," *Canadian-American Slavic Studies* 8 no. 2 (Summer 1974) 198-221; McGrew, *Russia and the Cholera,* 25-38.

5. A. I. Il'inskii, "Za polstoletiia: 1841-1892. Vospominaniia o perezhitom," *Russkaia Starina* 81 no. 3 (March 1894) 42-43.

6. Walter M. Pintner, "The Russian Higher Civil Service on the Eve of the 'Great Reforms'," *Journal of Social History* (Spring 1975) 55-68.

7. *Polnoe sobranie zakonov rossiiskoi imperii,* Series 2, no. 8337 (July 26, 1835), articles 160-63; no. 8688 (December 28, 1838), article 95; Series 3, no. 2404 (August 23, 1884); and no. 5211 (March 17, 1888).

8. Il'inskii, "Za polstoletiia," *Russkaia Starina* 82 no. 1 (July 1894) 12.

9. I. A. Mitropol'skii, "Iz vospominanii vracha," *Russkii arkhiv* 33 no. 9 (1895) 100-101.

10. V.I. Grebenshchikov, "Opyt razrabotki rezul'tatov registratsii vrachei v Rossii," *Spravochnaia kniga dlia vrachei,* 1 (Pbg., 1890), 123.

11. Social background of physicians is recorded in annual reports of the provincial medical administration. See, for example, Tsentral'nyi gosudarstvennyi istoricheskii arkhiv-SSSR, fond 1297 (Meditsinskii departament ministerstva vnytrennykh del), opis' 244-1857 god, delo 703 (Kursk), delo 718 (Poltava) delo 771 (Saratov). Hereafter TsGIA-SSSR and the customary form of notation: f. (fond), op. (opis'), g. (god), d., dd. (delo, dela), l., ll. (list, listy).

12. *Sovremennik* 89 (October 1861) 596.

13. *Meditsinskii vestnik,* 1864, no. 5, 42.

14. Two Soviet works on this period are M. M. Levit, *Stanovlenie obshchestvennoi meditsiny v Rossii* (Moscow, 1974), and A. P. Zhuk, *Razvitie obshchestvenno-meditsinskoi mysli v Rossii v 60-70 gg. XIX veka* (Moscow, 1963); they stress the radical and social service aspects of medical careers.

15. Joseph Frank, *Dostoevsky: The Seeds of Revolt, 1821-1849* (Princeton, 1976) 6-13, gives a fine description of the ambiguous social status of Dostoevsky's physician-father.

16. *Polnoe sobranie zakonov,* Series 2, no. 31453 (January 26, 1857), reform of the Medical Surgical Academy; no. 31815 (May 10, 1857), a liberalization of regulations on

students' uniforms; no. 35985 (June 28, 1860), an increase in the number of departments and professors in the medical faculties. Laws decreeing better pay, pensions, and care of families of physicians who died in service, were no. 29632 (August 31, 1855), no. 32681 (January 14, 1858), and no. 33783 (November 18, 1858). For a memoir describing the changes at the Medical Academy, see A. I. Il'inskii, "Za polstoletiia, 1841-1892," republished in *Memoirs of Russian Physicians, 1855-1870,* compiled by Nancy Frieden (Cambridge, England: Oriental Research Partners, Forthcoming).

17. Nancy Frieden, "The Roots of Zemstvo Medicine," Twenty-fifth Congress of the International Society of the History of Medicine, Quebec, 1976, *Proceedings.*

18. For the discussions in the Committee of Ministers regarding the zemstvos' superior capabilities, see TsGIA-SSSR, f.1263-,op. 1-1879g., d. 4025, 11. 307-37, "O predostavlenii zemskim uchrezhdeniiam prava isdavat' obiazatel'nye dlia mestnogo naseleniia uezdov postanovleniia v vidakh preduprezhdeniia i prekrasheniia poval'nykh i zarazitel'nykh boleznei," and d. 4024, 11. 487-522, "Osobyi zhurnal Komiteta ministrov, 21 i 27 fevrialia." The zemstvos acquired responsibility for insane asylums and epidemic controls in 1879.

19. P. A. Dobichina, "Zemskaia meditsina na iuge Rossii," *Meditsinskii vestnik,* 1884, no. 37, 601; V. Sviatlovskii, "Po povodu otnosheniia zemstva k postanovleniiam s'ezdov zemskikh vrachei," *Zemskii vrach,* 1888, no. 1, 2-4.

20. *Zdorov'e,* 1876, no. 44, 321; *Vrach,* 1881, no. 24, 403; Obshchectvo russkikh vrachei v pamiat' N. I. Pirogova, *Trudy vtorogo s'ezda russkikh vrachei* (Moscow, 1887), 1:28.

21. D. N. Zhbankov, "Zemskaia meditsina i eia protivniki," *Meditsinskoe obozrenie* 16 no. 3 (1889) 360-79, discusses the social tensions, noting that the physicians are not entirely blameless, for they tended to flaunt their educational attainments; the author, an outspoken advocate of improved public health and zemstvo medicine, was himself the illegitimate child of a landowner and a serf woman.

22. B. Lenskii, "Illiutsii zemskoi meditsiny," *Slovo,* 1880, no. 10, 49.

23. D. N. Zhbankov, *O deiatel'nosti sanitarnykh biuro i obshchestvenno-sanitarnykh uchrezhdenii v zemskoi Rossii* (Moscow, 1910) 14-18, 66-67.

24. Peter F. Krug, "The Debate over the Delivery of Health Care in Rural Russia: The Moscow Zemstvo, 1864-1878," *Bulletin of the History of Medicine* 50 no. 2 (Summer 1976) 226-41, discusses Moscow zemstvo medicine. Krug is now engaged in research on the Moscow zemstvo and will undoubtedly clarify the reasons for Moscow's unusual performance. See V. A. Bazanov, *E. A. Osipov* (Moscow, 1974), for interesting background on some of the people who established the medical-statistical bureau in Moscow.

25. D. N. Zhbankov, "Itogi zemskoi meditsiny," *Vrach,* 1894, no. 18, 513-19; no. 19, 546-51.

26. John M. Eyler, "William Farr on the Cholera: The Sanitarian's Disease Theory and the Statistician's Method," *Journal of the History of Medicine* 28 (April, 1973) 79-100, describes work in England after 1854 when cholera and impure water supply were shown to be closely related. Russian physicians knew the need for environmental controls, that the excreta of cholera patients carried the "bacteria," and that those who had an adequate diet rarely succumbed to the disease; for a typical discussion see Prof. E. E. Eikhval'd, *Chto delat' v ozhidanii kholery i pri pervom eia poiavlenii?* (Pbg., 1886), a speech delivered to the first public meeting of the First Congress of the Pirogov Society, the national medical society, December 26, 1885. Proof that the cholera vibrio caused the disease would not be conclusive until after the Hamburg epidemic of 1892. For an example of the administrative

obstacles to cholera controls, see the meetings of the Kazan medical society when cholera threatened in 1885: *Dnevnik Kazanskogo obshchestva vrachei pri Imperatorskom universitete,* 1885, nos. 1, 5.

27. M. Ia. Kapustin, "Zadachi gigieny pri bedsviiakh neurozhai," *Dnevnik obshchestva vrachei pri Imperatorskom Kazanskom universitete,* 1892, no. 1, 195, republished in *Vrach,* 1891, no. 41,931-32. Richard G. Robbins, Jr., *Famine in Russia, 1891-1892* (N.Y., 1975), expertly analyses the food crisis that preceded the cholera epidemic.

28. M. Timarenko, "O merakh preduprezhdeniia zabolevaemosti, kak sistem v zemsko-meditsinskoi organizatsii," *Zemskii vrach,* 1891, no. 25, 501-03.

29. *Vrach,* 1892, no. 11, 270-71.

30. Extensive data on physicians sent to cholera-infected areas are in TsGIA-SSSR, f. 1297, op.243-1892g., dd. 10, 24, 40, 72-73, 75, 89, 93, 131.

31. K. Pashkov, "Epidemiia kholery v derevne," *Zemskii vrach,* 1893, no. 4-5, 56.

32. M. I. Arustamov, "Kholera v Astrakhan gubernii v 1892 gody," Obshchestvo russkikh vrachei v pamiat' N. I. Pirogova, *Trudy piatogo s'ezda* (Pbg., 1894), 1:657-66, the report of the physician in charge of the harbor medical checkpoint, discussed below. The mortality rate was exceptionally high: between June 14 and July 31 in Astrakhan province 3151 of the 4499 cholera victims died, a rate of seventy percent. Rosenberg, *The Cholera Years,* 2-3, gives a classic description of the manifestations of the disease. See also William H. McNeill, *Plagues and Peoples* (New York, 1976), 261-74.

33. S. Ia. Elpat'evskii, *Vospominaniia za piat'desiat let* (Leningrad, 1929), 235.

34. V. G. Korolenko, "Kholernyi karantin na deviati-futovam reide: Stranichka iz nedavnogo proshlogo," *Russkoe bogatstvo,* no. 5 (May 1905), 58-76. *Russkaia mysl'* rejected this article when submitted in 1892; it is part of "V kholernye god," *Polnoe sobranie sochinenii* 9 vols. (Pbg., 1914), 3:369-421.

35. *Vrach,* 1892, no. 28, 771; no. 29, 738.

36. Ibid, no. 29, 742.

37. "Iz obshchestvennoi khroniki, August 1, 1892," *Vestnik evropi* 27 no. 8 (August 1892) 901.

38. A. Paevskaia, "Komandirovka na kholeru iz zapisok zhenshcheny-vracha," *Rosskoe bagatstvo,* no. 7 (July 1903), 125. The author is listed among the cholera physicians sent out by the Medical Department: TsGIA-SSSR, f. 1297, op. 243-1892 g., d. 131, 11. 35-37.

39. V. M. Rozhanskii, "Iz nabliudenii nad kholernoi epidemiei 1892 g. v Nizhnem Novgorode," *Dnevnik obshchestva vrachei pri Imperatorskom Kazanskom universitete,* 1893, no. 3, 184. See also E. D. Kuskova, "Davno minuvshee," *Novyi zhurnal* 49 (June 1957) 163.

40. Dr. D. L. Mandelshtam, *Dnevnik obshchestva vrachei pri imperatorskom kazanskom universitete,* 1893, no. 3, 36: Report to the meeting of December 5, 1892. A. P. Stolypinskii, "O kholernoi epidemii v Kazani 1892 g.," ibid., no. 1, 7, gives the following data on the social status of 420 cholera victims:

Gentry	5	Merchant	2
Bureaucrat	7	Artisan	91
Clergy	2	Peasant	313

A. V. Smirnov, "Kholera vo Vladimirskoi gubernii v 1892 g.," *Zemskii vrach*, 1893, no. 18, 313, reported that only five of his 346 cholera patients were people of the upper classes, and of those only one died.

41. Jean Mayer, "Famine Relief," *Famine: A Symposium dealing with Nutrition and Relief Operations in Times of Disaster* (Uppsala, 1971), 180; Chevalier, *Le cholera*, xv, 17-20.

42. Korolenko, "Kholernyi karantin," *Russkoe bogatstvo*, no. 5 (May, 1905) 70.

43. A. Anikin, "Kholernyi god," *Vestnik evropi* 49 no. 1 (January, 1913) 116.

44. V. P. Neboliubov, "Nabliudeniia iz poezdki na epidemiiu kholery v g. Simbirsk v 1892 godu," *Dnevnik obshchestva vrachei pri Imperatorskom kazanskom universitete,* 1894, no. 4, 165.

45. N. N. Vnukov, "O kholernom barake na Bakaldinskoi pristan v gorode Kazani," ibid., 1893, no. 1, 53.

46. Neboliubov, "Nabliudeniia iz poezdki," 166 n.1; see also Korolenko, "V kholernye god," 387-88.

47. Korolenko, "Kholernyi karantin," p. 75, cites the decisions of the military court in Astrakhan: 20 death sentences (commuted to hard labor for life), 22 sentences of hard labor for 12 to 20 years, and 33 lesser sentences. See also S. Anikin, "Kholernyi god," 126.

48. V. Kolpenskii, "Kholernyi bunt v 1892 godu," *Arkhiv istorii truda v Rossii,* Book 3 (1922) 111, cites police records to show that 170 people were jailed in Astrakhan for participation in the cholera disorders.

49. Ibid., 111, n.1.

50. S. Iaroshevskii, "Otchego v Samare tak sil'no svirepstvovala kholera," *Meditsina,* 1892, no. 47, 644.

51. *Vrach,* 1892, no. 28, 711.

52. Vnukov, "O kholernom barake," 53.

53. Ibid.

54. This summary of cholera legends is based on the contemporary medical reports and the articles cited above by Korolenko, Kolpenskii, Kuskova, Paevskaia, and A. K., "Vospominaniia o kholere." *Istoricheskii vestnik* 114 (November 1908) 570-75.

55. Elpat'evskii, *Vospominaniia,* 242. See also V. Veresaev, "Bez dorogi," *Russkoe bogatstvo,* no. 8 (August 1895), 15, describing a cholera physician who is initially distrusted as a government official but finally accepted as a "genuine" *(nastoiashchii)* physician.

56. September 20, 1892, reported in *Vrach,* 1892, no. 40, 1020-21.

57. Chekhov to A.S. Suvorin, *Polnoe sobranie sochinenii,* 15, 416.

58. Veresaev, "Bez dorogi," *Russkoe bogatstvo,* no. 8 (August 1895) 22.

59. Neboliubov, "Nabliudeniia iz poezdki," 166, n.1; Vnukov, "O kholernom barake," 55.

60. Korolenko, "V kholernyi god," pp. 385, 388; Elpat'evskii, *Vospominaniia,* 235-43; *Vrach,* 1892, no. 29, 738; S.I. Mitskevich, *Na grani dvukh epokh,* (Moscow, 1937), 112.

61. The most common rumor that physicians "brought" cholera, might easily arise out of circumstantial evidence as interpreted by the uneducated: the physicians arrived first, "tested" (poisoned, some thought) the wells, supervised the building of cholera barracks, and when all was ready "discovered" (fabricated, so the rumor went) a cholera patient, giving the physician an excuse to begin the murderous plot of luring patients into the barracks to kill them.

62. Chekhov to N. M. Lintareva, July 22, 1892, *Polnoe sobranie sochinenii,* 15:411. E. B. Meve, *Meditsina v tvorchestve i zhizni A.P. Chekhova* (Kiev, 1961) 185-207, is an interesting account of Chekhov's work during the epidemic.

63. D. N. Zhbankov, "Neskol'ko zametok o kholere 1892-1893 gg.," *Vrach,* 1893, no. 50, 1378, records only 654 cases of cholera in Moscow province in 1892, out of a national total then estimated as 433,643. In the neighborhing province of Tver' there were 29,332 cases of cholera, a morbidity rate of 37.46/1000 in contrast to Moscow's of 0.87/1000.

64. The profession's great pride in its performance during the epidemic is evident in the proceedings of the Fifth Congress of the Pirogov Society; a thorough account of the Congress was immediately available to all Russian physicians in *Vrach,* 1894, no. 1, 16-29; no. 2, 47-55; no. 3, 76-91; no. 4, 116-19; no. 6, 181-83.

65. TsGIA-SSSR, f.1297, op.243-1892 g., d.131, ll.1-37, 65-66, records governors' answers to the Medical department's confidential request for information on the cholera physicians, paramedical personnel, and medical students; these are full of praise for their devotion to duty and sensitive handling of the frightened peasantry. Ibid., d.24, ll.387-90, contains a report from the governor of Samara that the 118 peasants of the village of Maksimovka of their own volition gathered to vote a message of gratitude to the medical student and his sanitary squadron who had helped them during the epidemic. *Vrach,* 1894, no. 1, 31-32, reported that when the Pirogov Society met in Petersburg at the end of 1893 the city Council held a reception for the attending physicians "as an expression of gratitude for their work during the cholera epidemic."

66. *Obshchii obzor deiatel'nosti ministerstva vnuternnykh del za vremia tsarstvovaniia Imperatora Aleksandra III* (Pbg., 1901) 149.

67. TsGIA-SSSR, f.1297, op.243-1893 g., d.9, l.209.

68. Zhbankov, *O deiatel'nosti sanitarnykh biuro,* 20-24, 29-35.

69. Circular of the Medical Department, October 30, 1892, *Vestnik obshchestvennoi gigieny, sudebnoi i prakticheskoi meditsiny* 16 no. 2 (November, 1892), Section I:16. O. V. Aptekman, "Partiia 'Narodnogo Prava': Vospominaniia," *Byloe* 7/19 (July 1907): 191-96, recounts the author's participation in the meeting.

70. K. Tolstoi, "S'ezd vrachei prinimavshihkh neposredstvennoi uchastie v borbe s kholernoi epidemiei 1892 g.," *Vestnik obshchestvennoi gigieny* 17 no. 1 (January, 1893), Section VII:3.

71. G. I. Arkhangel'skii, *Kholernye epidemii v evropeiskoi Rossii v 50-ti letnii period, 1823-1872 gg.* (Pbg., 1874), was the standard reference for the statistics; D. N. Zhbankov relied on it for his *Kholernye epidemii v smolenskoi gubernii, 1831-1872 gg.* (Smolensk, 1893), to show that Russia's previous cholera epidemics were more severe in the second year. M. S. Onitsanskii, *O pasprostranenii kholery v Rossii* (Pbg., 1911), gives data on morbidity and mortality for cholera epidemics to 1910.

72. "Khersonskoe gubernskoe soveshchanie zemskikh vrachei i predstavitelei uezdnykh uprav po voprosu o kholere, 12-18 marta 1893," *Zemskii vrach,* 1893, nos. 14-17. For the

medical-food supply stations see V. V. Khizhniakov, *Polozhenie rabochikh v sel'skom khoziaistve v sanitarnom otnoshenii* (Kherson, 1899), and K.I. Idel'chik, *N. I. Teziakov i ego rol' v razvitii zemskoi meditsiny i stroitel'stve sovetskogo zdravookhraneniia* (Moscow, 1960).

73. *Vrach*, 1893, no. 50, 1379. According to Onitsanskii's work of 1911 (see above, n.71), there were 620,051 cases of cholera in 1892, with a mortality of 300,324; in 1893 there were 106,600 cases and a mortality of 42,250.

74. *Vrach*, 1893, no. 50, 1380-81. See above n.64 for citation of material on the Fifth Congress of the Pirogov Society; the full transcript of the "Cholera" sessions is in Obshchestvo russkikh vrachei v pamiat' N. I. Pirogova, *Trudy piatogo s'ezda* (Pbg., 1894), 1:626-712.

75. News items cited in Korolenko, "V Kholernyi god," 393-96. See also the sources listed above, n.65, for very positive approval from officials who supervised the physicians.

76. The development of these programs is discussed in my article, "Medical Reform in a Traditionalist Culture," *The Family in Imperial Russia*, ed. David L. Ransel (Urbana: University of Illinois Press, 1978).

77. *Vrach*, 1893, no. 41, 1157-58 and *Syn otechestvo*, October 8, 1893. Two were found guilty and sentenced to four years in jail.

78. Veresaev, "Bez dorogi," *Russkoe Bogatstvo*, no. 7 (1895) 45.

79. *Vrach*, 1894, no. 2, 51-52.

80. *Nikolai Ivanovich Pirogov i ego nasledie: Pirogovskie s'ezdy, iubileinoe izdanie*, M. M. Gran', Z. G. Frenkel, and A. I. Shingarev, eds. (Pbg., 1911).

81. *Polnoe sobranie zakonov*, Series 3, no. 6027 (June 12, 1890), articles 72, 73, 105, 108; moreover, the sanitary controls were shifted from the district to the province level, a decided advantage for the coordination of preventive measures and general medical policies. TsGIA-SSSR, f. 1287, op. 27-1894 g., d.2889. "Po khodataistvo zemskikh sobranii ob uchrezhdenii . . . meditsinsko-sanitarnykh sovetov," shows the senate's support of zemstvo efforts to establish medical bureaus; the senate cited the Zemstvo Statute of 1890 against the interference of governors who objected to the zemstvo technical bureaus.

82. Zhbankov, *O deiatel'nosti sanitarnykh biuro*. TsGIA-SSSR, f. 1287, op.27, d.470. "Po zhalobe tverskoi gubernskoi upravy . . . ob uvol'nenii doktora Sovetova," shows the ability of the zemstvos to block gubernatorial control of the zemstvo employees. For physicians' employment patterns, see Grebenshchikov, "Opyt razrabotki resul'tatov registratsii vrachei," 105. The great enthusiasm for zemstvo medicine is obvious in even a cursory scanning of the Pirogov Society's Journal and Proceedings, and of the popular weekly newsletters *Vrach* (1880-1901) and *Russkii vrach* (1901-1918).

83. For several official investigations of zemstvo medicine see TsGIA-SSSR, f. 1282, op.2, d.1842, "Sekretno. Obozrenie uchrezhdenii tverskoi gubernii, 1903," 11.27-37; f.1287, op.27, dd.3746, 3747, 3748, "O revizii moskovskoi gubernii, 1904"; and Kurskoe zemstvo, *Otchet po revizii Zinov'evym* (Kursk, 1904). On April 6, 1902, the Ministry of the Interior began an extensive correspondence with the governors to prepare a thorough overhaul of the empire's medical-sanitary administration: TsGIA-SSSR. f. 1287, op. 15, dd. 1970, 1971, "Po voprosu ob organizatsii vrachebnogo i sanitarnogo dela v imperii." Drastically changed "cholera regulations" of 1903 removed physicians from their former position of authority during emergencies and placed them under the jurisdiction of non-medical administrators. Increasingly severe repression of the Pirogov Society began in 1902; see TsGIA-SSSR, f. 1284, op. 188-1900g., d.77, "O rasreshenii uchredit' meditsinskoe obshchestvo v pamiat' Pirogova."